T0358201

EMBLEMATIC MONSTERS
UNNATURAL CONCEPTIONS AND DEFORMED BIRTHS
IN EARLY MODERN EUROPE

THE WELLCOME SERIES IN THE HISTORY OF MEDICINE

Forthcoming Titles:

*New Medical Challenges
during the Scottish Enlightenment*
Guenter B. Risse

*Medicine by Post in Eighteenth-Century Britain:
The Changing Rhetoric of Illness in Doctor–Patient
Correspondence and Literature*
Wayne Wild

The Wellcome Series in the History of Medicine series editors are
V. Nutton, C.J. Lawrence and M. Neve.
Please send all queries regarding the series to Michael Laycock,
The Wellcome Trust Centre for the History of Medicine at UCL,
210 Euston Road, London NW1 2BE, UK.

www.ucl.ac.uk/histmed

EMBLEMATIC MONSTERS
UNNATURAL CONCEPTIONS AND DEFORMED BIRTHS
IN EARLY MODERN EUROPE
A. W. Bates

Rodopi

Amsterdam – New York, NY 2005

First published in 2005
by Editions Rodopi B. V., Amsterdam – New York, NY 2005.

Bates, Alan W. © 2005

Design and Typesetting by Michael Laycock,
The Wellcome Trust Centre for the History of Medicine at UCL.
Printed and bound in The Netherlands by Editions Rodopi B.V.,
Amsterdam – New York, NY 2005.

Index by Indexing Specialists (UK) Ltd.

British Library Cataloguing in Publication Data
A catalogue record for this book is available from the British Library
ISBN 90-420-2115-2

'Emblematic Monsters:
Unnatural Conceptions and Deformed Births in Early Modern Europe' –
Amsterdam – New York, NY:
Rodopi. – ill.
(Clio Medica 77 / ISSN 0045-7183;
The Wellcome Series in the History of Medicine)

Front cover:

Conjoined twins, born on the borders of England and Normandy.
From *Histoires Prodigieuses* (1560). Courtesy: Wellcome Library.

© Editions Rodopi B. V., Amsterdam – New York, NY 2005
Printed in The Netherlands Transferred to digital printing

All titles in the Clio Medica series (from 1999 onwards) are available to
download from the IngentaConnect website: http://www.ingentaconnect.com

Contents

For
Ann

List of Illustrations

Abbreviations

BL	British Library
NBG	Nouvelle Biographie Générale
OED	Oxford English Dictionary

Introduction

This book is concerned with the written and artistic records of human monstrous births published in Europe between 1500 and 1700. It presents several arguments concerning the description of monstrous births in the early modern period rather than a narrative survey. The central claim is that early modern accounts of monstrous births were usually representations of individual cases rather than generalised or allegorical monsters, and that the descriptive accuracy and credibility of their accounts were among the writers' chief concerns. The starting point of this history is the beginning of the sixteenth century, roughly the time at which accounts of monstrous births began to appear in print. This is not meant to imply that attitudes to monsters changed markedly at this time, but to acknowledge the difficulty of building up a complete picture from the relative paucity of surviving accounts from before the age of print. Likewise, there was no sudden change at the end of the seventeenth century, but to extend the survey into the early part of the eighteenth century would increase the material quantitatively but not qualitatively. The end point of 1700 does, however, exclude almost all 'scientific' study of monsters as natural experiments. The rationalisation of monsters in the enlightenment, and the emergence of the science of teratology, are outside the scope of this book.

The present work attempts to integrate historical and medical approaches, as to adopt a single viewpoint is perhaps too restrictive. Although it is possible to treat the monster literature as a literary genre without considering whether it had a factual basis, and impossible to draw an absolute distinction between descriptive and creative accounts, our reading of the sources cannot be uninfluenced by whether we believe them to describe actual events. It will be argued, for example, that popular sixteenth-century printed broadsides show similarities of purpose and structure with observations in seventeenth-century learned journals, a meaningless claim if the latter were accounts of actual cases and the former were not. Despite the lists of witnesses and masses of circumstantial details that reports of monstrous births provide, there is very little documentary corroboration for the authenticity of these monsters. Indeed, any attempt to substantiate them by means of documentary evidence is likely to fail because of the difficulty in showing that different accounts were based on independent observations and because invented accounts might well be expected to have utilised real people and places. The approach adopted here will be to use internal evidence to demonstrate the observational basis of descriptions and illustrations of monstrous births from the early modern period by comparing them with birth defects that are seen today. Comparison with modern birth defects is open to criticism as inappropriate retrospective diagnosis, a point that will be considered in some detail later on (Chapter 7). The modern diagnostic categories are not however presented as equivalents to the original descriptions (though they are useful when the latter are too lengthy to quote in full) but are used in order to show that, to the modern student of birth defects, the early modern landscape of monsters looks strangely familiar.

The use of retrospective diagnosis is not intended to medicalise the history of monsters. The monster literature was more often theological than natural philosophical in type and indeed, by comparing historical and modern medical accounts, the ways in which the description of monstrous births was adapted to their uses is more clearly shown. It will be argued that these uses were more complex than the widely held view of monsters as portents or warnings to sinners. Representations and descriptions of them invited the early modern reader to contemplate superficially hidden levels of meaning that will be explored in the context of the language of emblems, of which it is suggested that many sixteenth- and seventeenth-century descriptions of monstrous births formed a part. The social history of monstrous births, still relatively unexplored, touches on many areas: childbirth, attitudes to disposal or preservation of the body, and attitudes to bodily deformity. In particular, the view of monsters as objects of fear, ridicule or exclusion will be challenged.

The decision to restrict this study to Europe has excluded a few cases reported by settlers in the New World, only one of which seemed to me to provide significant extra information, and for which I have made an exception. For the rest of the world, I can only say that I have been unable to locate significant materials on monstrous births from the sixteenth and seventeenth centuries outside Europe, and that colleagues from the Middle East, India, the West Indies and South-East Asia have not been aware of any relevant literature from their own countries. It remains to be seen whether the reporting of monstrous births was truly a Western phenomenon, but I shall be very grateful to any reader who can draw my attention to source materials from outside Europe or to European accounts that I have overlooked.

In quotations, the use of u, v, i and j has been modernised and some contractions expanded in the interests of readability. Place names and countries have been modernised according to the Times Atlas.

This work is based on an MD thesis written at The Wellcome Trust Centre for the History of Medicine at UCL. It is my pleasure to thank Professors Christopher Lawrence and Harold Cook for accepting me as a student and for their very learned and sympathetic advice in guiding me through the writing of the thesis, and Mr Michael Laycock for his expertise and courtesy during the production of this book. Dr Jason Davies kindly supplied a pre-publication copy of his book *Rome's Religious History* (Cambridge: Cambridge University Press, 2005). Thanks are also due to the staff of the Wellcome Library, the Library of the Royal Society of Medicine, the British Library, the London Library, the Wallace Collection, and the Bavarian State Library. My wife provided information on monstrous births in Vietnam, as well as much encouragement in the writing of this book, and in everything else.

1

Truth Under the Veil

The ancients concealed the secrets of nature not only in writings but also
with various pictures, characters, ciphers, monsters and animals diversely
depicted and transformed; and within their palaces and temples they painted
these poetical fables, the planets and the celestial signs, with many other
signs, monsters and animals; and they were not understood by anyone except
by those who had knowledge of those secrets...[1]

The sixteenth and seventeenth centuries have been seen as a 'golden age' of
monsters,[2] a period of unprecedented interest during which popular ballads
and pamphlets carried news of monstrous births, and books on monsters,
written by prominent physicians and natural philosophers, were widely read
and went through many editions.[3] When, towards the end of the seventeenth
century, learned societies began to publish their proceedings, it is not
surprising that descriptions of monstrous births were among the commonest
subjects chosen for communications. There is ample evidence that this
interest in human malformations continued into more recent times; one
need only think of *the* Siamese twins, and of subsequent 'Siamese'
(conjoined) twins, which have been the subject of books, films and television
programmes, or of the preserved foetuses that were exhibited in fairground
'freak shows' and pathology museums. Now that freak shows no longer find
favour with public opinion (which, post Alder Hey, has also succeeded in
closing many pathology museums), it is easy to dismiss pre-scientific
accounts of monstrous births as no more than sensational 'curiosities' for the
unlearned that became the subject of 'misguided' and rather aimless activity
among scholars. The argument of this book is that accounts of monstrous
births were descriptions of actual events that were of interest not merely as
news, as wonders or as part of the historical record, but because they were
thought to have a deeper meaning; the question of why monstrous births
attracted such interest will be approached by considering what they meant
for those who described them and those who saw them. The plainest
example of the quest for meaning is the belief that monstrous births were
messages from God, or moral warnings, to those who were able to 'read'
them. This 'warning' interpretation of monsters has been linked by
historians to the idea that the monstrous was characteristically seen as

outside the natural order, but to infer from this that monstrous births were anomalous outsiders and objects of loathing is to apply modern judgements too freely. This was only one of many meanings, and it will be argued that, as monsters were incorporated into the language of emblems, it was possible, and perhaps inevitable, to read them in more than one way.

The primary sources on which our interpretations will be based fall into three groups – popular literature, books and journals – and although their common subject matter, literary borrowings and overlapping readership bring these different formats into close contact, there is not in my opinion a single corpus of 'monster literature.' If we set aside the motive of selling publications, the author of a ballad did not write about monstrous births for the same reasons as a Jesuit scholar or a provincial German physician. One feature common to all these sources however is that monstrous births were not usually presented as isolated curiosities but were assigned a place in the wider scheme of things. The early modern reader was concerned not simply with the occurrence of monstrous births but with their significance, in how they fitted into the world. It seems that neither general nor professional audiences tired of fresh accounts of well-known monsters. There is something excessive in the detail and thoroughness with which commentators discussed questions such as the possibility of hybrids between humans and animals, or between humans and demons, and whether and how to baptise them. Monstrous births could not be predicted, prevented or treated; they were not thought to reveal anything about the development of the foetus, and observers were not concerned about (though as we shall see they were not unaware of) their physical causes. The sheer extent of the early modern literature on monstrous births, certainly as large as that on surgery or midwifery in the same period, calls for explanation and raises the question of how the mass of information gathered about them was used.

Monsters and prodigies

What did the words *monster* and *monstrous* signify to the early modern reader? The Latin *monstrum* means a portent or warning, and Lewis and Short in their Latin dictionary derived *monstrum* from *monere*, to warn. The Italian natural philosopher Ulisse Aldrovandi (1522–1605), in his book *Monstrorum Historia* (not published until 1642), offered a perhaps etymologically flawed but nonetheless interesting alternative derivation from *monstrer*, to show, as a monster was something customarily shown to others.[4] The Oxford English Dictionary (OED) gives as the first meaning of *monster:* 'something extraordinary or unnatural; a prodigy, a marvel'. Other meanings for which it gives examples from the seventeenth century or earlier are: 'an animal or plant deviating in one or more of its parts from the normal type', 'an imaginary animal' and 'a person of inhuman and horrible cruelty and wickedness'. *Monstrous* is defined as: 'deviating from the natural order', 'strange or unnatural' and 'abnormally formed'. The meaning of the Latin root, a portent, is not given in examples of early modern English usage in the OED, but most scholars were writing in Latin, where *monstrum* signified both a portent and an abnormal birth.[5] Phrases in sixteenth-century English texts such as 'a monstrous deformed infant'[6] and 'a straung and monsterous Child'[7] suggest that *monstrous* signified to the reader something more than just strangeness or deformity. Especially in the popular literature *monster* and *monstrous* appear to have been used in an imprecise way and may have carried several meanings simultaneously; there is no reason why a monstrous birth could not have been thought of as unnatural, strange and horrible all at the same time. *Monster* later became a technical term within medicine, signifying a child with severe congenital malformations, in which context it is now obsolete,[8] having largely been replaced by the terms *congenital malformation* or *birth defect*, both of which significantly refer to the medical condition, not the individual, and carry a sense of failure to attain a particular result, which *monster* does not.

The well-known work on monsters published in 1575 by the French surgeon Ambroise Paré (*c.*1510–90) is now generally known under the title of *Des Monstres et Prodigies*, usually translated into English as *On Monsters and Prodigies* or *Monsters and Marvels*. For Paré and for most writers of his time, monsters and prodigies were different, though the boundary between them was not always distinct. Essentially, a monster was within the compass of nature while a prodigy was totally outside it. The recognition of this distinction became a standard part of the preamble to scholarly accounts of monstrous births for over a century, and the French physician François Bouchard began a description of a monstrous child in 1672:

> A monster is anything that appears outside the usual course and order of nature, such as a child with two heads, or which has three or more arms or other superfluous members, mutilated or maimed.

> A prodigy is that which goes totally against nature, such as if a woman gives birth to a beast, whether four-footed, aquatic, flying, reptilian, or of some other kind.[9]

A birth could be natural, outside the usual course of nature or totally against nature, and for convenience I shall refer to these three groups, which correspond to 'normal' births, monsters and prodigies as *natural*, *unnatural* and *supernatural*.[10] If the distinction between monsters and prodigies now seems unclear, it was probably always so, since the division between what

13

was or was not within the bounds of nature was a subjective one. Lorraine Daston has compared the relationship between natural, unnatural and supernatural in the early modern period with pre-existing theological concepts of the miraculous; some theologians, for example St Thomas Aquinas, considered some miracles to be impossibilities in nature, whereas others, including St Augustine, questioned how anything done by the will of God could be contrary to nature.[11] Similarly, some early modern commentators such as Nicholas Remy (*c.*1525–1612) questioned whether any monstrous birth could be against nature.[12]

Daston has argued that the supernatural was the invention of thirteenth-century theologians such as Aquinas, and that it became gradually 'naturalised' during the sixteenth and seventeenth centuries when there was a growing distrust of supernatural events as diabolic. During this period, she suggests, there was a shift in interpretation of monstrous births from signs to facts: '[monstrous births] began as signs par excellence and ended as stubbornly insignificant.'[13] The issue is a complex one, but I may start by saying that in my view monstrous births were never considered supernatural. Monsters were not prodigies or miracles: they were outwith the normal course of nature, and so were unnatural, without transgressing the bounds of what was possible in nature and passing into the supernatural sphere. In the sixteenth and seventeenth centuries, the authors of descriptions of deformed foetuses assigned them to the 'monstrous' category in order to distinguish them from prodigies, which were supernatural or miraculous events. Furthermore, the division between unnatural and supernatural (and between monsters and prodigies) was in my view distinct from that between facts and signs. Both monsters and prodigies (and many other things) could serve as signs, since God colluded in the production of natural births and 'unnatural' monsters just as much as in supernatural prodigies:

> They are shewed that they may shew the speciall handyworke of God, and though, peradventure dead, yet speake, and tell the forgetful worlde, that God himself hath a speciall hand in forming and featuring the births conceived in the wombe.[14]

Monsters were outside the normal course of nature or, as some preferred to say, they transgressed its laws. This is another potential source of confusion to the modern reader, since when writers such as Paré referred to the natural 'law' being transgressed in the generation of monsters, they envisaged not the immutable 'laws of nature' as we might think of them (such as, say, the laws of motion) but usual types of occurrence. The natural law as posited in the early modern period resembled human law in that it could be broken. The natural law was also, as Aquinas had written, 'the mind and will of God', and as we shall see later, some deliberate blurring of the distinction between natural and human law enabled the moralising writer to imply that law breaking violated a divinely-established natural order.[15]

Probably we do not need to look beyond the availability of printing for an explanation of the apparent upsurge of interest in monstrous births at the beginning of the sixteenth century.[16] For the first time, it was possible to disseminate written accounts quickly enough and in sufficient numbers that readers could hope to go and see a monster for themselves. Monstrous births were news, and they featured in ballads and canards, which included not only descriptions and pictures but also dates and locations that particularised the monster in time and place. The delay between the birth of a monster and publication was short (broadsides describing monsters that were still to be seen indicate a publication time of at most a few weeks),[17] often intentionally so, because the printed matter acted as an advertisement.[18] Some historians have suggested that the increase in reports of monstrous births in the sixteenth century was due to an upsurge of interest in signs,[19] but this connection can be turned around; it was, I suggest, only because monsters could be reported relatively promptly and widely that it was feasible to use them in this way: interest in monstrous births grew *because* printed accounts of them were more readily available.[20] The monster, promptly reported, assigned to a time and place, became a chronological marker (everyone remembered things that happened at the time the monster was born), a sign of the times. Timing was an important feature in sixteenth century 'wonder books', which were arranged in chronological order and some of which, such as Conrad Lycosthenes' *Prodigiorum ac Ostentorum Chronicon* (1557), included blank pages for the reader to add further significant events as they occurred.[21]

When the printing press made it possible to produce accounts of monsters quickly and relatively cheaply, they found a ready audience. Because their appearance was out of the ordinary they suggested, as they had since antiquity, that all was not right with the world; the changing and uncertain religious, political and social climate of early modern Europe was for many people a state of affairs in which monsters could be expected to occur. The rise of Protestantism offered unprecedented numbers of people a significant religious choice, and by the sixteenth century there were relatively large numbers of educated laity who were able to choose, at least privately, what faith to follow. Many of them would have been glad of a sign that God approved of the new religion. They were also capable of being persuaded, at first by Protestant preachers and writers but later by the Catholic church as it attempted to reconvert the growing numbers of dissenters who were its neighbours, and monstrous births became agents of religious controversy.

Increasing contact with non-European peoples provided a fresh source of converts and in 1622 the Congregation for Propagating the Faith was set up to oversee Catholic missions abroad, its name providing a term for the increasingly subtle business of persuading people to change their religious allegiances: *propaganda*. Secular powers too were constantly changing and as states became increasingly territorial (many mapped their boundaries for the first time) and alliances were formed and broken, they, like the church, could no longer take loyalty for granted, while their subjects were not always sure where their allegiances lay. To the upheaval caused by endless religious and secular wars were added financial problems due to price rises in some parts of Europe after a long period of stability that left many people destitute and made many more think that the millennium might be at hand. In this mood of uncertainty, those on the look out for signs of instability turned their attention to events traditionally associated with a breakdown in the natural order.

'Hideous' monsters are found among us, wrote Cornelius Gemma (1535–79) in 1575, 'now that the rules of justice are trampled underfoot, all humanity flouted, and all religion torn to bits',[22] and many accounts of monsters in the popular literature associated them with worrisome departures from the norm: religious reform or heresy, wars and battles, and sudden changes in the price of commodities.[23] These associations do not mean that descriptions of monstrous births were a sort of literary panic attack, written as a horrified reaction to change or even as an incitement to disorderly behaviour. They were a *response* to disorderly events, but one that was intended to promote order. When we examine the primary sources in more detail it will become apparent that those who wrote of monsters were often most concerned with the preservation of order. They depicted monsters that transgressed the 'laws of nature' as punishments or warnings for sinners as a means of exhorting the reader to keep to societal norms by showing him that human and natural laws were interrelated. These laws derived their ultimate authority from God, who permitted monsters to be born:

> It is certain that most often these monstrous and marvellous creatures proceed from the judgement of God, who permits fathers and mothers to produce such abominations from the disorder that they make in copulation, like brutish beasts, in which their appetite guides them, without respecting the time, or other laws ordained by God and Nature.[24]

So religious, human and natural laws formed a mutually supportive structure under which transgressive behaviour such as bestiality and sodomy was at the same time a sin, a crime, and against nature.[25] The Lutheran physician Jacob Rueff (1500–58) wrote of one deformed foetus: 'It is said that this monster was caused of God's making; nonetheless, through the sin of Sodomy, this detestable monster was of our own making' and the professor of medicine at Paris, Jean Riolan (1580–1657), writing in 1614, called hermaphrodites: 'a perversion of the order of natural things, people's health and King's authority.'[26]

One-in-two

The question of what kinds of births were considered monstrous can be best answered by example; monstrous births are what the ballads, books and journal articles listed in the appendix were about. It is quite striking that, despite the many arguments over the causes and meaning of monsters, no writer, popular or scholarly, seemed to question what *was* a monster;[27] the same types of monsters, and often the same individual monsters, were accepted by many authors. They were monstrous because they were outside the normal course of nature. At least one 'monstrous Chyld' would now be considered morphologically normal,[28] but all monsters were thought be deformed; Fortunio Liceti (1577–1657), for example, did not consider pygmies to be monsters because although they differed from other men, it was in size only and not in form.[29] For early modern observers the two recognised characteristics of monsters were deformity, sometimes expressed by saying that they were not as they 'ought' to be, and rarity. Historians have however attempted to find other common properties that, in retrospect, unite early modern monsters. The suggestion that the monstrous (which included a whole range of unnatural events from monstrous births to meteors) was that which defied classification is a significant one,[30] and once one is aware of this argument examples of monstrous births that resist normal categorisation are readily found: for every apparent dichotomy – male/female, human/animal, single/twin – there are monstrous births that seem to possess both elements together. Nor were ambiguities and the crossing of boundaries limited to their form: monstrous births were also, as we have seen, associated with the transgression of religious and societal norms and the breaching of moral boundaries. Christians who strayed into heresy, or parents who behaved too much like animals and failed to exercise the control over sexual behaviour thought proper to humanity, were all associated with monstrous births.

The theory that monstrous births are intermediates is perhaps most clearly applicable to double monsters (conjoined or 'Siamese' twins), which were by far the most common type of monstrous birth described in the sixteenth and seventeenth centuries. Double monsters account for just over a third of all records of monstrous births during this period, yet in the present day (and there is no reason to believe their incidence has significantly changed) they are rare among congenital malformations.[31] This suggests that these rarities were favoured for description over less infrequent monstrous forms; indeed, they were the archetypal 'monstrous birth', and the illustrator of a ballad whose author mentioned monstrous births without describing them drew a double monster.[32] Because they were neither one nor two individuals, it can be argued that they were necessarily outside the natural order.[33] Writers of both popular and scholarly accounts often concerned themselves with the individuality of double monsters, a problem that had practical implications because if they were to be baptised it was necessary (as baptism ought not to be repeated) to decide whether they were one or two children. In practice, despite much theoretical discussion on this subject, they were almost always baptised twice, regardless of the numbers of heads and limbs present, and even if one half was much smaller than the other (what we would now call a 'parasitic' twin).

In antiquity, higher numbers of multiple births (quadruplets or greater) had been considered monstrous,[34] and there was known to be an association between multiple births and other monstrous births, of which Aristotle had written: in man monstrosities occur more often in regions where women give birth to more than one at a time'.[35] Twins, which in many cultures are regarded as less individual than other siblings, can be seen, like double monsters, as ambiguous – two and yet one – and as an extreme example the Nuer people of Southern Sudan treated twins as one social person:

> *Like a historical event,* their birth is a sign of the intervention of *Kwoth* (spirit). Because of this, and to distinguish them from ordinary men, Nuer call human twins birds, because birds are the creatures closest to the primary abode of Spirit, which is the sky.[36]

These anthropological observations have several parallels with the interpretation of monsters in the sixteenth century. Monsters were signs of the intervention of God, yet at the same time they were historical events, and there was assumed to be a reason why they occurred at a particular time. In his studies of the Nuer, Sir Edward Evans-Pritchard speculated on *why* they saw twin births as a special revelation of spirit, concluding that it was because they were unusual events.[37] The Nuer did not compare twins to birds, they called them birds, a practice that puzzled anthropologists and which is curiously similar to some animal/human comparisons found in the literature of monstrous births. Anthropological evidence links twin births with animals: 'Men who have begotten twins are held to have an intimate connection with animals (who also reproduce by multiple births).'[38] Monstrous births were also linked with animals, because they were thought

18

to be hybrids, or the result of changes in the foetus brought about by mental images in pregnant women frightened by animals ('maternal impressions'), or a consequence of 'degeneration' of the human seed. The many descriptive comparisons between monstrous births and animals, while not usually intended to suggest a causal link, tended to reinforce an association between them, although cases where women actually gave birth to an animal, if they occurred, were considered prodigies rather than monsters.

The unease concerning anything that blurred the distinction between animals and men was deep rooted. In fifth-century Britain, rituals that involved men pretending to be animals, by putting on skins and masks, were considered 'devilish' by Christian writers, who found it difficult to understand why men created in the image of God would want to make themselves resemble animals. 'Is there any sensible man', wrote St Caesarius of Arles (470–542), 'who could ever believe that there are actually rational individuals willing to put on the appearance of a stag and to transform themselves into wild beasts?'[39] Since the time of Pliny monstrous races had been thought to exist at the periphery of the known world,[40] but prior to the sixteenth century men were seen as a single group, equal before God, a concept that the Catholic church struggled to preserve in subsequent centuries. The exploration of the world outside Europe brought Europeans into contact not with the fabled monstrous races (Columbus recorded his failure to find 'human monstrosities, as many expected' in his exploration of the Caribbean[41]), but with men whose appearance and language were very different from European norms and who were considered by some to be 'beastly' (in 1537 it was necessary for Pope Paul III to declare explicitly in the bull *Sublimis Deus* that the natives of the New World were fully human and possessed souls).[42] In making Caliban 'as disproportion'd in his manners as in his shape', Shakespeare was reflecting contemporary anxieties about the 'savages' of the New World,[43] and when monsters that were common in distant lands were born closer to home, this was a sign that the behaviour of Europeans was no different from that of savages:

I read how Affrique land was fraught,
For their most filthy life,
With monstrous shapes confuzedly,
That therein wer full rife.

But England now pursues their vyle
And detestable path
Embracyng eke all mischeefs greet,
That moves Gods mightie wrath.[44]

19

At the same time, travellers were also encountering animals that were different and perhaps more human in appearance than any seen in Europe, and the distinction between men and animals was becoming increasingly difficult to maintain – by the eighteenth century some non-European races were classified with apes and in 1758 Linnaeus (Carl von Linné, 1707–78) included in his classification the semi-human species *Homo monstrosus*.[45]

In his consideration of the relationship of animals to human society, *Man and Beast*, Roy Willis examined the dualistic nature of animals as fellow-creatures yet outside humanity[46] and found that animals that defied classification acquired a particular importance: 'There is an animal, half-bird, half-animal, the flying squirrel or scaly tail, which seems to the Lele [of the present-day Democratic Republic of Congo] uncanny because it defies normal classification, and so this too is avoided by women'[47] because 'they are not sure what it is, bird or animal.'[48] Daston and Park made this claim about 'wonders' in general, of which they used monstrous births as a key example: 'As theorized by mediaeval and early modern intellectuals, wonder was a cognitive passion, as much about knowing as about feeling.' To register wonder was to register 'a breached boundary, a classification subverted.'[49] Clearly, there had to be a classification for a creature to subvert it, and it can be argued that any attempt at categorisation necessarily created monsters in the gaps between categories:

> No doubt the first essential procedure for understanding one's environment is to introduce order into apparent chaos by classifying. But, under any very simple scheme of classification, certain creatures seem to be anomalous. Their irregular behaviour is not merely puzzling but even offensive to the dignity of human reason. We find this attitude in our own spontaneous reaction to 'monstrosities' of all kinds.[50]

The theory that monsters are intermediates has been used to explain responses to them. Salisbury noted that 'humans are uncomfortable with ambiguity', citing the disgust often felt about bats, which are 'neither bird nor beast';[51] and in the Christian tradition the Mosaic laws, which forbade practices such as allowing cattle to mate with different breeds or even sowing a field with mixed seed,[52] provided a foundation for the dislike of intermediates in general. If monsters were seen as intermediates, one might expect a similar emotional response towards them. Daston and Park[53] refer to 'horror' of monsters and even 'repugnance', due to moral as well as aesthetic outrage: 'The horror did not spring simply from the confusion of categories – animal and human, for example, or male and female – that anthropologists have placed at the heart of ideas of pollution; its roots lay rather in the perceived violation of moral norms.' Some of the reactions to monstrous births from many periods support this view: the Spartans exposed hermaphrodites and left them to die, and the Norman–Welsh chronicler Gerald of Wales (*c*.1146–*c*.1223) reported that the supposed offspring of a bitch and a monkey were killed because: 'their deformed and hybrid bodies revolted this country bumpkin'.[54] Even Paré, usually eager to tell a good story, balked at illustrating or even describing supposed human–animal hybrids:

> Now I shall refrain from writing here about several other monsters engendered from such grist, together with their portraits, which are so hideous and abominable, not only to see but also to hear tell of, that, due to their great loathsomeness I have neither wanted to relate them nor to have them portrayed.[55]

Horror and repugnance are undoubtedly responses to deformity that have occurred throughout history, but do such reactions explain the widespread interest in monstrosities in the early modern period? Monsters were routinely exhibited in the public view and were seldom killed or concealed, and unless we suppose that observers enjoyed being horrified and wanted opportunities to show their disgust – and there is no evidence for behaviour of this kind – other explanations for why people were prepared to travel and pay to see monsters, and then to buy and keep images of them must be sought. The reaction to monsters was more complex than terms such as 'horror' and 'repugnance' suggest, and attitudes to them were as ambivalent as the monsters themselves. Comparative anthropology shows that human–animal intermediates, hermaphrodites and physical deformities have all been revered as well as tabooed.[56] 'One-in-two' could be at the same time: 'scandalous, unthinkable, and much to be desired.'[57]

Important though the theory of monsters as intermediates is as a retrospective explanation for their importance, we must be cautious of imposing it universally. There was an alternative early modern view, represented in Montaigne's essay *On a Monstrous Child* (1580), of the monster as part of an orderly creation, a view encountered particularly in the book literature. From this standpoint, the monstrous provided evidence of the works of God not by its exceptional character but by its place in the 'great chain of being'.[58] Although many monsters can be seen as intermediates there were many others – 'a child without a head', 'a shapeless mass', a child whose abdomen was 'transparent' – that it is difficult to read in this way. Moreover, intermediates are not necessarily outsiders: green is a mixture of blue and yellow but it is also part of a spectrum. Aristotle considered creatures such as seals, bats and sponges not as uncategorisable but as belong to two categories at the same time.[59] In this sense, intermediates, rather than being incongruous exceptions, could point to the fullness of creation in which every possible creature was represented. I shall argue that the concept of monsters as part of a greater order underpinned much of the scholarly effort that was devoted to their description, collection and classification, and that through these classifications monstrous births were presented to the reader as symbols of order.

Reading the monster of Ravenna

Some of the issues surrounding monstrous births may become clearer by examining an example. Perhaps the best known of all monstrous births is the monster of Ravenna, illustrations of which are often reproduced on the covers of books and in articles dealing with monstrous births and the history of teratology (Figure 1.1). Although perhaps not entirely typical, this much-discussed case illustrates some approaches and difficulties to reading early modern accounts of monstrous births.[60] According to one early source, this monster was born at Bologna on 22 March 1512. News of it soon spread by letters, broadsides and pictures, the Florentine apothecary Luca Landucci saw a painting of it and wrote a description in his diary,[61] and it was illustrated in a woodcut of 1513.[62] A German broadside of 1512 apparently depicting the same monster stated that it was born in Florence on 27 February and it has been suggested that these illustrations all had a common source, now lost, perhaps in a monster born in Florence in 1506,[63] which became known as the monster of Ravenna because its birth was linked with the battle of Ravenna in 1512, when the city was taken by the French and sacked and its citizens massacred.[64]

Dates and locations of the different versions of the monster seem to have been arranged to provide a sign for a specific purpose (not a portent, as the connections were made after the event). The text of two early Protestant woodcuts stated that it was born in a Florentine convent to a nun impregnated by the Pope, but by 1512 it had been re-located nearer in place and time to the battle of Ravenna[65] (though even then the closest birthplace, Bologna, was over forty miles away). The form of the Ravenna monster also changed between the various accounts, perhaps because of exaggeration to emphasise its monstrous nature, or by descriptions of several monstrous births becoming conflated as the tales were passed around. A poem about the battle described a different monster, which had two heads. The variety of illustrations as artists attempted to match the text, or copied and embellished earlier images, acquired a life of their own, distinct from the prose descriptions,[66] and by 1557 the monster illustrated in Lycosthenes' *Prodigiorum* had one leg rather than two and bird's wings rather than the bat's wings of earlier illustrations. Some later versions of the monster show it

Figure 1.1

The evolution of the monster of Ravenna as illustrated in Caspar Schott's
Physica Curiosa *(1662). The older form (upper left) has two lower limbs,*
male external genitalia and facial clefts; the later (upper right) has a single
lower limb with an eye in the knee, and is an hermaphrodite.
Below is a cacodemon.

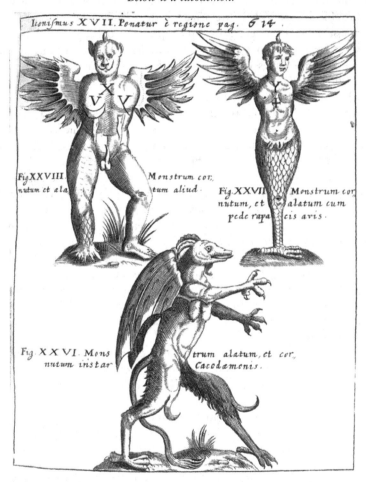

as an hermaphrodite, depicted in the conventional manner not as sexually
indifferent but with male and female external genitalia side by side. The
monster's anatomy appears to have been changed for a purpose. Rather than
being 'forced to fit',[67] monsters in the sixteenth and seventeenth centuries

often seem to have been made to stand out; thus hermaphroditism ('participating both of the man and woman'),[68] which was said by some early modern commentators to be against 'Natural Reason',[69] was imposed on the monster of Ravenna in order to emphasise its exceptional status.

Bizarre though the Ravenna monster appears, many modern interpreters have risen to the challenge and offered retrospective diagnoses of various combinations of sirenomelia, cyclopia and hemiamelia.[70] Although it appears impossible to make a definitive diagnosis, there has at least been agreement amongst most commentators with experience of teratology that the descriptions of the monster may have been derived from an actual birth.[71] The term 'birds' wings' for example, was, I suggest, no more intended to be taken literally than 'hare lip' or 'pigeon toes' are today. Some illustrators of the Ravenna monster drew a bird-like or bat-like wing, but the intended comparison was probably with the wing of a plucked bird. This was how the arms of the eighteenth-century foetus later known as the 'chicken man' (and still preserved in Waldenburg museum) were described in 1737.[72] Feet described as being like those of birds or animals[73] were usually depicted literally but may have been references to absence of digits or clefting giving a resemblance to a bird's foot. The condition seems to have been relatively common (Caspar Schott would later devote an entire category to monsters with the feet of 'evil beasts') and may have referred to the deformity now known as talipes. The prevalence of 'hermaphrodites' amongst monstrous births is misleading as many were originally described as *sexum utroque* or *utriusque generis*,[74] which suggests that 'sexual indifference' (lack of differentiation of the external genitalia) shown by foetuses in the first months of their development was being described, rather than 'true' hermaphroditism (the presence of both male and female genitalia) in the modern sense.

Accounts of the Ravenna monster circulated as cheap broadsides of the kind produced to carry news or religious, political or moralising messages. Monstrous births were a significant subject for the popular presses of Italy, Germany, France and England, and their use in popular prints as 'warnings from God' has received much attention from historians. This was certainly how the Protestant authors of the Ravenna broadsides and many ballads and books of wonders from the sixteenth and seventeenth centuries presented them, juxtaposed to contemporaneous events as signs of divine intervention. One well-known example, the so-called monk–calf published by Martin Luther, has become a prototype of the use of monsters in theological arguments. By contrast, accounts of monstrous births in natural philosophical books and theses and in early proceedings of learned societies have received less attention from historians, perhaps because they are perceived as 'medical curiosities'[75] that did not contribute significantly to scientific progress.

The traditional historical emphasis on a progress from 'superstition' to 'science' reflects the contributions to the history of medicine made by scientists such as the French zoologist and embryologist Isidore Geoffroy Saint-Hilaire (1805–61), who developed his father's pioneering interest in teratology into a vast taxonomy of monsters that was in its time unequalled. He was keenly aware of the history of his subject and set a pattern for historians of monstrous births when he divided their study into three periods, the earliest of which, characterised by 'vague, incomplete and chance observations', extended until the end of the seventeenth century when it was superseded by a more enlightened attitude based on exact and careful study.[76] Although historians who are not also scientists have taken more balanced views, descriptions of monstrous births in the sixteenth and seventeenth centuries have often been read in the context of a progress towards the modern science of teratology and away from superstition.[77] An alternative view, proposed by Daston and Park, is that readings of monstrous births changed as a consequence of the separation of popular and scholarly culture that occurred in the early modern period, so that while in the early sixteenth century they were generally accepted as signs, by the end of the seventeenth this reading was only to be found in 'popular' literature.[78] The fall in 'portentous' uses of monsters coincided with an increase in descriptive natural philosophical accounts, a change of emphasis which, they suggested, may have been brought about by a 'conspiracy' of social and intellectual elites to diminish the role of portents because they were socially dangerous: 'Disorderly nature could be used by disorderly people'.[79] However, early modern observers may not have been as alarmed by monstrous births as is sometimes supposed. Monsters were signs of divine intervention that could serve as reminders that every birth was dependent upon divine providence. The occasional monstrous birth was a reminder that God was always active behind the scenes. The author of an Elizabethan ballad on a 'Childe with Ruffes' reproved himself for the suggestion that it was merely a sport of nature:

By nature's spite, what do I say?
Doth nature rule the roost?
Nay God it is say well I may
By whom nature is tost[80]

In any discussion of the interpretation of monstrous births, it is necessary to distinguish signs from portents. A portent, from *protendere*, to stretch forth, is a prediction of the future, and to portend something is to 'point to or indicate beforehand' (OED). The portentous use of natural phenomena is rooted in an assumption that *if* a particular thing is observed *then* a certain event will happen in the future: if we pass a sign pointing to a place, then we shall eventually arrive there. The use of monstrous births as portents, which was responsible in no small part for the care with which they were observed, has a long history. They were studied (in considerable anatomical detail) for their prophetic significance in ancient Babylonia, and methods of divination such as teratoscopy (also called fetoscopy) that foretold the future through monsters helped to make them worthy of record even if their appearance was similar to that of earlier monsters. These methods seem to have been of comparatively minor importance in the constellation of different techniques for divination (using everything from incense to onions) that was available in the ancient world, probably because monsters could not be produced when required. Anatomical peculiarities were more predictably available for inspection by haruspicy, the complex Etruscan discipline of divination by means of entrails that survived in the Roman Empire until the sixth century. It has been argued that the belief in monstrous births as portents was still in existence in Europe, among the uneducated, as late as the nineteenth century,[81] and in south east Asia, they have retained their portentous reputation until the present day; as one observer, who remembers large numbers of people visiting a Vietnamese hospital to see a child born with sirenomelia, put it: 'God does not allow such things to happen unless there is going to be a disastrous time ahead.'[82]

Belief in portents has been considered to be widespread in early modern times: 'From the Dissolution of the Monasteries to the Revolution of 1688 there was scarcely any important event which educated men did not believe to have been presaged by some occurrence in the natural world',[83] and Protestants, who denied the possibility of purgatory and the efficacy of intercession for the dead, may even have expected God to warn men of their impending damnation. As the puritan William Greenhill (1591–1677) wrote: 'God doth premonish before he doth punish',[84] and comets and other rare phenomena had reputations as auguries of the (usually calamitous) future. We cannot know what people, particularly those who left no written records, *believed* about monstrous births in the early modern period, but it is an oversimplification to say that published accounts of monsters presented them as portents. Edward Fenton, writing in 1569, regarded the portentous interpretation of monstrous births as a historical curiosity:

> The auncients of olde time had these monstrous creatures in so greate horrour, that if they fortuned to meete any of them by chaunce in their way, they judged it to be a foreknowledge of their misfortune.[85]

26

Monsters such as the Ravenna monster were often reported after the event of which they were a sign and could not possibly have been supposed to predict it. They were signs of another kind, in that they coincided with, and so drew attention to (or, one might say, pointed to) important contemporary events. The monster was a sign of the times rather than a portent of the future and, like a sign, needed a specific location and appearance in order to be useful. For a monstrous birth to be read properly it was necessary for the reader to know when and where it was seen and what form it took, information that printed accounts usually provided.

Emblematic monsters

The stereotyped way in which the Ravenna monster was presented, and its resemblance to earlier 'composite images' used as visual *aides-mémoire*, emphasised to readers that they were to consider the monster not just as news but also as having a hidden meaning. The contemporary French chronicler Joannes Multivallis and many later writers treated the monster as an emblem in whose anatomy could be read the sins purported to have given rise to it, so that the horn represented pride; the wings, inconsistency; the eye on the knee, worldliness; and the bird's foot, rapacity.[86] The way in which the monster was depicted placed it in the emblem tradition; it has been shown to resemble earlier images of *Frau Welt*, the sinful world represented as a human figure,[87] and it is also similar to an early fifteenth-century personification of the seven deadly sins.[88]

We will need to consider the relationship between signs and emblems, for monsters were used as both. Images such as the pictorial device on a banner or the board outside an inn show how 'signs' (*signum*, a mark or token) could not only physically point out where something was but also represent it symbolically (*symbol*, from Greek, also means a sign or token). In modern usage a symbol has come to mean 'a material object representing or taken to represent something material or abstract' (OED), but a symbol did not have to be a picture: the archetypal symbol was the creed, the 'mark' or 'sign' of a Christian,[89] and the term was applied by Catholics to the Eucharistic elements. Monstrous births were signs of events with which they coincided in time (a famine or a battle, for example) but also symbols ('outward and visible signs' like the Eucharist and other sacraments) of the invisible workings of the Creator, examples of providence that served to demonstrate divine authority – as Moses had through the power to 'do signs'.[90]

The terms *symbol* and *emblem* were not distinct in early modern usage – emblems were sometimes known as *symbolum* and sometimes as *devices*, *impressa*, *hieroglyphs*, *icons* or *posies* – but nor were they identical. An emblem is difficult to define,[91] but a typical 'emblem' of the type printed in emblem books of the period consisted of a title, epigram and picture. Emblems did not have to include pictures; there was also emblematic language, an allusive way of expressing ideas that was a desirable attribute in fashionable society and an amusing game for Renaissance courtiers: 'often "emblems" as we nowadays call them, were devised; in which discussions a marvellous pleasure was had.'[92] Emblems emerged as a literary form early in the sixteenth century,[93] probably, I suggest, for the same reason that monsters did: that it was technically feasible to produce illustrated books in relatively large numbers. It has been estimated that, between 1531 and 1700, over a thousand emblem books by more than six hundred authors, and containing over a million emblems, were published.[94] Each emblem had a self-contained meaning for the reader to work out. They were meant to entertain and instruct: 'at least half the point, if not the pleasure, of emblem books was puzzling through the cunning (or plodding) analogies between the exterior world [as shown in the emblem] and their meanings for the interior life of the spirit.'[95] Printed emblems were not confined to emblem books but also appeared in other works, such as those on alchemy, where they did not simply illustrate the text, but were interpretable apart from it, as 'an independent pictorial language'.[96] Even the humble placenta could be part of the language of emblems: the engraved additional title leaf from the Swedish man-midwife Johan von Hoorn's (1662–1724) *Jorde-Gumma* depicted a placenta as (we are told in the accompanying verse) the rose of Jericho, a plant thought to expedite parturition.[97]

Popular accounts of monstrous births resembled the emblems of emblem books in their arrangement; there was a title, a picture and verses or text, which sometimes supplied clues to the monster's interpretation, as in the descriptions of the Ravenna monster that suggested a meaning for each part of the monster's body. Martin Luther's (1483–1546) pamphlet describing a 'monk–calf'[98] presented a malformed calf resembling a monk as an emblem of the supposed corruption of the monasteries. The purpose of such tracts was to use the monster to convey a theological or moral message, not to use theology to explain a monster. Writers such as Luther realised that they could use monsters as emblems to convey religious or moral arguments to people who would not read a theological tract but who might read an account of a monster.[99] Emblems were also messages and in emblem books the message was that intended by their author. For Luther and his contemporaries, God was the author of monsters and the search for their meaning can be seen as a quest for signs of the creator in the creation that preoccupied early modern writers. The doctrine of signatures, revived in the early sixteenth century by Paracelsus (Theophrastus Bombast von Hohenheim, 1493–1541), maintained that God had placed signs in the created world for the benefit of men: '…by the outward shapes and qualities of things we may know their inward Vertues, which God hath put in them for the good of man.'[100] This doctrine was adopted by writers of herbals, such as Giovanni Battista della Porta in Italy (1588), Johann Popp in Germany (1625), and William Cole (1657) and Robert Turner (1664) in England.[101] Turner, for example, wrote that: 'God hath imprinted upon the Plants, Herbs, and Flowers, as it were in Heiroglyphics, the key signature of their Vertues'.[102] Signatures could be very simple; for example, liverwort and kidneywort looked like the parts of the body that they were used to treat, but they could also be more complex, depending upon the names of things rather than their appearance, and requiring an explanation. Also, mercury was used to treat venereal disease and Mercury was the god of the marketplace, where prostitutes were to be found.[103]

Early modern scholars usually treated the names of things as part of their nature rather than as arbitrary designations, and hieroglyphics attracted interest as a novel means of naming. Hieroglyphs appealed to the Renaissance love of codes, hidden messages and secrets, as well as to the interest in *arcana*, the wisdom of the ancients. Horus Apollo's *Hieroglyphica*, a work purporting to explain Egyptian hieroglyphs discovered in 1419 by a Florentine monk and circulated in manuscript before being printed in 1505 by the Aldine press, was an important text in Renaissance emblematics. It was translated into many languages and, it has been suggested, inspired Francesco Colonna's *Hypnerotomachia Poliphili.*[104] In a 1600 edition of *Hieroglyphica* under the title of *Le Tableau des Riches…* François Béroalde wrote:

> This Author… follows the manner of the Ancients who veiled any kind of philosophical truth with certain agreeable figures which attracted mens hearts, either to detain them upon the husk of what offered itself, or to strive to open that which hid the inner beauty in order to enjoy it, thus both pleasing the vulgar and satisfying those desirous of perfection.[105]

Monstrous births undoubtedly pleased the vulgar, while offering a deeper meaning to those that sought it, and the iconography of monsters reflects their emblematic usage. The simplest illustrative material, used in some books and ballads, consisted of decorative figures added to the text. In Stephen Batman's *The Doome Warning All Men to the Judgement…* (1581),[106] for example, the same woodcuts appear more than once on different pages so that the description of a monstrous birth is accompanied by a picture of a monster, any monster, to draw the reader's eye to it. At the other extreme were illustrations made from life by artists who had seen the subject for themselves. There is documentary evidence of this mode of working[107] or it may be inferred from the result[108] that the illustration was intended to show the child 'just as it was.'[109] More commonly, illustrations represented a specific monster but not in a realistic way: newborn or stillborn babies (their ages given in the text) were shown alive, older than their actual years and standing or walking.[110] They were sometimes depicted with characteristic attributes, for example feathered wings or an animal's head or symbols on their bodies, which, at a time when emblem books and visual allegories were commonplace, invited emblematic interpretation. The final, 'standard' image of the Ravenna monster had characters and symbols added to it, one way of creating emblems from pictures. Goossen van Vreeswijck (1626–c.1689) provided emblems for his alchemical work *De Goude Leeuw…* by adding symbols to existing and unrelated illustrations.[111]

Representations of monsters and alchemical emblems drew on the same iconography, with which readers would have been familiar. The letter Y shown on the breast of the Ravenna monster was seen by many people, who offered 'diverse judgements' of it, but to 'learned and holy men [who] began… to decipher the misery of this infant' meant that 'by this figure Y, & the crosse, they were two figures of salvation, for *Ypsilon* signifieth vertue: the Crosse sheweth that al those… wil returne to Jesus Christ'.[112] In Michael Maier's *Symbola Aureae Mensae* (1617) the androgene, like the Ravenna monster, holds the letter Y, this time as a sign that: 'The androgene or Rebis [double thing] results from the conjunction of the twin Principles, obtained with the help of the double saline mediator of which the Y is a symbol.'[113] The hermetic tradition suggests meanings for the hermaphrodite. The Greek god Hermes (Mercury, who holds the Caduceus)[114] united with Aphrodite, the goddess of femininity, who bore the man–woman Hermaphrodite: alchemists represented the union of masculine and feminine by the so-called hermetic androgene or rebis. The *Rosarium Philosophorum* of 1550 illustrated the androgene, the product of the union of *sol* and *luna* (sulphur and mercury), as a two-headed human body with concealed, and therefore ambiguous, genitalia. This type of image would have been as familiar as the depictions of double monsters, which were often said to combine male and female. A double monster born in Brussels in 1588 was represented as half male and half female, with the sun and moon beside each.[115] A later alchemical work, *Atlanta Fugiens*[116] depicted the hermaphrodite as a twin with one male and one female head and male and female external genitalia. Théophraste Renaudot (1586–1653), writing in 1664 of animals that possessed the attributes of both sexes, referred to the alchemical tradition to show that Nature could imitate fable:

And though 'tis a fiction of the Poets that the son begotten of the Adultery of Mercury and Venus was both male and female... yet we see in Nature some truth under the veil of these Fables. For the greatest part of insects and many perfect animals have the use of either sex.[117]

The emblematic image can 'almost by definition, be interpreted in more than one way'[118] and descriptions of monstrous births drew attention to their dual nature not only anatomically, for example through emphasis on shared organs in double monsters, but emblematically, using symbols of duality from the world of alchemy or from among the animals. Accounts of monsters often alluded to the combination of two natures. One (perhaps an anencephalic in which the brain had failed to develop) was described as having the head of a frog, a creature that, being amphibious, combined elements of earth and water (the Egyptian god Nau, represented as frog-headed, was also androgynous, shown sometimes as male and sometimes as female),[119] while another (with a facial cleft?) was said to have a leopard's head. This unusual choice of comparison with an animal that most readers would never have seen (why not a cat?) may be explained by the dual nature of the leopard (leo-pardus, a hybrid between a lion and a panther):

Amongst beasts, Leopards, Mules, Doggs, and many others, partake of two different natures; the Bat is between a beast and a bird, as Frogs, Ducks, and other amphibious creatures, partly fish, and partly Terrestrial Animals. The Bovaretz [vegetable lamb] is a plant and an animal; the Mushrome is between earth and a plant.[120]

The use of monsters as emblems does not imply that they were fables. In his study of seventeenth century imagery, Praz has emphasised that emblems (for which he uses the term 'devices') were expected to utilise genuine properties of their constituent elements: 'one would, however, be mistaken in thinking that the device-writers were ready to take up any fable; on the contrary they insist upon the exclusion of the fabulous.'[121] He quotes the Italian scholar Scipione Bargagli (d. 1612), 'one of the chief authorities on devices' in sixteenth century Italy:

In the main subject of the devices there can be no room, according to my firm belief, for mere fictions; since we must deal with real things and we have to explain and prove them... those will be rightly blamed who have made and will continue to make use of the false properties of things universally known to be false.[122]

An effective emblem normally required a factual basis: the pelican feeding its brood with its own blood is a valid emblem only if this is, or is believed to be, what a pelican actually does.

Figure 1.2

A 'manne chylde, having three armes, three legges and very terrible to beholde' (Batman, 1581).

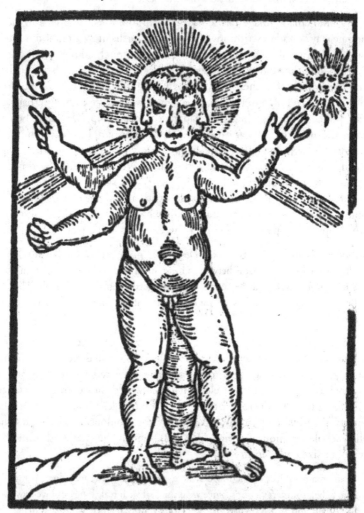

Although emblems were mostly derived from facts, the emblematic use of monstrous births is especially well seen in those few accounts that were not intended to represent actual monsters but which were created especially to serve as emblems. Early modern writers made a distinction between actual cases and stories, the latter sometimes being referred to as 'poetical' accounts:

There was a mayden childe borne, having foure legs, foure armes, two bellies, proportionable joyned to one back, one head with two faces, the one before, & the other behind, like to the picture of Janus: the like of this with two several faces under one scull, I never read before in any Chronicle, except by way of a Poeticall report.[123]

The following example, from Batman's *Doome* is, like all emblems, not an attempt to deceive, but an invitation to discover a hidden meaning, and the account opens with improbable details that signal immediately its 'poetical' nature:

A maid named *Ida*, aboute the age of 77 yeares, never suspected by the inhabitantes for any stayne or dishonestye, she was at this age married to one *George*, of the age of 60 yeres. Being married aboute 12 moneths, shee was found with child to the great admiration of many: at the laste shee was delivered of a manne chylde, having three armes, three legges and very terrible to beholde, he hadde three faces, as it were in one head, and in the one of his hands a bloody crosse: In the night tyme there was a shyning lighte aboute the Childe, and aboute his heade a bloodye Sunne and a half moone. There resorted to see this straunge Chylde a verye great multitude, among whiche pressed a blynde Mayde of the age of fifteene yeres, that was borne blind, who by the touching of this sayd monster was presentlye healed, and hadde her perfecte sighte: and another that was born dumme, at the sighte of the Chylde was restored to hys speeche. Some sayde it was an illusion of the Devill: some sayde it was done by sorcerye or witchcrafte. The Chylde at the laste opened hys mouth and sayde: *You unbeleevers greate plagues shall fall on you all, O wo that you received life.* He sayde moreover that in the yere one thousand five hundred eightie and eight the worlde shall stand in so extreame a state, that the people which live in those dayes shall tremble and quake for feare, and having ended these wordes he departed and spued forth flames of fyre, in so muche that the standers by were hurte and scorched therewith, whereupon ensued such a pestilence, that in three dayes there died 8 of the beholders: they carying the Child to the burial, it sodainly vanished from them, no man knew which way.[124]

The monster was depicted with three faces, surrounded by an aureole of the sun's rays (Figure 1.2). The symbolic sun and moon on either side of its head, sol and luna, recall the elements of the hermetic androgene. The monstrous child has a threefold anatomy suggesting the Trinity, and its very presence is sufficient to work miracles (a good reason for going to see it). A person born blind is healed (recalling John 9:13, a key text in interpretations of monstrous births)[125] and a final fiery assumption and vanishing away (as on the road to Emmaus) point even the least perceptive of readers to the monster as an emblem of Christ.

Notes

1. G. Bracesco da Iorci Novi, *La Espositione de Geber Philosopho* (Venice: G. Giolito, 1544), quoted in S. Klossowski de Rola, *The Golden Game: Alchemical Engravings of the Seventeenth Century* (London: Thames and Hudson, 1988), 17.

2. A phrase originally used of monsters by J. Céard, *La Nature et Les Prodiges* (Geneva: Droz, 1977).

3. For an overview of monstrous births in Europe from mediaeval times to the present see D. Wilson, *Signs and Portents: Monstrous Births from the Middle Ages to the Enlightenment* (London: Routledge, 1993).

4. *Ibid.*, 73.

5. An extensive linguistic discussion of *monster* and related words is to be found in the first chapter ('Definitions') of Wilson, *op. cit.* (note 3).

6. R. J[ones], *A Most Strange and True Discourse of the Wonderfull Judgement of God...* (London, 1600).

7. Anon., *A True Report of a Straung and Monsterous Child...* (London: T. Gosson, *c.*1580).

8. Except as a diagnostic category in the Systematised Nomenclature of Pathology, still in use in some hospitals.

9. *Monstrum est omne id, quod praeter cursum & ordinem Naturae apparet; Velut infans biceps, vel qui habet tria aut plura brachia seu alia membra superflua mutila vel manca. Prodigiorum est, quod prorsùs contra naturam venit, velut si mulier pariar brutum, sive sit quadrupes, aquatile, volatile, reptile, sive prodigiosum aliud:* F. Bouchard, 'Infante Monstroso Lugduni in Viam Publicam Die V Martii A. MDCLXXI Exposito', *Miscellanea Curiosa*, series 1, iii (1672), 14–16.

10. The alternative nomenclature of natural, supernatural and praeternatural is more consistent with early modern usage but ambiguous for modern readers.

11. L. Daston, 'The Nature of Nature in Early-Modern Europe', *Configurations*, vi (1998), 149–72.

12. See Chapter 5, 124–5.

13. L. Daston, 'Marvelous Facts...', in P.G. Platt (ed.), *Wonders, Marvels and Monsters* (Newark: University of Delaware Press, 1999), 76–104.

14. T. Bedford, *A True and Certain Relation of a Strange Birth...* (London: A. Griffin, 1635), 12.

15. Daston, *op. cit.* (note 13).

16. For mediaeval monsters see D. Williams, *Deformed Discourse: The Function of the Monster in Mediaeval Thought and Literature* (Exeter: University of Exeter Press, 1996); K.E. Olsen and L.A.J.R. Houwen (eds), *Monsters and the Monstrous in Medieval Northwest Europe* (Leuven: Peeters, 2001) and

A. Bovey, *Monsters and Grotesques in Medieval Manuscripts* (London: British Library, 2002).

17. Some foetuses and neonates had their life as an exhibit extended by artificial preservation; see Chapter 6, 160–1.

18. For an overview of monstrous births in popular literature, especially of France and England, see Wilson, *op. cit.* (note 3). A.W. Bates, 'Birth Defects Described in Elizabethan Ballads', *Journal of the Royal Society of Medicine*, xciii (2000), 202–7, briefly reviews the Elizabethan literature.

19. T. Anderson, 'Documentary and Artistic Evidence for Conjoined Twins from Sixteenth-Century England', *American Journal of Medical Genetics*, cix (2002), 155–9: 158.

20. This is a personal view, but the alternative, that increased survival of printed compared with manuscript accounts does not reflect increased interest, remains open.

21. See L. Daston and K. Park, *Wonders and the Order of Nature, 1150–1750* (New York: Zone Books, 1998), 187.

22. *Ibid.*, 175, their translation.

23. For increased reports of monsters in times of war see Daston and Park, *op. cit.* (note 21), 187–8; for a monstrous birth associated with a change in corn prices see Appendix, 1541a.

24. A. Paré (ed. and transl. J.L. Pallister), *On Monsters and Marvels* (Chicago and London: University of Chicago Press, 1982), 5.

25. B.J. Shapiro, *Probability and Certainty in Seventeenth-Century England…* (Princeton: Princeton University Press, 1983), 164–6, argues that in the sixteenth century an increasingly historical approach to law was adopted in Europe, partly as an appeal to the Renaissance ideal of an 'ancient constitution' and partly because of the growing requirement to establish the reliability of documents and witnesses since, because of population growth and social changes, juries could no longer be relied upon to have first-hand knowledge of the circumstances of a case. As Shapiro observes, both law and 'science' shared similar ideas of credibility and concern for truth; Bacon for example claimed that the proper method of obtaining knowledge was the same in both spheres of enquiry. Both canon and civil laws were concerned with monstrous births, as shown by debates concerning their baptism.

26. J. Rueff, *De Conceptu et Generatione Hominis…*(Basel: C. Waldkirch, 1586), I, 383; Daston and Park, *op. cit.* (note 21), 203.

27. Except for some rhetorical thesis writers, see Chapter 3, 85.

28. See Appendix, 1562a.

29. F. Liceti, *De Monstrorum Caussis, Natura, & Differentiis* (Padua: C. Crivellarium, 1616), 38.

30. K. Park and L.J. Daston, 'Unnatural Conceptions: The Study of Monsters in

Sixteenth and Seventeenth-Century England and France', *Past & Present*, xcii (1981), 20–54: 25, argued that monstrous births 'straddled the boundaries' between the natural and supernatural.

31. 1 in 50,000 to 1 in 100,000 births.

32. Anon., *A Lamentable List, of Certaine Hidious, Frightfull, and Prodigious Signes…* (London: T. Lambert, 1638), reprinted in H.E. Rollins (ed.), *The Pack of Autolycus…* (Cambridge: Harvard University Press, 1927), 22–5. On the history of conjoined twins see also J. Bondeson, 'The Biddenden Maids: A Curious Chapter in the History of Conjoined Twins', *Journal of the Royal Society of Medicine*, lxxxv (1992), 217–21. The tendency to 'over report' conjoined twins has continued to the present day: see the remaks of K.R. Winston, 'Craniopagi: Anatomical Characteristics and Classification', *Neurosurgery*, xxi (1987), 769–81: 769.

33. Park and Daston, *op. cit.* (note 30), 34.

34. Pliny the Elder, *The History of Nature*, book VII, ch. 4.

35. *The Generation of Animals*, book IV, ch. 4.

36. R.G. Willis, *Man and Beast* (St Albans: Paladin, 1975), 20, my italics.

37. *Ibid.*, 55.

38. M. Douglas, *Implicit Meanings: Essays in Anthropology* (London: Routledge and Kegan Paul, 1975), 18.

39. Quoted in M. Summers, *The Geography of Witchcraft* (London: Routledge and Kegan Paul, 1927), 69.

40. Some of these monstrous races resemble modern categories of birth defect and H. Schierhorn, 'Die Terata auf der Weltkarte des Richard de Haldingham (um 1280): Versuch einer Deutung', *Gegenbaurs Morphologisches Jahrbuch*, cxxviii (1982), 137–67, suggested that they had been derived by generalization from monstrous births. C.A. Bos and B. Baljet, 'Cynocephali en Blemmyae: Aangeboren Afwijkingen en Middeleeuwse Wonderbaarlijke Rassen', *Nederlands Tijdschrift voor Geneeskunde*, cxliii (1999), 2580–5, identified each type with a modern class of birth defects: hippopodes with lobster claw syndrome, cynocephali with anencephalics, arimaspi with cyclopia, blemmyae with acardia, the double-faced with diprosopus twins, sciopods with polydactyly and antipodes with sirenomelia. Pathologists who attempt such demythologising comparisons are in distinguished company; the eminent nineteenth-century pathologist von Recklinghausen proposed that Satyrs were based on descriptions of spina bifida: F. von Recklinghausen, 'Untersuchungen über die Spina Bifida', *Archiv fur Pathologische Anatomie*, cv (1886), 243–330.

41. D.J. Boorstin, *The Discoverers* (New York: Random House, 1983), 629.

42. R. Hakluyt, *The Principal Navigations, Voyages, Traffiques and Discoveries of the English Nation…* (Glasgow: Maclehose, 1903–5), VI, 167.

43. A. de Waal Malefijt, 'Homo Monstrosus', *Scientific American*, ccxix (1968), 112–8: 117.

44. Anon., *The True Discription of Two Monsterous Chyldren Borne at Herne in Kent...* (London: T. Colwell, 1565), reprinted in Philobiblon Society (eds), *Ancient Ballads & Broadsides...* (London: Whittingham and Wilkins, 1867), 321. J. Riolan, *De Monstro Nato Lutetiae anno Domini 1605: Disputatio Philosophica* (Paris, O. Varennaeum: 1605), fo. 6v, wrote that the monsters rare elsewhere were common in Africa.

45. Malefijt, *op. cit.* (note 43).

46. Willis, *op. cit.* (note 36), 9.

47. *Ibid.*, 15.

48. *Ibid.*, 30.

49. Daston and Park, *op. cit.* (note 21), 14.

50. Douglas, *op. cit.* (note 38), 32.

51. J.E. Salisbury, *The Beast Within: Animals in the Middle Ages* (New York: Routledge, 1994), 139.

52. Leviticus 19: 19.

53. Daston and Park, *op. cit.* (note 21), 176.

54. Salisbury, *op. cit.* (note 51), her translation.

55. Paré, *op. cit.* (note 24), 73.

56. Sir J.G. Frazer noted that some animals were regarded as both 'unclean' and 'divine': *The Golden Bough: A Study in Magic and Religion* (London: Macmillan, 1913), part 5, II, 24.

57. J. Gélis, *History of Childbirth: Fertility, Pregnancy and Birth in Early Modern Europe* (Oxford: Polity Press, 1991), 269.

58. See A.O. Lovejoy, *The Great Chain of Being: A Study of the History of an Idea* (Cambridge: Harvard University Press, 2001).

59. Apes were considered as 'participating in the nature of both man and quadrupeds', *ibid.*, 56–7.

60. Appendix, 1512a. For a meticulous analysis of its history, the reader is referred to: O. Niccoli (transl. L.G. Cochrane), *Prophecy and People in Renaissance Italy* (Princeton: Princeton University Press, 1990), 35–51.

61. Daston and Park, *op. cit.* (note 21), 177.

62. Niccoli, *op. cit.* (note 60), 39.

63. *Ibid.*

64. The battle, fought on 11 April 1512, arose out of an attempt by the Spanish and Italian forces to relieve Ravenna, besieged by the French under Gaston de Foix, Duke of Nemours, and was noted for the heavy casualties inflicted by artillery.

65. R. Schenda, 'Das Monstrum von Ravenna: Eine Studie zur Prodigiensliteratur', *Zeitschrift für Volkskunde*, lxvi (1960), 209–15; A.J.

Schutte, '"Such Monstrous Births": A Neglected Aspect of the Antinomian Controversy', *Renaissance Quarterly*, xxxviii (1985), 85–106.

66. Daston and Park, *op. cit.* (note 21), 179, observed that the monster resembles composite 'memory images' that were used to help learn texts; E. Holländer, *Wunder Wundergeburt und Wundergestalt...* (Stuttgart: F. Enke, 1921), 314, 317–9 reproduces various illustrations from 1506, 1512, and 1514.

67. See K.P. Long, 'Sexual Dissonance: Early Modern Scientific Accounts of Hermaphrodites', in P.G. Platt (ed.), *Wonders, Marvels, and Monsters in Early Modern Culture* (Newark: University of Delaware Press, 1999), 145–63.

68. E. Fenton, *Certaine Secrete Wonders of Nature...* (London: H. Bynneman, 1569), fo. 139v.

69. T. Renaudot, *A General Collection of Discourses of the Virtuosi of France...* (London: T. Dring and J. Starkey, 1664), 578.

70. See M.T. Walton *et al.*, 'Of Monsters and Prodigies: The Interpretation of Birth Defects in the Sixteenth Century', *American Journal of Medical Genetics*, xlvii (1993), 7–13: 12: '[The Ravenna monster] appears to be an example of the sirenomelia sequence: severe caudal "regression," fusion of the lower limbs, hydrocephalus with bulging of the anterior fontanelle, upper limb deficiencies, and pterygium.' As with most attempts to diagnose the 'Ravenna monster' it is based on Lycosthenes' illustration rather than the earlier two-legged versions.

71. See, for example, M.-L. Martinez-Frias, 'Another Way to Interpret the Description of the Monster of Ravenna of the Sixteenth Century', *American Journal of Medical Genetics*, xlix (1994), 362.

72. A.W. Bates, 'A Case of Roberts Syndrome Described in 1737', *Journal of Medical Genetics*, xxxviii (2001), 565–7.

73. Appendix, 1554a, 1578b.

74. For example, Appendix, 1555b, 1556a, 1617c.

75. A.R. Hall, 'Medicine in the Early Royal Society', in A.G. Debus (ed.), *Medicine in Seventeenth Century England* (Berkeley: University of California Press, 1974), 421–52.

76. I. Geoffroy Saint-Hilaire, *Histoire Générale et Particulière des Anomalies de l'Organisation chez l'Homme et les Animaux...* (Paris: J.B. Baillière, 1832–7), I, 4.

77. For example Wilson, *op. cit.* (note 3), 172–4, writes of monsters in the eighteenth century: 'Perhaps the main advance was the increasingly professional nature of the approach', while E. Geoffroy St Hillaire's classification of birth defects is: 'not much better than the displaying of monsters in cabinets of curiosities.'

78. Park and Daston, *op. cit.* (note 30), 35, argue for a shift from 'horrible' and

'terrible' to 'wonderful' and 'strange'. They subsequently revised this view and recognised three emotional responses; 'horror', 'pleasure' and 'repugnancy': Daston and Park, *op. cit.* (note 21), 176.

79. Daston and Park, *op. cit.* (note 21), 208.
80. H.B., *The True Discription of a Childe with Ruffes...* (London: J. Allde, 1566); see Appendix, 1566b.
81. See J.W. Ballantyne, 'The Teratological Records of Chaldea', *Teratologia*, i (1894), 127–42: 140.
82. A. Pham, in conversation with the author, 11 June 2002. These events took place just before the communist takeover of South Vietnam.
83. K. Thomas, *Religion and the Decline of Magic...* (London: Weidenfeld and Nicolson, 1971), 90.
84. *Ibid.*
85. Fenton, *op. cit.* (note 68), fo. 14v. The classical basis of prodigies as portents is also equivocal: Livy alleged that people no longer believed them to herald future events, but Tacitus, a century later, accepted them as omens; see J.P. Davies, *The Articulation of Roman Religion in the Latin Historians Livy, Tacitus and Ammianus Marcellinus* (PhD, University College London, 1999), 59.
86. Rueff, *op. cit.* (note 26), I, 384; see also Daston and Park, *op. cit.* (note 21), 181–2. It has been argued that in ancient Rome prodigies functioned as warnings of a particular outcome expressed metaphorically: see B. MacBain, *Prodigy and Expiation: A Study in Religion and Politics in Republican Rome* (Brussels: Collection Latomus, 1982), 122–4.
87. Niccoli, *op. cit.* (note 60), 44–5.
88. *Biblia Pauperum* (Bavaria, 1414), Munich Staatsbibliothek MS cod. lat. 8201, fo. 95.
89. This use is traceable to St Cyprian, Bishop of Carthage (*c.*250 AD), and the OED furnishes numerous examples from the sixteenth and seventeenth centuries.
90. Exodus, 4: 17.
91. According to one recent account of emblems, an exact definition is not possible: J. Manning, *The Emblem* (London: Reaktion Books, 2002), 13–21.
92. B. Castiglione (transl. C. Singleton), *Book of the Courtier* (New York: Anchor Books, 1959), 17.
93. Manning, *op. cit.* (note 91), 14.
94. On the significance of the emblem as a means of communication during the sixteenth and seventeenth centuries see M. Bath, 'Recent Developments in Emblem Studies', *Bulletin of the Society for Renaissance Studies*, vi (1998), 15–20.
95. S. Schama, *The Embarrassment of Riches...* (Bath: Fontana Press, 1987), 491.

96. Klossowski de Rola, *op. cit.* (note 1), 8.

97. Stockholm: N. Goldenau, 1697; reproduced in O. Hagelin, *The Byrth of Mankynde...* (Stockholm: Svenska Läkaresällskapet, 1990), 80.

98. P. Melanchthon and M. Luther, *Deuttung der Zwo Grewlichen Figuren, Bapstesels zu Rom und Munchkalbs zu Freyburg in Meyssen Funden* (Wittenberg: N. Schirlentz, 1523).

99. The symbolism in Luther's tract seems to be at odds with his statements about the unambiguousness of divine revelation, for example: 'the Holy Spirit... cannot have more than one most simple sense' – see T.H. Luxon, '"Not I, but Christ": Allegory and the Puritan Self', *English Literary History*, lx (1993), 899–937 – however it is perhaps unreasonable to expect Luther to have presented a single coherent view.

100. Paracelsus, quoted in A. Arber, *Herbals: Their Origin and Evolution, A Chapter in the History of Botany, 1470–1670* (Cambridge: Cambridge University Press, 1986), 250–1.

101. *Ibid.*, 252–5.

102. *Ibid.*, 254–5.

103. H.M. Pachter, *Paracelsus: Magic Into Science...* (New York: Schuman, 1951), 80.

104. F. Colonna, *Hypnerotomachia Poliphili* (Venice: Aldus, 1499).

105. Klossowski de Rola, *op. cit.* (note 1), 12.

106. S. Batman, *The Doome Warning All Men to the Judgement...* (London: Ralphe Nubery, 1581).

107. Appendix, 1555a, 1593a, 1624, 1684a.

108. For example see Appendix, 1576b, 1628.

109. Paré, *op. cit.* (note 24), 33, see Appendix, 1573.

110. See, for example, Appendix, 1511a, 1544b, 1605.

111. G. van Vreeswijck, *De Goude Leeuw...* (Amsterdam: J. Jansson van Waesberge, 1675).

112. Fenton, *op. cit.* (note 68), fo. 139v.

113. Klossowski de Rola, *op. cit.* (note 1), 114.

114. The snake is another symbol of duality; see the discussion of dualistic animal symbols in C. Lawrence, 'The Healing Serpent – The Snake in Medical Iconography', *Ulster Medical Journal*, xlvii (1978), 134–40: 138–40.

115. Anon., *Erschroeckliche und Warhafftige Contrafaytung* (Brussels: Johann Wollaert, 1588).

116. M. Maier, *Atalanta Fugiens...* (Hessen: H. Galler, 1618), emblem 33.

117. Renaudot, *op. cit.* (note 69), 578.

118. D. Russell, *Emblematic Studies in Renaissance French Culture* (Toronto: Toronto University Press, 1995), 238.

119. A. de Vries, *Dictionary of Symbols and Imagery* (Amsterdam: North-Holland, 1984), 204–5.
120. Renaudot, *op. cit.* (note 69), 578.
121. M. Praz, *Studies in Seventeenth-Century Imagery* (Rome: Edizione di Storia e Letteratura, 1964), 68.
122. The quotation is from his *Delle Imprese* (Sienna, 1578).
123. E. Howes, *Annales, or, A Generall Chronicle of England / Begun by John Stow...* (London: A. Mathewes, 1631), 1006.
124. Batman, *op. cit.* (note 106), 406.
125. See Chapter 2, 54.

2

Resembling Sins:
Monstrous Births as Moralising Emblems

Some lowzy ballad? I cannot choose but laugh
At these poor squitter pulps.[1]

Printed sources on monstrous births in early modern Europe can be divided into scholarly publications such as books, theses and sermons, and popular prints such as broadsides, ballads, chapbooks and advertisements. These two categories are by no means independent as they shared content (many monsters in the popular literature subsequently appeared in books) as well as, potentially, readers. Although some later commentators assumed readers of ballads to have been poorly educated, the audience for 'popular' literature of the period is far from clear, and the whole concept of 'popular' and 'elite' cultures has been criticised for ignoring the multi-stratified nature of society, with its large numbers of middling groups, and for making the assumption that particular types of culture necessarily correspond to particular social groups.[2] Popular culture is perhaps best defined simply as being open to everybody,[3] and the potential readership was probably wide.

Broadsides, so called because they were printed on a single unfolded sheet, came into existence around the end of the fifteenth century, perhaps as a development from bulls and other official notices that were cheaply printed and widely distributed. Monstrous births were the subject of some of the earliest of these publications, appearing around the beginning of the sixteenth century in Germany[4] and Italy.[5] In England, the first broadsides, possibly derived from French chapbooks,[6] were printed in the 1540s and the first to describe a monstrous birth appeared in 1552, while France was producing popular accounts of monstrous births from the 1570s.[7] Broadsides had a variety of formats but the usual layout included a title and a large woodcut illustration with subjoined verses and/or prose text (Figure 2.1, overleaf). They were sold by itinerant ballad-mongers or chapmen at a halfpenny or a penny a sheet. Readers probably expected a familiar format, and the rhyming and scanning verse might have helped the less literate to follow the text. Some ballads suggested a tune to which the verses could be sung, probably by the seller in order to attract customers. Given the subject matter these performances cannot have been very cheerful, but their doleful mood would have echoed that of the melancholy ballads popular at court.

Figure 2.1
Two monstrous children, shown in an English ballad of 1566,
embracing one another.

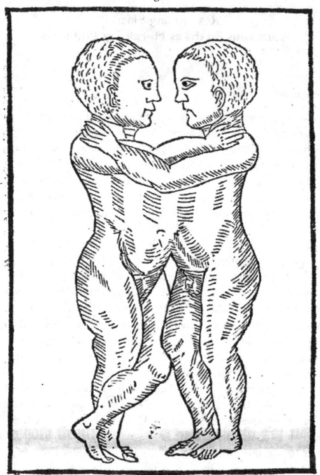

Broadsides were not publications to cherish; only a single copy now remains of some, which suggests that many others failed to survive. From 1557, ballads printed in London had to be registered with the Stationers' Company, whose records provide a complete list of all registered titles.[8] This shows the relative importance of monstrous births compared with other subject matter in terms of the number of different ballads printed (but not the number of copies). The range of subjects was diverse and included stories, true crime and news;[9] each had to be sufficiently arresting to

44

persuade passers-by that the broadside was worth their time and money and in some respects they resembled modern journalism. Only seventeen out of a total of 3,081 (in the Stationers' register) described monstrous births, mostly those born in Britain, while none dealt with illness, accidents or medical matters (epidemics of the sweating sickness in 1551 and 1578 killed thousands without being mentioned in a ballad). There were no accounts of giants, dwarfs or other 'freaks', although these featured in advertisements for London fairs, so it was not as medical curiosities that monstrous births were chosen for publication. Tessa Watt has estimated that a third of the ballads in the Stationers' Company's registers were of a 'religious' or 'moralising' type,[10] but excluded from these accounts of 'deformed babies', which she placed in the secular category and for which she assumed a 'humble' readership. One thing that set monsters apart from sickness or accidents was their congenital nature: they were born monstrous, and were seen as having been so formed in the womb by the action of God,[11] who made nothing without a purpose. Ballads about monstrous births were read not because monsters were intrinsically interesting (although they may have been), but because they carried a message for the reader, a hidden meaning that had to be puzzled out with the writer's help. They were religious emblems (the English ones seem to have been specifically Protestant in nature – I am not aware of any printed during the reign of Mary I) that called for a degree of interpretation on the part of their readership. Ballad-writers did not intend monstrous births to be taken at face value and they left the reader in no doubt of what was required: monsters were 'tokens true and manifest', 'signes and tokens strange', 'wonderful tokens'[12] and 'lessons'; they were a 'monstrous Message sent from the King of Glorie' that the reader was enjoined to 'consider right' and to 'beh[o]ld with inward eyes'.[13]

Broadsides and chapbooks were usually anonymous and of the few writers that were named none had a significant literary output outside the ballad market. Most were probably town-based men in literate trades who earned extra money by writing ballads (some printers wrote their own), and they may well not have seen the monstrous birth they were describing. For the most part they seem to have been competent craftsmen who could turn a verse or provide a readable description, and despite the *de haut en bas* attitude of English scholar Sir Thomas Bodley (1545–1613) towards 'riffe raffe bookes',[14] modern judgements that popular accounts of monstrous births were aimed at the 'credulous and ill-educated individual'[15] are open to question. Ballad-writers took pains to provide supporting details to convince sceptical readers, and the punning use of language seems to have aimed at a readership who, though perhaps ignorant of childbirth, were no strangers to the printed word:

And monster caused of want or to[o] much store
Of matter, shewes the sea of sinne: whose storm
Oreflowes and whelmes vertues barren shore.
    Faultye alike in ebbe and eke in flowd,
Like distant both from meane, both like extreames.
Yet great excesse the want of meane doth shrowde
And want of means excesse from vertues meanes.
So contraryest extreames consent in sinne...[16]

One of the first broadsides to describe a monstrous birth, printed in Germany in 1511, was in Latin,[17] whereas later German examples almost all appeared in the vernacular. An early French example[18] was also partly in Latin, suggesting that publishers initially anticipated a learned audience for these publications but found them also to be of interest to those unable to read Latin. The reader likely to buy a ballad describing a monstrous birth was perhaps someone of moderate education, sufficiently well read to appreciate a verse, with a curiosity about monsters and an interest in theological speculation, such as any thoughtful churchgoer might derive from weekly sermons. Perhaps he relished a respectable excuse to read of 'incestuous copulation' and the like, but he also knew that God spoke through signs and that monstrous births were meaningful events.

Most broadsides included a large (even life-sized in the case of a foetus[19]) figure of the monster being described. Little is known about the illustrators and they were rarely named,[20] but the way in which they worked can be inferred from the results. In one early German broadside[21] a double monster (recognisable as what we would now call *parapagus tetrabrachius dipus* conjoined twins) appears to have been realistically drawn from life, or rather, from death (it is unusual in the early literature in depicting a monster as recognisably dead),[22] and although most illustrators did not show such technical skill (if we equate skill with the production of a realistic representation), I argue that the resemblance to birth defects seen today indicates that they drew from life, or from a description by an eyewitness. The illustration for *A Discription of a Monstrous Chylde...*[23] for example appears to show slippage of the skin and overlapping of the bones of the head, consistent with the child having been dead for some days *in utero* and even the quite crudely-drawn picture in *The True Description of a Monsterous Chylde...*[24] shows a resemblance to the condition now known as *fetus amorphus* (Figure 2.2).

Illustrators who had not seen a monster for themselves worked towards a representation that fitted the text, a method that sometimes gave rise to anatomically impossible monsters.[25] Occasionally they provided a picture of a standard type of monster if the text was not sufficiently detailed to serve as

Figure 2.2
A woodcut from an English ballad of 1564 showing a foetus consisting of trunk
and lower limbs (fetus amorphus), next to a normal twin.

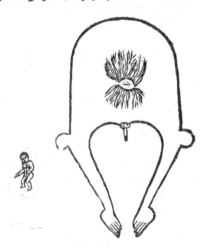

a model; headless monsters with faces in their chests (variations on the classical Blemmyae) and double monsters were popular in this respect, and were used where the text gave no clue to a monster's appearance.[26] Printers adapted existing blocks if possible; a disproportionately small normal twin shown next to a monster[27] was probably from a woodcut of a child already in the printer's stock. Another labour-saving device was copying from existing illustrations: a picture of a woman born without arms described in a German broadside of 1596 bears a striking resemblance to that of a similar case illustrated twenty years later.[28]

Of the thousands of sixteenth-century English ballads known only by title (from sources such as the Stationers' register and the Harleian Miscellany) only some 250 survive as black-letter copies.[29] Watt, who made a thorough study of English ballads from the period 1550–1640, concluded that an apparent glut of ballads dealing with birth defects between 1561 and 1571 reflected the survival of a particular collection, and argued that such ballads were a staple product of presses throughout the sixteenth and seventeenth centuries.[30] The evidence from the Stationers' register does not however suggest that ballads on monstrous births published during this decade survived preferentially; there seems to have been a genuine upsurge of publication in England around this time (this was perceived by chroniclers: 1562 was a year 'fertile in monsters' and 1556 was 'so fertile in prodigious accidents')[31] probably because monstrous births were particularly useful to Protestant writers. Sixteenth-century popular prints on monstrous births were produced in centres of Protestantism such as Germany (especially Lutheran Wittenberg), Switzerland and Elizabethan England. Ballads offered, it has been suggested, exegetical models for the masses, in which monstrous births were used as figurative expressions of human sinfulness.[32] The anatomy of a monstrous birth gave substance to the abstract concept of sin, 'brassed out' in human form, and the reader was exhorted to: '[l]et it to you a preaching be…'.[33]

A sermon published in 1635 by an English Protestant minister, Thomas Bedford,[34] shows that the seventeenth-century clergyman could still be expected to preach at the burial of a monstrous birth and to use its appearance as a guide to morals. Bedford (d. 1653) was rector of St Martin Outwich in the City of London when a Mrs John Persons of Plymouth gave birth to 'concorporate' twins after a fourteen-hour labour. He made an external examination and found them to have a common sternum and a single umbilical cord, which finding led him to speculate that there was a shared liver and that the twins were two infants coalesced into one by external pressure. Some of Bedford's remarks applied to monstrous births in general, but he saw the twins as having a specific as well as a general meaning: '[It] speaketh something in common with the rest of strange and misshapen Births: and if I deceive not my selfe over-much, something in peculiar by it selfe.'[35] His account indicates that although he had not seen the illustration when he wrote it (a situation in which we may suppose ballad-writers also found themselves) he expected a realistic picture: 'Not the mere fiction of an over-daring picturer dost thou here behold, but, if he hath done his part, the true portraiture of the work of God, presented to the world to be seen and admired.'[36] The monster's form was important because it spoke of particular sins. As Bedford wrote:

> If God hath (as it were) spit in the face, and laid the black-finger of Deformity upon the body, ought it not to be entertained with sorrow of Heart and, Humiliation? Hath God written in great Letters the guilt of Sin, and in a deformed body drawn a resemblance of the Soules deformity; drawn it (I say) so; that others may see and know…[37]

God's handy-worke in wonders

In the classical tradition the birth of a monster was said to precede or to coincide with a significant social upheaval; as Cicero succinctly put it: 'monsters, signs, portents, prodigies are so called because they indicate, show, portend and predict.'[38] Later, they were reported after the event of which they were a sign; the well-known English twins the Biddenden maids were said to have been born in 1100, thus coinciding with the untimely death of William II, shot by an arrow whilst hunting in the New Forest. Although their actual year of birth may have differed from this, it was arranged, like that of the Ravenna monster, to coincide with an important event.[39] Ballads continued the tradition of monsters as 'signs from God' but in a form in which the monster was to be interpreted emblematically rather than as a portent. The design of a typical broadside on a monstrous birth was similar to that of an emblem in an emblem book, with a title, picture and text. Sometimes the description and circumstances of a case were printed in prose while the verse pointed to the monster's meaning; sometimes the text made no mention of a specific monster, the illustration alone serving to particularise it. That illustrations often contained information not found in the text suggests that both were considered as a single unit of meaning, as emblems were. Monsters were presented after the events with which they were associated and were not used to foretell the future but to show in retrospect that something important had occurred, a sign of the times rather than a signpost to the future. Whereas in the book literature individual monsters tended to be subservient to the writer's wider concerns (see Chapter 3), in the popular literature the singularity of monsters as events was emphasised, partly because the value of a monster as a sign lay in its particularity. Monsters had been produced over thousands of years in many places but their appearance at a specific time and place was local evidence of divine intervention ('this monstrous shape to thee England'),[40] a place-specific manifestation of God.

Broadsides continued the association between monstrous births and social upheaval; they were expected to appear, providentially, when and where they were most needed.[41] An early German description of a child with two heads linked it to schism in the church:

He who has ears, let him harken to this:
  He will readily see from the picture displayed
That they are indeed separate: head, groin, legs and hands
  The bodies and viscera alike are joined.
If the heads of the boy were joined one to another
  It had survived body and members joined for a long time

But in fact the heads were separate; it was monstrous;
 The ruin of the body and the cause of a horrible death.
Alas the heads, O heads; through the head

 It will begin. But it will not soon finish
The church and the faith though you became divided
 Which will spread to the arms and feet and members.
Thus far they were sewn together like lovers; and now
 Head and members that were hidden are revealed
Oh, I hope these sad things are not the image of Germany
 And the men of the Rhineland divided;
I wish this monster had existed elsewhere
 And not of Germany born, boding ill.[42]

It has become commonplace for historians to describe monstrous births as 'God's punishment for the wickedness of the parents',[43] however, as monstrous births were rare and sin common, the relationship was more subtle than this. A monstrous birth was not a warning of what would happen if one sinned – daily observation would have shown that adulterers, fornicators, heretics and blasphemers did not give birth to monsters – but a reminder that God was watching from behind the scenes, to discover 'our false dissembling' and 'our secret sins'.[44] It was the reader, not the child's parents, that ballads addressed ('The sayde childe was borne alyve, and lyved xxiiij houres, and then departed this lyfe, – which may be a terror as well to all such workers of filthyness and iniquity.')[45] and even when the parents of monsters were said to have been guilty of sexual misconduct, usually by producing offspring illegitimately or incestuously, the reader was supposed to apply the message to his own morals. These displays of 'the anger of God'[46] would, it was hoped, be sufficient 'to affright us from our sinnes'.[47] Reports of monstrous animals also show that monstrous births were not causally attributed to parental sin but were presented as a call to moral self-examination amongst those who witnessed them ('Our filthy lives in Pigges are showed').[48] The description of a pig farrowed near Hampstead in 1562 (Figure 2.3) used the animal's deformity as an emblem of spiritual malaise:

And loke what great deformitie,
In bodies ye beholde:
Much more is in our mindes truly,
 an hundredth thousande folde.[49]

A few lines from *The True Reporte of the Forme and Shape of a Monstrous Childe, Borne at Muche Horkesleye* (1562) indicate that physical causes of

50

Figure 2.3
A monstrous pig, farrowed in Hampstead, London, 1562.

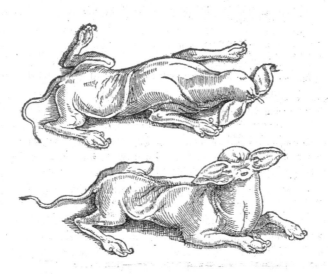

monsters such as excess or deficiency of material were recognised, but were not considered relevant to their message:

> I meane not this as though deformed shape
> Were alwayes linkd with fraughted mind with vice
> But that in nature god such daughters doth shape
> Resemblyng sinnes that so bin had in price,
> So grossest faultes brast out in bodyes forme
> And monster caused of want or too much store
> Of matter, shewes the sea of sinne…[50]

The message of a monstrous birth was read from the emblematic interpretation of its form; the description of *The Forme and Shape of a Monstrous Child, Borne at Maydstone in Kent…* (1568) shows the monster both as a place-specific sign of divine intervention ('This monstrous shape to thee England', suggests that it might have appeared elsewhere had the English not been so corrupt) and an emblem, each part of its anatomy being representative of a particular type of sin, so that the gaping mouth denoted 'poysoned speech', the misshapen hands idleness, the distorted legs refusal to be led, and the 'hinder part', where there arose a mass of flesh with a central hole, sodomy[51] (Figure 2.4). In a society capable of interpreting almost everything as a symbol of something else, the form of a monster could even be used to express puritan disapproval of the fashion for wearing ruffs. The accompanying verses made the connection between deformity, showy costume and vanity: 'Deformed are the things we were [wear] / Deformed is our hart / The Lord is wroth with all this geere / Repent for fere of smarte.'[52]

By the seventeenth century, monsters were no longer used as moralising emblems in the popular literature except in a rather debased way in formulaic accounts that involved a rash expression of heresy by the mother during her labour followed by an appropriate monstrous birth; the form of the monster was appropriate to the mother's impiety, but there was not the interpretative complexity of older accounts. An Englishwoman who stated that she would rather her baby had no head than have it be baptised was surprised when it suffered just such a deformity,[53] and in Catholic France an impious woman cried that she would rather give birth to a calf than pray to St Margaret (the traditional intercessor for pregnant women), again with predictable results.[54] These may represent actual cases to which the details of the mothers' conduct were added after the event in order to enable their use as propaganda. During the English Civil War, when it was discovered that a Mrs Haughton of Kirkham in Lancashire, who had given birth to 'a Monster, which had no head',[55] was a Catholic, the news was passed to Parliament who caused it to be published, with the ingenious claim on the title page that she had wished rather to have a child with no head than a Roundhead.

Lutheranism has been described as the child of the printed book[56] and in general, Protestants were quick to take advantage of the potential of print. Monsters such as Luther's 'monk–calf' were a convenient way to represent the error of opposing views. After showing the reader that the monk–calf (probably a deformed calf rather than a human monstrous birth[57]) was a real happening rather than a fable (by giving its date of birth), Luther referred to the bestial nature of religious orders in order to point the casual reader attracted by the picture of the calf (standing on its hind legs looking almost human) in the right interpretative direction to ensure that the emblem was not misinterpreted (Catholics wryly commented that it symbolised Luther's own abortive monastic career). This was more than just consideration for the reader; Protestant theology required that emblems, which were sent to warn men of their imminent damnation, conveyed their message plainly: there was no room for 'allegorical fancies' because the Holy Spirit was 'the very simplest writer and speaker there is', and men should 'have but one sense and

Figure 2.4
A Warning to England. An anonymous English broadside of 1568.

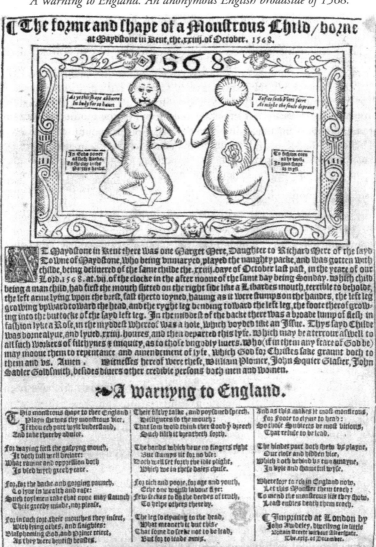

meaning in their mindes'.[58] However, the creation of such emblems was practically impossible, and no effort could render them unambiguous, because, 'almost by definition' they could 'be interpreted in more than one way.'[59] Arnaud Sorbin (1532–1606), Bishop of Nevers, wrote a tract in response to Luther's, in which he used the monk–calf to represent the sin of the Reformation;[60] and later, when stories of Luther's unnatural parentage made him into a kind of monstrous birth himself, the monk–calf was used to represent him, at the root of a tree of Protestant heresies.[61]

The popular literature of Catholic states tended not to concern itself with the position of monsters in the theological scheme of things; they were shown as a direct consequence of unnatural behaviour, as in the case of a supposed half-human, half-monkey born in Paris in 1600,[62] and consequently the birth of a monster could result in the mother's execution for bestiality or even, at least in fictional works, sorcery.[63] But for Protestants, the Creator himself was the architect of monsters and texts such as: 'In Gods power all flesh stands, /As the clay in the potters hands, /To fashion even as he will, /In good shape or in yll',[64] a paraphrase of Romans 9:21,[65] were used to show that monstrous births were tokens of providence, the direct action of God in the natural world. For Protestant ballad-writers, monstrous births were not only convenient emblems for moral and theological instruction, but also tangible signs of religious experience, all the more conspicuous since many of the sacraments, ceremonies and objects that had once formed part of the religious landscape had been proscribed by the reformers. Even at a time when emblems were fashionable and where the interpreting of such devices gave a 'wonderful pleasure', the idea of using monsters to inculcate morality still seems curiously oblique, suggesting that this approach may have been adopted because there were good reasons to avoid a more straightforward one. Before the Reformation, devotional images had been one of the most popular forms of printed material. Afterwards, the permissibility of images was a complex issue, but printers may have been reluctant to use overtly religious illustrations in case they were misinterpreted as icons. Under these restrictions, emblems came into their own; Christ who could no longer be depicted plainly was present in emblems: the *chi-rho* in the reredos above the Creed, the pelican carved on the font, walnuts and cheeses in Dutch still lifes,[66] and monstrous births. A difficulty for Protestant writers wishing to employ monstrous births as emblems was that the scriptures made no mention of them;[67] the nearest thing was the story in St John's gospel of the man born blind 'that the works of God should be made manifest in him', and this solitary example of a congenital condition apparently produced for the edification of witnesses was often referred to in ballads describing monstrous births.[68]

Because the value of a sign lay in its appearance at a specific time and place – and also to give their accounts veracity – broadside writers usually took pains to give details of the date and place of birth of a monster, sometimes so precisely as to include the time of birth or the name of an inn:

One Marget Mere, daughter to Richard Mere, of the sayd towne of Maydstone, who, being unmaryed, played the naughty packe, and was gotten with childe, being delivered of the same childe the xxiiij daye of October last past, in the yeare of our Lorde 1568, at vij of the clocke in the afternoone of the same day, being Sonday...[69]

Both as news and as emblems, reports of monstrous births were expected to be descriptions of actual events: 'a Trouth and no Fable, But a warninge of God'.[70] Broadsides depended for sales on the reader believing the account to be true and new (both favourite words in their titles) and their writers took pains to provide details that lent their account immediacy and verisimilitude. If the monster was false then the reader might suppose its proffered meaning to be false also. Concerns over the 'truth' of these accounts were as old as the ballads themselves; expectations from '[s]ome lowzy ballad' were probably low and only the gullible such as Mopsa in *The Winter's Tale* were 'sure they are true'.[71] One means to achieve credibility was by emphasizing the number and status of eyewitnesses ('it is approved to be true, by the attestation of many godly, honest, and religious women')[72] – an approach comparable to that used subsequently in learned periodicals, and in contrast to the reliance of book writers on textual authorities. A common factor in the appeal to either printed sources or eyewitnesses as authorities was the social standing of those involved, those from the higher social groups, who were often affiliated with the academic or ecclesiastical establishment, forming part of a tradition of gentlemen 'truth-tellers'.[73] In the mid-seventeenth century, when the means of substantiating truth claims were questioned, it was scholarly reliance on written sources – of which Bacon was the great critic[74] – that was most criticised. Thomas Browne wrote in 1646:

But the mortallest enemy unto Knowledge, and that which hath done the greatest execution upon Truth, hath beene a peremptory adhesion unto Authority, and more especially, the establishing of our beliefe upon the dictates of Antiquity. For (as every capacity may observe) most men of Ages present, so superstitiously do look on Ages past, that the Authorities of the one, exceed the reasons of the other. Whose persons indeed being farre removed from our times, their works which seldome with us passe uncontrouled, either by contemporaries or immediate successors, are now become out of the distance of envies: And the farther removed from present times, are conceived to approach the nearer unto truth it selfe.[75]

By the eighteenth century, a vigorous debate over the comparative values of textual and eyewitness authority was in progress. In 1727, for example, James Blondel (c.1666–1734) ridiculed the reliance on ancient authority shown by supporters of the theory of maternal impressions. He argued that cases had to be supported by direct (eyewitness) evidence, and that credit given to earlier accounts should therefore diminish '[i]n Proportion of the Distance of Places and Times' of the occurrence. The surgeon Daniel Turner (1667–1741) responded that written authorities, like gentlemen of his own time, were to be taken on the 'credit' of their word. If one slavishly followed Blondel's approach, he argued, one would credit nothing that one had not seen, and if the double monster then being exhibited in London had been 'presented one hundred Years past, it [would]... have been reckoned by Dr. B[londel] as a fiction'.[76]

From a historical perspective the claims made in early modern accounts of monstrous births are hard to substantiate through external evidence – the existence of different reports of the same monster is of little value in this respect, as these accounts are more likely to have been copied than written independently; and though some broadsides can be corroborated by reference to registers of births and deaths,[77] the names of parents and witnesses are also unhelpful in substantiating truth claims, as an invented or exaggerated account might well make use of real people. The strongest evidence that broadsides were attempts at accurate description is that the monsters described usually correspond with types of birth defects recognised today. Anatomical impossibilities such as a boy with seven heads and seven arms, which found their way into the books of more scholarly authors,[78] seldom occurred in broadsides. Another point in favour of accuracy is that some of the monsters are not especially interesting; anyone wishing to invent a monster would have surely come up with something more remarkable than the macerated baby of Chichester.[79]

As we have seen, not all accounts of monstrous births were representations of actual events. One Scottish monster allegedly had two heads, one hairy and one 'effeminate' (another example of hermaphroditic imagery), each with a single eye, long ears like an ass's, a body like a barrel, and long thin arms growing from 'several places'. It was said to have been born alive and to have uttered the words: 'I am thus deformed for the sins of my parents.' This, along with the illustration, a child-like outline of a doubly smiling monster, and the mother's elaborate confession (she had allegedly desired 'the utter ruin and subversion of all church and state government', though it is not clear how she intended to bring about this lofty objective), signal the 'poetical' nature of the account.[80] A few popular pamphlets mentioned monsters but made no attempt at description; *The Ranters Monster*, for example, tells the story of one May Adams, an alleged Anabaptist who went about calling herself the Virgin Mary. The account of her becoming mad, developing boils and scabs, giving birth to a monster of unspecified type and finally killing herself reflects the writer's view of her deserved fate rather than an actual sequence of events; it is a morality play in which the monster is one of the actors.[81] Although the monster was not described, the minister, churchwardens, constable and other witnesses were named in order to attest to the truth of the story, and it is possible that her pregnancy did have an abnormal outcome.

The tradition of descriptions of monstrous births in popular literature did not come to an end in the early modern period and, as birth defects are still reported in tabloid newspapers, can be seen as ongoing; but the elaborate emblems of the sixteenth century disappeared and their influence must be followed elsewhere, into the orderly classifications of the counter-reformation and into the work of learned societies with their preoccupation with hidden knowledge. In the sixteenth and seventeenth centuries, book writers were not particularly concerned with the presentation of new cases and relied primarily on existing, often classical, literature for examples of monsters; they preferred to cite each other and rarely mentioned the ballad literature, although popular literature was often the unacknowledged source of monsters that appeared in books.[82] They also had less reason to worry about the accuracy of individual cases: books of monsters were, like modern textbooks, intended to give an overall account of the subject, which did not depend on the authenticity of each individual case, and to present the whole of a subject, including fables and stories rather than just a collection of facts.[83] Paradoxically, the use of monsters as signs or emblems in popular literature required a greater emphasis on the individual case than did medical or natural philosophical works, which could afford to generalise. If it were to act as a sign, the monster had to have a particular location and meaning, and an emblem had to possess a distinctive form. An unexpected legacy of the broadside literature was the case report – the title provided a short introduction, the illustration and prose text the description, and the verse the discussion – foreshadowing the scholarly observations that would appear in journals towards the end of the seventeenth century.

Notes

1. J. Day, *The Parliament of Bees* (London: W. Lee, 1641), l. 445.
2. T. Watt, *Cheap Print and Popular Piety 1550–1640* (Cambridge: Cambridge University Press, 1991), 2.
3. P. Burke, *Popular Culture in Early Modern Europe* (London: Temple Smith, 1978), 28.
4. See E. Holländer, *Wunder Wundergeburt und Wundergestalt...* (Stuttgart: F. Enke, 1921).
5. See O. Niccoli (transl. L.G. Cochrane), *Prophecy and People in Renaissance*

Italy (Princeton: Princeton University Press, 1990), 35–65.

6. Philobiblon Society (eds), *Ancient Ballads & Broadsides Published in England...* (London: Whittingham and Wilkins, 1867), xvii.

7. D. Wilson, *Signs and Portents: Monstrous Births from the Middle Ages to The Enlightenment* (London: Routledge, 1993), gives the most comprehensive account of the French literature pertaining to monsters.

8. H.E. Rollins, 'An Analytical Index to the Ballad-Entries (1557–1709) in the Register of the Company of Stationers of London', *Studies in Philology*, xxi (1924), 1–324.

9. For a bibliography of English ballads see C.R. Livingston, *British Broadside Ballads of the Sixteenth Century: A Catalogue of the Extant Sheets and an Essay* (New York: Garland Publishing Inc., 1991).

10. Watt, *op. cit.* (note 2), 48–9.

11. Congenital conditions are those present at birth. A few monstrous adults had conditions that a modern observer would recognise as acquired, for example lymphoedema (see Holländer, *op. cit.* [note 4], 144–5), but they were probably thought to be congenital.

12. Anon., *The Description of a Monstrous Pig...* (London: A. Lacy for G. Dewes, 1562).

13. Anon., *A Wonder Woorth the Reading...* (London: W. Jones, 1617), sig. A1v; J. Mellys, *The True Description of Two Monsterous Children...* (London: A. Lacy, 1566).

14. Wilson, *op. cit.* (note 7), 32.

15. S. McKeown, *Monstrous Births: An Illustrative Introduction to Teratology in Early Modern England* (London: Indelible, 1991), 8.

16. Anon., *The True Reporte of the Forme and Shape of a Monstrous Childe Borne at Muche Horkesley...* (London: T. Marshe, 1562), one of the more eloquent English ballads.

17. Anon., *Monstrificus Puer...* (n.p.: S. Brant, 1511); see Holländer, *op. cit.* (note 4), 343.

18. Anon., *L'Androgyn né a Paris...* (Lyon: M. Jove, 1570).

19. Anon., *The True Reporte...* (1562) see Philobiblon Society, *op. cit.* (note 6), 38–42.

20. The anonymous *A True Report of a Straung and Monsterous Child, Born at Aberwick...* (London: T. Gosson, 1580) was illustrated 'by Raphe Cooke, Paynter, of Berwick upon Tweed'.

21. Anon., *Am XXIIIII Tag des Mai, Also am Sankt-Urbans-Tag, Zwischen Fünf und Sechs Vormittags, hat Eine Siebenundzwanzigjöhrige Frau in der Stadt Landshut an der Donau in Bayern...* (n.p., *c.*1517); see Holländer, *op. cit.* (note 4), 65.

22. As do those in Anon., *Warhaffte Abconterfectur* (Augusberg, 1560).

23. J.D., *A Discription of a Monstrous Chylde, Borne at Chychester in Sussex...* (London: L. Askel for F. Godlyf, 1562).

24. J. Barkar, *The True Description of a Monsterous Chylde...* (London: W. Gryffith, 1564); reproduced in A.W. Bates, 'Birth Defects Described in Elizabethan Ballads', *Journal of the Royal Society of Medicine*, xciii (2000), 202–7.

25. See Appendix, 1511b. Perhaps no monster is theoretically impossible but experience shows that some anatomical arrangements never occur.

26. See, for example, J. Locke, *A Strange and Lamentable Accident...* (London: R. Harper and T. Wine, 1642). Two anonymous English Civil War pamphlets, *A Declaration of a Strange and Wonderfull Monster...* (London: 1646) and *The Ranters Monster* (London: G. Horton, 1652) used the same illustration for different monsters.

27. Barkar, *op. cit.* (note 24); Appendix, 1564.

28. Both are using a key to open a chest, with three books on a shelf in the background: Holländer, *op. cit.* (note 4), 123, 126.

29. C.R. Livingston, 'The Provenance of Three Early Broadsheets', *The Library*, series 6, ii (1980), 53–60.

30. Watt, *op. cit.* (note 2), 145.

31. According to the chronicles of Hollinshed and Stow: see Philobiblon Society, *op. cit.* (note 6), xvii; E. Fenton, *Certaine Secrete Wonders of Nature...* (London: H. Bynneman, 1569), fo. 148r.

32. H. Razovsky, 'Popular Hermeneutics: Monstrous Children in English Renaissance Broadside Ballads', *Early Modern Literary Studies* 2.3 (1996), 1.1–34.

33. Barkar, *op. cit.* (note 24).

34. T. B[edford], *A True and Certain Relation of a Strange Birth...* (London: A. Griffin, 1635).

35. *Ibid.*, 15.

36. *Ibid.*

37. *Ibid.*, 17.

38. *Quia enim ostendunt, portendunt, monstrant, praedicunt, ostenta, portenta, monstra, prodigia dicuntur.* quoted in D. Cressy, *Travesties and Transgressions in Tudor and Stuart England...* (Oxford: Oxford University Press, 2000), 44.

39. For some interpretations of this fascinating and much discussed case see: J.D. Heaton, 'United Twins', *British Medical Journal*, i (1869), 363; J.W. Ballantyne, 'The Biddenden Maids – The Mediæval Pygopagous Twins', *Teratologia*, ii (1895), 268–74 and J. Bondeson, 'The Biddenden Maids: A Curious Chapter in the History of Conjoined Twins', *Journal of the Royal Society of Medicine*, lxxxv (1992), 217–21.

40. Anon., *The Forme and Shape of a Monstrous Child, Borne at Maydstone in*

Kent, the xxiiij of October, 1568 (London: J. Awdeley, 1568); Appendix, 1568b.

41. The 'Christian doctrine of God's providence' led sixteenth-century physicians to look for a cure wherever there was a disease: see, for example, T. Bright, *A Treatise, Wherein is Declared the Sufficiencie of English Medicines, for Cure of All Diseases, Cured With Medicine* (London: H. Middleton for T. Man, 1580), 9. This disarmed any criticism that new cures appeared as and when they were needed, and spas in particular tended to do just that: A.W. Bates, 'Cures at Newnham Regis Spa, 1579', *Warwickshire History*, x (1996), 19–25.

42. Audiat hec/ aures quisquis habet: & facile inde
    Conijciet: presens quid sibi schema velit.
    Sunt seiuncta quidem capita: inguina: crura: manusq[ue].
    Corporis ac iuncti viscera iuncta manent.
    Si capita in puero hoc mansissent iuncta bimembri
    Vixisset corpus/ membraq[ue] cuncta diu.
    Sed capita in partes distracta. Immane fuere
    Corporis exitium. causaq[ue] dira necis.
    Heu capita. O capita. hec capitum discessio per vos

    Incipiet. sed nec dum cito finis erit.
    Ecclesie & fidei per vos discrimina cepta:
    In brachia/ atq[ue] pedes/ membraq[ue] cuncta fluent.
    Hactenus assimiles fueratis amantibus/ at nunc
    In capite & membris/ que latuere patent.
    Ah saltem hec tristis non Theutona corpora Imago
    Disiungi faciat: Rhenicolasq[ue] viros.
    Quam vellem monstrum hoc. Alio sub sole. fuisse
    Et non Germano progenitum orbe, minax.
    (Appendix, 1511a).

43. T. Anderson, 'Documentary and Artistic Evidence for Conjoined Twins from Sixteenth-Century England', *American Journal of Medical Genetics*, cix (2002), 155–9: 158.

44. Mellys, *op. cit* (note 13).

45. Anon., *op. cit.*, (note 40).

46. A. Paré (ed. and transl. J.L. Pallister), *On Monsters and Marvels* (Chicago and London: University of Chicago Press, 1982), 3.

47. Anon., *A Wonder Woorth the Reading…* (London: 1617), sig. A2r.

48. H.B., *The True Discription of a Childe with Ruffes, Borne in the Parish of Micheham in the Coñtie of Surrey, in the Yeere of Our Lord MDLXVI* (London: J. Allde, 1566).

49. W.F., *The Shape of ii Monsters, MDlxii* (London: J. Alde, 1562).
50. K. Park and L.J. Daston, 'Unnatural Conceptions: The Study of Monsters in Sixteenth and Seventeenth-Century England and France', *Past & Present*, xcii (1981), 20–54, argued that in the mediaeval world, enquiry into the physical causes of monsters was perceived as a waste of time if 'nature was merely a cipher, a mirror of God's will', and that this attitude persisted in early modern popular culture.
51. McKeown, *op. cit.* (note 15), 36.
52. H.B., *op. cit.* (note 48); Appendix, 1566b.
53. Locke, *op. cit.* (note 26); Appendix, 1642.
54. Anon. *Histoire Miraculeuse, Advenue dans la Ville de Geneve...* (Lyon: C. Farine, 1609).
55. Anon., *A Declaration, op. cit.* (note 26), 7.
56. A.G. Dickens, *Reformation and Society in Sixteenth-Century Europe* (London: Thames and Hudson, 1966), 51.
57. It has been interpreted as a calf with anencephaly and a posterior encephalocoele or nuchal oedema: M.T. Walton, R.M. Fineman and P.J. Walton, 'Of Monsters and Prodigies: The Interpretation of Birth Defects in the Sixteenth Century', *American Journal of Medical* Genetics, xlvii (1993), 7–13.
58. T.H. Luxon, '"Not I, but Christ": Allegory and the Puritan Self', *English Literary History*, lx (1993), 899–937.
59. D. Russell, *Studies in Renaissance French Culture* (Toronto: Toronto University Press, 1996), 238.
60. A. Sorbin, *Tractatus de Monstris...* (Paris: H. de Marnef and G. Cavellat, 1570).
61. An anonymous woodcut in the Ashmolean Museum, reproduced in Watt, *op. cit.* (note 2), 155. On Luther's demonic parentage see, for example, F.M. Guazzo, *Compendium Maleficarum* (Secaucus: University Books, 1974), 31.
62. Anon., *Discours Prodigieux et Veritable, d'Une Fille de Chambre, Laquelle a Produict un Monstre...* (Paris: F. Bourriquant, c.1600).
63. For example the anonymous *Traite Merveilleux d'un Monstre Engendre dans le Corps d'un Homme...* (Rouen: J. Petit, 1606), a fanciful account of a man giving birth to a monster; see Wilson, *op. cit.* (note 7), 58–60.
64. Anon., *op. cit.* (note 40).
65. 'Shall the thing formed say to him that formed it, Why hast thou made me thus? Hath not the potter power over the clay, of the same lump to make one vessel unto honour, and another unto dishonour?'
66. Cheese was an emblem of the transubstantiated Body of Christ, and walnuts represented His dual nature (God and man = flesh and shell). Nuts also symbolised Christ's flesh (kernel) and the wood of the cross (shell). S.

Schama discusses these perhaps overenthusiastic interpretations in *The Embarrassment of Riches...* (Bath: Fontana, 1987), 161. P. Camporesi devotes a chapter to the symbolism of cheese in *Anatomy of the Senses* (Cambridge: Polity Press, 1994), 37–63.

67. Protestants did not accept the books of Esdras as canonical.

68. John 9:1–3: 'And as Jesus passed by, he saw a man which was blind from his birth. And his disciples asked him, saying, Master, who did sin, this man, or his parents, that he was born blind? Jesus answered, Neither hath this man sinned, nor his parents: but that the works of God should be made manifest in him.' The man subsequently undergoes a miraculous cure. The story was often referred to in the popular literature, for example by Mellys, *op. cit.* (note 13), and was identified as one of three key biblical passages in the monster literature by Wilson, *op. cit.* (note 7), 27–8.

69. Anon., *op. cit.* (note 40); Appendix, 1568b.

70. Anon., *The True Fourme and Shape of a Monsterous Chyld...* (London: 1565).

71. IV, iii, 261; see Wilson, *op. cit.* (note 7), 40.

72. Anon., *op. cit.* (note 47), sig. A3r.

73. See S. Shapin, *A Social History of Truth* (Chicago: University of Chicago Press, 1994) for a discussion of the significance of social status as a guarantee of probity.

74. In *The Great Instauration* (1620) he wrote that he would accept nothing 'but on the faith of my eyes': F. Bacon, 'The Great Instauration', in J. Spedding, R.L. Ellis and D.D. Heath (eds), *The Works of Francis Bacon* (London: Longman, 1857–74), IV, 30. As we have seen, readers of the ephemeral monster literature were of the same opinion, as, later, were the learned societies.

75. R. Robbins (ed.), *Sir Thomas Browne's* Pseudodoxia Epidemica (Oxford: The Clarendon Press, 1981), 32.

76. This controversy is discussed in P.K. Wilson, *Surgeon 'Turned' Physician: The Career and Writings of Daniel Turner (1667–1741)* (PhD, University College London, 1992).

77. R. Hole, 'Incest, Consanguinity and a Monstrous Birth in Rural England, January 1600', *Social History*, xxv (2000), 183–99.

78. Appendix, 1579e.

79. Appendix, 1562a.

80. Anon., *Strange news from Scotland...* (London: E.P. for W. Lee, 1647).

81. Anon., *The Ranters Monster...* (London: for G. Horton, 1652); see McKeown, *op. cit.* (note 15), 67–9. It was illustrated without a head and with a face in its chest.

82. See, for examples, Appendix, 1552a, 1562a, 1570b, 1576a, 1578b, 1579a, 1580b.

83. A point that has been well made elsewhere: W.B. Ashworth, Jr, 'Emblematic Natural History of the Renaissance', in N. Jardine, J.A. Secord and E.C. Spary (eds), *Cultures of Natural History* (Cambridge: Cambridge University Press, 1996), 17–37.

3

The Divine Works of God

[In] Olaus Magnus, and Aldrovandus, and Conrad Lycosthenes, with his
magnificent Prodigiorum ac Ostentorum Chronicon... facts are either kept
in their proper subordinate position, or else entirely excluded on the general
ground of dullness.[1]

By comparison with broadsides and the publications of learned societies, the
book literature, composed of often-repeated cases derived mostly from
written authorities rather than eyewitness accounts, appears relatively
intellectually stagnant. The period of the Reformation saw a striking rise in
book production; between 1436 and 1536 an average of 420 new titles
appeared each year, but between 1536 and 1636 this rose to 5,750.[2] Though
expensive, printed books were more affordable than manuscripts and were
aimed at an increasingly wide readership. Books that included substantial
references to monstrous births fall into two groups: 'wonder' books, which
presented monsters as signs in the same way as the popular literature, though
necessarily with less immediacy, and natural philosophical and medical
books (and theses), which had a stronger analytical or synthetic component.
The latter were less concerned with individual cases – and therefore with
signs, which were by their nature particularised – than with generalizations:
natural philosophers grouped monstrous births together according to form
or cause, while writers of wonder books listed them separately and
chronologically. Although wonder books resembled emblem books in a way
that medical books did not, both were capable of being read on more than
one level, and I will argue that both made theological use of monsters,
though in natural philosophical texts this was less overt. It is also possible to
divide the book literature according to religious allegiances: wonder books
were generally written by Protestants of various persuasions, whereas the
writers who dealt most extensively with the natural properties and
classification of monsters were Catholics. Protestants emphasised divine
intervention, signs and morality, and Catholics tidied everything away into
categories, which were themselves emblematic of an orderly, created world.
All were largely dependent upon patronage and presented monstrous births
in ways that suited the religious and other expectations of their patrons:[3] the
Protestant Pierre Boaistuau (d. 1566) travelled to England to present his

warnings of the ire of God – specially illustrated for the occasion – to Elizabeth I, while Ulisse Aldrovandi's meticulous natural histories earned him a chair at the university of Bologna and the patronage of three popes.[4]

Books of wonders

'Wonder' books were compendia of natural (or more usually unnatural) phenomena of interest for their rarity as well as their meaning. The first to contain new material collected after 1500 was the work of Conrad Lycosthenes (Conrad Wolffhart, 1518–61). In 1552, Lycosthenes had published an edition of Julius Obsequens' (fl. *c.*fourth century A.D.) *Prodigiorum Liber,* a late-classical list of prodigies that derived much of its information from Livy. Lycosthenes supplemented Obsequens' chronological tables of prodigies, of which only those for 190–112 B.C. survived,[5] adding prodigies from the foundation of Rome onwards. *Prodigiorum Liber* enjoyed considerable popularity in the sixteenth century, and the 1720 edition listed some eighteen previous editions between 1508 and 1703, of which Lycosthenes' is the best known.[6]

In 1557, Lycosthenes published a new work, *Prodigiorum ac Ostentorum Chronicon,* bringing Obsequens up to date with descriptions of monsters and other phenomena up to the time of publication. The book was a collection of 'all the strange prodigies hapned in the Worlde', which apart from monstrous births included earthquakes and meteorites, animals and men from distant lands, and a history of the world presented as a sequence of key events from classical Rome to the sixteenth century. A passage chosen more or less at random illustrates its style, which sacrificed literal accuracy for a sense of historical immediacy:

> Charles the great first king of France & after emperor of the Romanes, as saith our histories, was seemly of body, fierce in countenance, his stature was 8 of his feete in length, which was very large, nere to 11 foote of our measure, brode backed, clean bellied, big armes & thighes, he was a fierce & skilful souldier, & very strong in al his lims, his face 18 inches compas breadth & length, his nose half a foote long, his foreheade a foote brode, his eyes were like a lions, round & sparkling, so y on whome he frowned he greatly feared.[7]

The book is a history of the unusual, told vividly and anecdotally, and while it adheres to a relatively strict chronology there is no attempt to identify underlying trends, draw conclusions (the job of the reader), or even to note similar incidents that occur in the course of the work. It is certainly not a book of monstrous births, which represent only a small part of the whole; they are not discussed or compared one with another, and their inclusion is due to their being unusual, and datable, phenomena.

In the threefold division, postulated by Park and Daston, of 'scientific', 'cosmographical' and 'portentous' interpretations of monsters,[8] Lycosthenes' work sits most appropriately in the last group. However, because not all of the events described in his *Chronicon* were interpreted as portents I prefer to describe the monstrous births as 'wonders' as, even if they had at one time been seen as portents, this was not necessarily how they were read in the sixteenth century.[9] Like most books of the time, which were expensive to produce, Lycosthenes' *Chronicon* had to appeal to a fairly wide readership in order to sell sufficient copies to make a profit. Wonders were a subject of general interest and the Latin text could be translated and sold to a less well-educated market without any significant alterations. It had over 1,500 woodcuts (including repeats), three or more to a page, making it one of the best-illustrated books of its time: the range of sources consulted, mostly classical, was also unusually wide and the table of them occupies five pages of six-point type. Obviously, Lycosthenes' principal source was Obsequens, but he included a detailed list of additional Greek and Roman classical sources and scores of more recent ones such as Stow's annals and the 'chronicles' of Meissen, Polen, Brabant, Saxony and other parts of Germany. A source of illustrative material was Sebastian Münster's *Cosmographia*,[10] with which, as Wilson pointed out, *Chronicon* shared a publisher.[11] The results of Lycosthenes' extensive reading were placed in chronological order and vividly recounted; his skill lay in selecting his material and admitting only that which he thought especially significant, but once admitted each piece of information was treated as equal. Like Aldrovandi, Lycosthenes presented a mass of information for the reader without distinction between fable, anecdote and widely agreed 'truths'.

Lycosthenes' overblown style is apparent (through Stephen Batman's translation) in his descriptions of monsters; for example a child born in Saxony:

> …with a grisly looke, having a whole body and well compacte, but all his limmes were brused, torne and loose, saving that his head was copped like a sugarloaf, and as it were set out with a Turkish cap.[12]

Or this from Damenwald, in which the post-mortem changes of a child that had died *in utero* are vividly described:

> Al the childs body was of a bright Bay, his heade had hornes, his eyes were greate and hanging out, he had no nose, his mouth broade a span long… a white tong… no neck… all his body was puffed up, and full of wrinckles, hys armes did sticke in his loynes… from his Nauill there hung down to his feete a kinde of loose bowel….[13]

A proper consideration of the historical basis of the monsters described by Lycosthenes would require a detailed comparison with potential sources, particularly the German ephemeral literature of the early sixteenth century, and in the absence of such correlation the extent to which he attempted to describe individual cases, rather than using them as types of monster in general, remains unclear; nevertheless, most correspond to malformations recognised today.[14] Lycosthenes was on the look out for monsters, and at a time when many people wanted to exhibit their own or their children's deformities for profit, it would not have been too difficult for someone collecting examples for a book to see a few for himself. 'I saw also the like monster in Bavaria,' Lycosthenes said of a two-headed woman.[15] Paré wrote that this was the same monster seen by the Italian philologist Lodovico Ricchieri (1469–1525) and described in his *Antiquarum Lectionum...*,[16] which if correct indicates that she lived for at least twenty years, perhaps making a living by begging door-to-door, in which case many thousands of people might have seen her as she travelled around either in search of charity or because, as Lycosthenes related of her time in Bavaria, she was moved on by authorities fearful of further monsters being engendered in pregnant women who saw her.

Lycosthenes was born in Rouffach, a small town in Alsace, in 1518 and studied at the University of Heidelberg, proceeding MA in 1539. The university was already noted for its Protestant sympathies when he arrived and attempts in the early 1520s by Pope Adrian VI and Elector Louis V to suppress reformed teachings there had been ineffectual. The university did not collectively declare support for Luther until 1545, and after graduating, Lycosthenes, in common with many of his co-religionists, made his way to Basel, a centre of Protestant scholarship (and printing) where the Catholic faith had been declared abolished; here he became Professor of grammar and rhetoric and deacon of the Church of St Leonard.[17] Some of his books were condemned by the Council of Trent, and in his *Chronicon*, published in Basel in 1557, he reiterated his criticisms of the Church and the papacy. In some ways it can be seen as an apocalyptic or even a millenarian work, promoting the belief that the Last Days were approaching. Although Lutherans publicly disowned millenarianism (in the Augsberg confession of faith in 1530), they had other reasons to be interested in wonders, which were a legitimate means of investigating divine purpose in an age in which miracles were supposed no longer to occur. Nature was to Lutherans, and even Calvinists, 'God's great book in folio', and they mined its meaning as they did the holy scriptures,[18] although their approach to wonders, as to religion, was more often based on textual authority – a characteristic of the wonder book literature – than experience.

Of thirty-four sixteenth-century monsters mentioned in Lycosthenes' *Chronicon*, twenty-one occurred within the ten years prior to the book's publication; most of these were from Germany, and a few from Switzerland and Italy. It appears, not surprisingly, that it was easier for Lycosthenes to locate recent and relatively local cases. He is often apparently the first to have described them; however, those for which he did not give a source may have been taken from popular German literature that he did not cite, either because he disdained such sources or because he considered it pointless to name ephemera that his readers had little hope of consulting. In fact his list of sources did not include any named works in German, but the number of cases given without reference to existing scholarly literature suggests that he may have drawn on popular prints, as Park and Daston claim. Had Lycosthenes seen a monster himself he would presumably have said so, as he did of the woman in Bavaria, but it is also possible that he obtained accounts, at first, second, or third hand, from eyewitnesses.

The English cleric Stephen Batman's additions to Lycosthenes certainly drew on the English ballad literature, though he did not acknowledge these sources.[19] When Batman (or Bateman, d. 1584) came to prepare *Prodigiorum ac Ostentorum Chronicon* for translation he updated the work, principally with cases from his own country. Some of these were derived from broadsides, suggesting either that he had been collecting them in anticipation of his work, or that he had access to a collection (comparison with the ballads listed in the Stationers' Company records – see Chapter 2 – shows that he missed some interesting monsters). Batman was a prolific author who was chaplain to Mathew Parker (Archbishop of Canterbury 1559–75). His very readable translation is thought to have been the source for the descriptions of cannibals and 'men whose heads / Do grow beneath their shoulders' in *Othello*,[20] although it was not intended for scholars, who could have read the original, but for interested readers who had not had a university education, his corrigenda demonstrate that he took pains to ensure textual accuracy and made a point of showing this. Wonder books were presumably read for pleasure, and the appearance of monsters in the vernacular literature has been described as part of their 'secularization'.[21] Batman was however just as concerned with the theological context of his subject as Lycosthenes had been, as the book's new title, *The Doome Warning All Men to the Judgement*, indicated.

By retitling the work, Batman showed that it was to be read as an apocalyptical warning, in which the overwhelming weight of examples indicated to the reader that the established order was fragile and liable to descend into chaos. Indeed the excess of cases close to the publication date, albeit explicable by the recent literature being the most accessible, did give an impression of increasing divine intervention in the world. Everyone reading the book would have known that a doom was a representation of the day of judgement, traditionally placed prominently on the wall of a church as a *memento mori* to the congregation (though most did not survive the reformation): Lycosthenes' collection of wonders was another kind of doom, the contemplation of which offered a similar sense of the order of the world dissolving in the *dies irae*. However, Batman faced a problem: Lycosthenes' orderly chronology of wonders, rather than conveying an impression of a breakdown of the natural order, showed that they had occurred throughout history. This being far from the desired effect, he used the opportunity of updating the work to append (and to invent) a succession of striking monsters to conclude it. He added thirteen for the years 1562–80, mostly from England but also from Germany and elsewhere, including at least one (Chapter 1, 33) that was clearly not intended as a description of an actual event. The sins with which these monsters were associated were shown by the behaviour ascribed to their parents, so for example one was illegitimate, while the father of another was: 'a lewd minstrel or idle vagabond' (synonyms rather than alternatives), perhaps the sort who sold ballads.

Batman used these monstrous characters as mouthpieces (some literally had words put into their mouths but all 'spoke' in a metaphorical sense) for theological discourse. The most striking is the triple monster described in Chapter 1: this monster was an emblem of Christ, and Batman's account of its brief existence reads like a bizarre parody of the gospels, culminating in a curious ascension. Of course there could have been no intention of parody on Batman's part; the monster as Christ had been foreshadowed throughout the work in the association between human sin and divine intervention in the form of monstrous births, for without sin, there would have been no Incarnation: 'O happy fault which merited such and so great a Redeemer' as the Catholic liturgy put it.[22] The concepts of 'happy fault' and 'necessary sin' had been expunged from Protestant liturgies, and images of sin and salvation fitting together in a unified whole were superseded by a more alarming eschatology. Towards the end of the book (if not the end of the world) one Alice Perin, a 60-year-old from Yorkshire, gives birth to a creature:

> ...whose head was like to a sallet or head piece, the face somewhat small, onely the mouth long as a Rat, the fore parte of the body like unto a man, having eight legges, and the one not like the other, a taile in length half a yard, like to the tayle of a Rat.[23]

Even more alarming was the 'uggly monster' born at Arnheim:

> [The] woman very unadvisedly said, I woulde I might beare a Divell, so should I once be rid of this wo and misery, &c. not long after she broughte

forth a wonderfull Monster. As soone as the neighbours and Midwife were
come, shee began for very gret pains to cry out fearfully, & not long after was
delivered, but sodainley the Monster ranne under the bed. The proportion
of his body and lims was as followeth, being seene of many both men and
women: a rough bodie hairie and blacke, except his belly which was like a
swan, the two feete like Peacockes, clawed, his eyes shined like fire and were
very great, he had a mouth like to a Storke or Crane, blacke, a tayle like an
Oxe, two bending hornes on his heade, in steade of handes clawes like a
Hauke. After this hideous Monster was thus seene, to the greate feare of
manye, among them it was smoothered to deathe betweene two beddes.[24]

This tale was a morality play similar to those told in some ballads, in
which the woman's impious utterance characteristically sealed her fate, and
the description and illustration of the monster was similar to
contemporaneous depictions of devils (according to the theory of maternal
impressions this was not unexpected as pregnant women might see such
pictures).[25] John R. McNair, in his introduction to the 1984 reprint of *The
Doome*, suggested that Batman's work was a topical attack on Elizabeth I's
proposed 'French marriage'; while this may well have been on his mind, the
warning message of his work is firmly in the tradition of the monster
literature in Protestant ballads of the period, with which he was familiar, and
of the work of Melanchthon and Luther, who had used monstrous births to
present reformed theology to a wider audience.

The inclusion of monsters in wonder books is explicable in the same
terms as their popularity in ephemeral literature: they were intrinsically
interesting, susceptible to interpretation as signs, and suitable emblems with
which to convey a theological message. Publishers would have known from
ballad sales that monsters were popular with readers. Despite the emphasis
on textual authority we cannot assume that readers found books more
believable than ballads, but they were useful, as an early reader of *The Doome*
noted in the margin: '*multa vera, multa falsa, sed omnia vere utilia.*'[26] ['Much
truth, much falsehood, but all very useful.'] Order is now a familiar basis for
scientific and theological arguments, and exceptions are seen as problematic;
evolutionists had to explain the peacock's tail, and creationists explained
antediluvian animals. Wonder books were composed entirely of exceptions
and, although on one level these would have entertained the curious, they
were also an attempt to use diversity and unpredictability as an indication of
continuous supernatural control of worldly affairs. They proclaimed that the
world is more complex than it looks, and this complexity was a sign of God,
to be documented and celebrated but never fully comprehended. Wonders
were important things to discover, as greater complexity in created things
argued greater glory for their creator. The ballad *Gods Handy-Worke in*

Wonders[27] reminded the reader that monsters were not to be viewed as if God were 'a bungler in some common trade', but as 'the great master, in whose hand it lies to make a beggar or a king, a beautiful body or a monstrous'.[28] The monster was a messenger, but needed to bring 'into the world no other news, but an admiration of the devine works of God'.[29]

Lycosthenes' *Chronicon* was the basis for another Protestant wonder book, Pierre Boaistuau's *Histoires Prodigieuses* of 1560.[30] Further volumes of which, by Claude de Tesserant (d. 1575), François de Belleforest (1530–85) and Rod Hoyer, augmented by additional woodcuts, appeared in 1566, 1571, 1574, 1576, 1594 and 1598. In all there were more than thirty-seven editions, with translations into English, French, Dutch and Welsh.[31] Boaistuau diligently collected material and supplied references to other printed books, in accordance with his stated intention 'not to commend thorowout this whole boke, anything which is not confirmed with sufficient credit by some notable author, eyther Greeke or Latine, Sacred or Prophane.'[32] The work was translated into English in 1569 by Edward Fenton, as *Certaine Secrete Wonders of Nature, Containing a Descriptiõ of Sundry Strange Things, Seming Monstrous...'.* As in other wonder books, monstrous births formed part of a chronology of mixed wonders and prodigies:

> [A]mongst all the thinges whiche maye be viewed under the coape of heaven, there is nothying to be seene, which more stirreth the spirite of man, which ravisheth more his senses, which doth more amaze him or ingendereth a greater terror or admiration in al creatures, than the monsters, wonders, and abominations, wherein we see the workes of Nature, not only turned arsiversie, missehapen and deformed, but (which is more) they do for the most part discover unto us the secret judgement and scourge of the ire of God by the things that they present.[33]

Boaistuau,[34] a native of Paris, known as a good talker and 'not without a certain erudition',[35] travelled to England in 1559 to present an illuminated manuscript version of his work to Elizabeth I. The text appealed to the less austere aspects of scholarship, devoting (separate) chapters to subjects such as famous courtesans and methods of torture. Boaistuau justified his inclusion of monstrous births by their value as a moralising message to sinners:

> It is most certaine, that these monstrous creatures, for the most part do proceede of the judgement, justice, chastisement and curse of God, which suffreth that the fathers and mothers bring forth these abhominations, as a horrour of their sinne, suffering themselves to run headlong, as do brute beastes without guide to the puddle or sinke of their filthie appetites, having

no respecte or regarde to the age, place, tyme or other lawes ordeined of Nature.[36]

Despite the harshness of the message the appropriate response was Christian compassion towards the messenger:

[The] auncient Romaines had these litle monstrous creatures in such abhomination, that as soone as they were born, they were immediately committed to the ryver Tyber, there to be norished. But we being better broughte up, and fostred in a schole of more humanitie, knowying them to be the creatures of GOD, suffer them to be brought to the church, there to receive the holy sacrament of Baptisme.[37]

The association in the sixteenth (and to a lesser extent the seventeenth) century between moral deformity on the part of parents and physical deformity in their offspring was commonplace, a probable reflection of the traditional association of deformity with sin.[38] The puritan divine and schoolmaster Thomas Beard's (d. 1632) *The Theatre of God's Judgements* (1597), a popular compendium of punishments for sinners based on a French original, told of a man who used to hunt every Sunday at sermon-time, and whose wife had a child with a head like a dog, and which cried like a hound. Boaistuau's puritanical text, which included a favourable review of ancient punishments for adultery, linked monstrous births with sexual immorality – the mother of one was 'a fallen woman, who prostituted herself to all and sundry'[39] – and those resembling dogs or other animals with bestiality.[40] Boaistuau's message was not that monstrous births were the physical result of 'unnatural' sexual acts (although he also discussed the vexed question of whether demons could beget viable offspring) but that they served as a warning of the 'secret judgement' that sinners must ultimately undergo.

Medicine and natural philosophy

The separation of medical and natural philosophical texts from wonder books in this chapter is not intended to obscure their similarities. The sources, textual and illustrative, were often the same, as ultimately were the monsters themselves, although the intended readership was not, and the authors' perception of their readers' interests influenced their approaches. In contrast to ballads, wonder books and journals of learned societies, which presented discrete units of pertinent information ('observations') selected by the author, natural philosophers such as Ulisse Aldrovandi and his contemporaries presented their readers with a large volume of material, which they were invited to assimilate into a complete picture. Aldrovandi's three-volume *Ornithologiae*, the beginning of a projected fourteen-volume natural history, described the moral lessons to be drawn from birds, as well as their uses in food, hunting and heraldry. He filled eighty pages with stories and fables about eagles before beginning a description of the eagle itself, but to Aldrovandi and his readers the fables were part of the description.[41]

In common with many early modern writers on natural history, Aldrovandi had a medical degree and was licensed to practice medicine, though there is no evidence that he did so. It is not my intention to 'medicalize' monsters, and medical men were so often natural philosophers that it is hardly reasonable to class their writings on every subject as medical. On the other hand, the limits of medicine in the early modern period are not easily defined; university-educated medical men had a wider range of scholarly interests than is usual today, and to confine medicine to the treatment of disease seems unnecessarily proscriptive. Monstrous births were associated with medicine, but the literature on them was not primarily 'medical' in purpose. Consider Jacob Rueff's *De Conceptu et Generatione Hominis* (1554),[42] an obstetrical work modelled on one of the earliest vernacular treatises on obstetrics, Eucharius Rösslin's *Der Swangern Frauwen und Hebammen Rosengarten* of 1508.[43] Rueff (1500–58) was city physician of Zürich, responsible for the teaching and examination of midwives, to whom his book was sent with instructions that parts of it should be read to them 'by a well-read woman'.[44] They are unlikely to have found the section on monstrous births especially useful, except as a warning that they might occasionally meet with such cases. Although *De Conceptu* was a 'medical' book intended for the instruction of practitioners, Rueff, a Lutheran at least to the extent that he had served with the troops of Zürich against the Catholic cantons,[45] presented monsters in the same way as Protestant ballads or wonder books did: they were a sign of the anger of God. Rueff's remarks on the monster of Kraków implied a typically Protestant linkage of human and natural laws: 'It is said that this monster was caused of God's making; nonetheless, through the sin of Sodomy, this detestable monster was of our own making.'[46] The inclusion of monsters seems to have been as much for the midwives' moral as medical instruction.

Perhaps the book that most obviously suggests a medical approach to monstrous births is *Des Monstres Tant Terrestres que Marines avec Leurs Portraits* (1573), part of Ambroise Paré's (*c.*1510–90) *Deux Livres de Chirurgie*. This is the best known of all such works from the early modern period – the only one still in print, and among the earliest books to include a classification of monstrous births.[47] As its title suggests it was abundantly illustrated and the simple but engaging woodcuts are frequently reproduced in works on the history of monstrous births. At the time of writing Paré was at the top of his profession and was probably the best-known surgeon in

74

France. He was famously at loggerheads with the hierarchy of the Parisian *Faculté de Médecine*, whom he had, probably deliberately, antagonised, by writing in French rather than Latin – making medical and surgical texts open to laymen (and even laywomen) – and by trespassing on traditionally medical preserves. But Paré's position as surgeon to Charles IX, and later to Henry III, usually ensured that he got his own way. In 1554, he had been rapidly advanced through the bachelor's degree and licentiate in surgery of the Confraternity of St Côme, 'since the King wished it', despite having given some perfunctory answers in his examination, and later in the year he presented a Latin thesis and so became a master Surgeon, entitled to wear not only the long robe of a 'scholar' of the *Faculté* but the square hat of a master. The *Faculté* resented his preferment, pointing out apparently correctly that he knew no Latin and had to have his thesis written out for him to read. While we might agree with the *Faculté* that the inclusion of monstrous births in Paré's book was 'completely off the subject', their dismissal of them as 'fit for amusing little children'[48] reveals a view that they were not even appropriate for serious study, which perhaps stemmed from their association with cheap prints and wonder books. This may also explain why Paré included them; although the popularity of monsters had resulted in a lowering of their scholarly credibility, they were *popular*, and Paré probably wrote about them with the intention of attracting a wider readership that a purely surgical book might have done. As we shall see in the next chapter, opposition among Paris physicians was relatively short-lived and by 1600 monstrous births were being studied in the university school of anatomy.

The opening chapter of *Des Monstres* is amongst the best-known writing on the subject and begins with a list of 'several things that cause monsters':

The first is the glory of God.
The second, his wrath.
The third, too great a quantity of seed.
The fourth, too little a quantity.
The fifth, the imagination.
The sixth, the narrowness or smallness of the womb.
The seventh, the indecent posture of the mother, as where, being pregnant, she has sat too long with her legs crossed, or pressed against her womb.
The eighth, through a fall, or blows struck against the womb of the mother, being with child.
The ninth, through hereditary or accidental illnesses.
The tenth, through rotten or corrupt seed.
The eleventh, through mixture or mingling of seed.
The twelfth, through the artifice of wicked spital beggars.
The thirteenth, through Demons and Devils.[49]

These were statements of generally accepted knowledge, many derived from classical sources, as Paré acknowledged when writing of causes such as the quantity and corruption of seed, maternal imagination and smallness of the womb; for example, his justification for 'mixture or mingling of the seed' as a cause of monsters was 2 Esdras 5:9: 'and menstruous women shall bring forth monsters' (that is, children conceived during menstruation shall be monstrous). Paré went on to write that there were other causes as yet unknown, because for some monsters, such as those 'with only one eye in the middle of the forehead', he was unable to give an explanation that was either sufficient or probable. In subsequent chapters he used this list of causes as the basis of a classification of monstrous births, assigning examples of monsters to each group. This was not a series of rigid compartments but a system of overlapping groups into which cases were placed so as to appear in an orderly fashion before the reader. The relationships between the categories are however more complex than they may first appear: the first and second presumably included the following eleven groups, as it does not appear that Paré supposed that any monsters were not the result of the actions of God.[50] In his chapter twenty, for example, on 'mixture or mingling of seed', he wrote of atheists and sodomites 'provoking the wrath of God against them[selves]', thereby acknowledging an overlap between the wrath of God and physical causes.

Paré's surgical background and his interest in collecting curiosities seems to foreshadow a modern approach to teratology. A number of monsters were seen by Paré and described by him for the first time, and in one or two cases he mentions that they were dissected and preserved at his house (the autopsy as a means of examining monstrous births had been practiced in Europe for at least fifty years),[51] though he did not publish any further observations on them. Some modern commentators have portrayed Paré as in effect the first teratologist, someone who treated monsters as 'from the outset a matter of "scientific" enquiry'[52] and whose 'basic concern' was 'his search for causes'.[53] But his interpretations of monstrous births were actually closer to those of ballads and wonder books in their outlook. He claimed an association between monstrous births and wars and other catastrophes and suggested that monsters were examples, like the man born blind in St John's gospel (which he cited), of the glory of God. In sixteenth-century France it cannot have been difficult to find conflicts with which to link monstrous births. During Paré's lifetime France had been almost continuously at war with Italy, England, Switzerland and Spain and in 1562 began over forty years of civil wars between Catholics and Protestants. Like many of his contemporaries, Paré had learned his trade as a military surgeon and, while this was an excellent training in the art of surgery (and provided material for books on his travels and on the treatment of the gunshot wounds he encountered), his personal experience of years of campaigning must have been conducive to a view of the world as troubled and confused. Another suggestion is that Paré's classification is evidence for the declining importance of the supernatural in theories of causation of monsters, as only three of his causes fall into this category.[54] However, this assumes that it was comprised of equal and mutually exclusive categories, and that having known physical causes precluded monsters from acting as signs of the power of God, neither of which was the case. It also overlooks Paré's own statement that: 'most often these monstrous and marvellous creatures proceed from the judgement of God, who permits fathers and mothers to produce such abominations from the disorder that they make in copulation, like brutish beasts...'.[55]

After Paré, no other writer published a classification of monstrous births until Caspar Bauhin (1560–1624), in his book *Hermaphroditorum Monstrosorumque* in 1600.[56] Bauhin's attempt to order all types of monstrous births by cause is a valuable summary of contemporary theories concerning their origin. A Calvinist whose father had been a Huguenot refugee, Bauhin studied theology at Basel and medicine at Montpellier, Heidelberg and Strasbourg, becoming professor of botany and anatomy at Basel, where his collection of over 4,000 plants is still preserved. He held the first public dissection there, and later replaced Felix Platter as professor of medicine and became rector of the university. He is now most noted for his anatomical work *Theatrum Anatomicum* (anatomists will be familiar with Bauhin's valve) and for his catalogue of plants *Pinax Theatri Botanici*, which introduced the system of binominal nomenclature later adopted by Linnaeus. Bauhin applied his enthusiasm for classification to monstrous births, devising a scheme that consisted of several 'levels' of causes of monsters, rather than overlapping groups, and placing the higher causes first, as had Paré. The concept of hierarchical causes of monstrous births, the higher encompassing the lower, can be traced to Aquinas:

> I answer that cognitive habits differ according to higher and lower principles: thus in speculative matters wisdom considers higher principles than science does, and consequently is distinguished from it; and so must it be also in practical matters. Now it is evident that what is beside the order of a lower principle or cause, is sometimes reducible to the order of a higher principle; thus monstrous births of animals are beside the order of the active seminal force, and yet they come under the order of a higher principle, namely, of a heavenly body, or higher still, of Divine Providence. Hence by considering the active seminal force one could not pronounce a sure judgement on such monstrosities, and yet this is possible if we consider Divine Providence.[57]

Bauhin presented a hierarchical tree (Table 3.1) of causes of monsters of the sort widely used in books of the time and perhaps derived from the dialectical classifications of the French academic Peter (Petrus) Ramus (1515–72). Many types of knowledge could be structured in this way, since almost anything can be divided into *x* or not *x*, then subdivided into *y* or not *y*, and so on. He did not allocate specific examples of monstrous births to categories he outlined, but his choice of dichotomies is of interest as a list of properties or causes that he believed some, but not all, monsters shared.[58]

Like many classifications this is not as straightforward as it seems: the categories were not necessarily mutually exclusive and there is the possibility both of multiple causes and multiple levels of causation. Did the anger of God or the influence of the stars act directly on the developing infant, or did they bring about their effects by, for example, altering the quantity of semen, or stimulating the maternal imagination? Although Paré and Bauhin did not describe multiple causation, the categories in their classifications do appear to overlap. While the 'higher' category in Bauhin's classification includes monsters due to the 'anger or judgement of God' because of 'errors of sexual union', another group appears in the 'lower' category under 'union contrary to nature'. These cases seem to have been subject to double jeopardy as they were against the laws of both God and Nature – an indication not only that 'higher' and 'lower' were not exclusive categories, but of the connection between natural laws and the laws of God.

Fortunio Liceti's *De Monstrorum* (1616) represents, I suggest, a change of emphasis in the way in which monstrous births were presented. Liceti (1577–1657) was one of the leading Italian scholars of his day. He is perhaps best noted for having survived extreme prematurity; his mother was some seven months pregnant when she went into labour on a stormy sea voyage and her newborn son fitted into the palm of a hand (a small 28-week baby in a foetal position just about fits onto a man's hand). His medical father used a primitive incubator based on a modified oven to rear Fortunio, who earned his name. He was a brilliant student, receiving his doctorate in medicine and philosophy at Bologna in 1600 before taking up the chair of logic at Pisa. He was an authority on Aristotle, and it may have been through *The Generation of Animals* that he acquired his interest in monstrous births. In 1609, he became professor of philosophy at Padua, where his reputation for encyclopaedic knowledge brought him many students. From there he moved to Bologna before returning to Padua as professor of theoretical medicine, a post that he held until his death. Throughout his academic career, Liceti wrote books at the rate of about one a year. The range of his learning was unusually wide even by the standards of the time and his output included everything from historical works such as *De Annulis Antiquis*, an erudite treatise on the history of finger-rings, to the

Table 3.1
Bauhin's Hierarchy of 'Monsters'

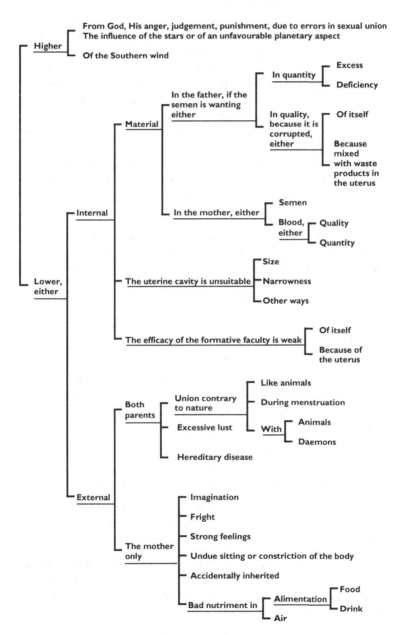

astronomical text *De Novis Astris et Cometis*. Books with a medical theme included a work on the spontaneous generation of animals and another on survival of long periods of fasting.[59]

After his death, his reputation was sustained for a time by reprints of his works but then suffered a decline, perhaps because of a perceived credulousness. In *De Lucernis Antiquorum Reconditis* (1621), for example, he advanced the theory that the ancients had placed perpetually burning lamps in their tombs, producing a peculiar glow on opening that Ottavio Ferrari explained away in his *De Veterum Lucernis Sepulchralibus* (1670) as nothing more than a momentary phosphorescence on exposure to air. Like many Catholics, Liceti opposed Harvey's account of the circulation of the blood, putting forward an alternative in accordance with his own interpretation of Aristotle's writings.[60] The structure of *De Monstrorum* owed much to its author's background in classical philosophy. Liceti began by setting out his motivation in dealing with the subject of monstrous births:

> No matter how widely these rare things that, to men's great astonishment, differ from the general order and condition of things of their kind, whether for good or ill, they are usually said, according to the sum of informed opinion, to be monsters; thus honourable and civilised men have, one might say, become more excellent and almost like gods, whereas men defiled by the sins of beasts have become gross and corrupt.[61]

De Monstrorum was clearly intended as a reference for other scholars (perhaps Liceti lectured on the subject) rather than a practical account for medical practitioners. He defined a monster thus:

> A monster is a being under heaven [ie. not supernatural] that provokes in the observer horror and astonishment by the incorrect form of its members, and is produced rarely, begotten, by virtue of a secondary plan of nature, as a result of some hitch in the causes of its origin.[62]

He portrayed the monster not in wonder book terms as an unusual occurrence but as Aristotle had, as something that was not as it 'ought' to be. The monster told the observer something about its own nature and origin:

> It is this field of physiology, at present lying fallow, which I intend to cultivate: where all monsters will be studied... their causes; their origins; their differences.[63]

Catholic theologians had been interested in Aristotle since the Middle Ages, partly because his concept of the fulfilment of purpose could be related to the purpose of the Creator.[64] Liceti addressed the problem of how Nature could be said to make a slip by referring to the idea of a 'secondary plan'. He emphasised 'natural' causes while rejecting the 'vulgar' concept that Nature simply made a mistake.[65] Liceti's interpretation of the place of Nature in monstrous births was carefully expressed: he used the Latin word *error* (going astray) to describe the process ('nature produces monsters in error...') but denied that nature sinned (*pecat*).

The first edition of *De Monstrorum* contained no illustrations. Most of the text was taken up with a classification of monsters, arranged first by morphology and then into subgroups by 'cause', for each of which Liceti supplied examples from antiquity to recent times. Although he probably started out with no practical experience of monstrous births, after the appearance of the first edition he became known in connection with them, and cases were referred for his opinion. In 1622 Auguste Princet, a Genoese physician, wrote to him describing a baby with an attached homunculus.[66] His letter, and Liceti's reply with remarks on the possible causes of the defect and the observation that such twins could live for a long time (he was correct in this case), was included in the second edition of *De Monstrorum* (Figure 3.1, overleaf), which appeared in Padua in 1634 with additional text and high-quality illustrations, most of which were adapted from Paré and Lycosthenes. Liceti seems to have been on the alert for new cases, and a cyclopic girl born at Fermo was another addition.[67] His approach is distinguishable from earlier writers on monstrous births by the confidence of his assumption that all monstrosities could be classified and explained. In the popular view of the time a monster was something almost miraculous, a sign of divine intervention, which of course was one of the reasons why they provoked such interest, but Liceti observed that, if God is the sole cause of everything, only by adding further levels of causation can a meaningful explanation be arrived at. *De Monstrorum* was primarily an analytical work and the former professor of logic assumed that monstrous births, just like anything else, could be classified systematically. The significance of this conceptual change can be shown by comparing Paré's statement, made forty-three years earlier: 'There are divine things, hidden, and to be wondered at, in monsters – principally in those that occur completely against nature – for in these, philosophical principles are at want, so that one cannot give any definite opinion in their case', with Liceti's magisterial dismissal of some of the earlier theories of their origin: 'Monsters are produced merely when nature makes a mistake, and sin cannot result in the appearance of a monster', '[a] monster does not foretell the future',[68] and 'a monster does not signify evil'.[69] 'It is unbelievable,' he wrote, 'that God produces monsters in order to warn men of imminent catastrophes. It is not what they presage, but their rarity that makes the world wonder at them.'[70]

Figure 3.1
The title page of Fortunio Liceti's De Monstrorum (Padua, 1634).

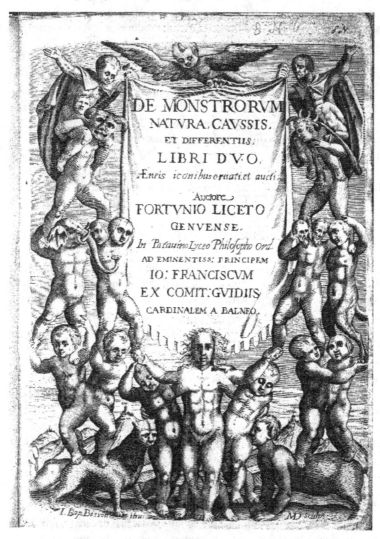

Liceti's elaborate classification system combined (intentionally, rather than just confusing the two) morphology and cause. Monsters were divided into two principal groups: 'uniform', of a single species and gender, and 'non-uniform', possessing elements of different species or sexes.[71] 'Uniform' monsters were then sub-divided into: deficient or mutilated (eg. lacking arms or feet), excessive (eg. two-headed), of two natures (deficit and excess combined), double (conjoined twins), unformed (eg. a child with its limbs bruised, broken and disarticulated) and extraordinary (morphologically complete but unusual in substance, eg. hirsute or pigmented). 'Non-uniform' monsters could be of the same or different species: the first category included hermaphrodites, the latter hybrids with demons as well as with animals. Liceti then applied the same set of causes (deficiency of material, quality of semen, compression within the uterus, etc.) within each morphological group.

The most extensive early modern taxonomy of monsters is that of Caspar Schott (1608–66), a Jesuit priest who studied at Wurzburg under Athanasius Kircher until forced to flee by the Swedish invasion in 1631. He later returned to teach natural philosophy and mathematics and wrote *Physica Curiosa* (1662), an exhaustive study of natural magic, including physics, music, mathematics and natural philosophy. 'Magic' was almost synonymous with 'knowledge', and from the outset the book made a distinction between 'licit and illicit magic' (*Magiae in licitam & illicitam*), the former being 'the knowledge of hidden things handed down from Adam to his descendents' (*ita reconditarum quoque rerum scientia ab Adamo posteris suis tradita*).[72] Book five dealt with monsters, their history and causes, in thirty chapters. Schott drew cases from earlier book literature and placed them in a classification that encompassed all known human monstrous births – he even created a category of seven-headed monsters, which had only one member.[73] Schott's classification consisted of a series of precise, morphologically based categories formulated to accommodate all the monstrous births that he knew of:

Human acephalics
Human polycephalics
  Two-headed
  Two-headed with one head in the belly
  Three and seven heads
Animal polycephalics
Human monsters with non-human heads
Animal monsters with heads of other species
Human monsters with abnormal heads
Human monsters without arms and compensating for their loss
Human monsters with arms
  Mutilated
  Transposed
Human monsters with supernumerary arms
Human monsters with imperfect hands, maimed or with superfluous digits

Human monsters with deformed bellies and genitalia
Human monsters without legs or feet
Human monsters with 3 or 4 feet
Human monsters with feet like those of evil beasts
Human monsters by reason of various affections of the skin
Human monsters born with the skin wounded or peeling off
Monsters born as stone
Human monsters double below, single above
Human monsters double above, single below
Human monsters with two bodies laterally conjoined
Human monsters with two bodies longitudinally conjoined
Human monsters made from perfect and imperfect bodies joined
Monsters with two bodies from human and animal foetuses combined
Monsters that differ from the progeny of all species
Rare kinds of monsters

Some monsters were included in more than one group but this implied not overlap but co-incidence, the equivalent of a patient with more than one disease. Although Schott's approach may appear less analytical than that of Liceti or even Paré, who sought to categorise monsters by cause, it had the advantage of practicality. Causes were often speculative and matters of dispute, but morphological features were susceptible to reproducible description. While classifications by cause provided information about the supposed origins of monstrous births, classifications by morphology were probably easier for the reader to navigate, since the morphology of a monster would be known even if the cause were not. The classification of monstrous births was in some ways analogous to that of animals and plants (Bauhin and Aldrovandi worked in both areas) and monsters were sometimes presented as though whole races rather than isolated examples were being described.[74] Morphological classification may have influenced the way in which monstrous births were seen and portrayed; as with taxonomic classifications of animals, description acquired fresh importance if classification depended on it. Schott made no attempt to endow individual monsters with any overt emblematic or theological significance, but he was the most thorough of classifiers, so much so that the classification itself is perhaps the real message of his work. Detailed and internally consistent, it reflected not only the intellectual discipline that characterised the Jesuit order but the orderly creation of an omnipotent creator.

Theses and universities

Most natural philosophical writers on monstrous births, like Bauhin, Liceti and Schott, taught in universities. It is likely that they, and others, taught on monstrous births and that students read their books, and the introduction of classifications may in part have been to make the subject easier to learn. In the seventeenth century, students began producing dissertations on monstrous births, the earliest of which, by Jean Riolan the Younger (1580–1657),[75] was seen by Wilson as something of a turning point: 'one of the first efforts towards a more scientific view of the monstrous birth.'[76]

Riolan graduated MD from Paris in 1604, and his doctoral dissertation was printed in the following year. The double monster that he described is particularly well-documented, appearing in at least three other contemporary publications.[77] Riolan's disputation was set out in a standard formal question-and-answer format. The first of his four questions was whether the twins were monstrous, which he argued they were. The second was whether they had two souls or only one: Riolan based his answer that they had two primarily on the differences in temperament between them; and, to support his claim that 'contrary to medical and Platonic opinion the brain is the seat of the rational soul,'[78] he used examples of the Oxford twins of 1552 and the Northumbrian monster of 1490 (conjoined twins who lived to the age of 28) to demonstrate that twins with two heads and shared viscera showed clear differences in behaviour if they lived to maturity. Such differences had long been accepted as evidence that double monsters were two individuals, as accounts from as early as 1533 show (see Chapter 6, 155), and Riolan's approach was not innovative. His third question was whether monsters should be killed at birth: he rejected this proposal, but favoured segregating them from society. The final proposition, that monsters were prodigies, he also rejected. Riolan and the three vernacular publications that he cited all put forward a physical cause for the monstrosity – nature had been obliged to 'sew together' the two embryos due to narrowness of the womb.[79] Like many dissertations, Riolan's questions and answers were largely rhetorical: the twins were self-evidently a monster, conjoined twins with two heads were invariably treated as two individuals, there is nothing to suggest that infanticide was ever openly performed in the early modern period, though unwanted children, monstrous or otherwise, may of course have been secretly destroyed (see Chapter 6, 158–9), and the distinction between monsters and prodigies was well accepted (see Chapter 1, 12–13). What makes his work stand out is his dissection of the twins. His monograph included an impressive intaglio engraving, which would have been expensive to produce, showing the arrangement of their abdominal viscera (Figure 3.2, overleaf). The twins shared a liver and a heart (or at least pericardial sac) and the artist arranged the viscera symmetrically, with one twin almost a mirror image of the other.[80] Although the engraving includes a high level of detail (and order), it was not a literal rendering: the dissected twins were shown alive and older than their years.

Figure 3.2
An engraving from Jean Riolan's De Monstro nato Lutetiae *(1605). The*
anatomised twins are shown alive and older than their years: C is the stomach,
E the liver, and F the heart (Appendix, 1605).

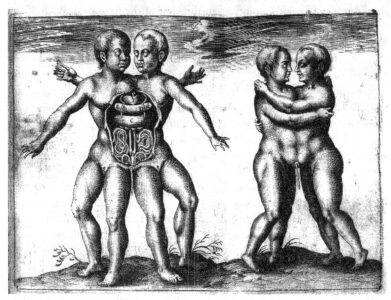

Riolan was only twenty-five at the time *De Monstro* was published and
had just been appointed to the chair of anatomy and botany at Paris. The
presentation of a thesis was a formal occasion[81] that we might regard as
resembling a modern inaugural lecture, with the faculty in attendance and a
rather reserved discussion afterwards. The audience was meant to appreciate
Riolan's use of logic and rhetoric rather than his conclusions; it was, in Roger
French's words: 'a specimen magisterial performance'.[82] We do not know if
Riolan delivered the disputation in the presence of the twins' dissected body,
but the dissection was clearly intended as a teaching tool and the high-
quality engraving required to do it justice suggests that Riolan hoped to
impress the faculty with his anatomical skill (he would become one of the
best known French anatomists, and the vessel that connects the superior and
inferior mesenteric arteries is still known as the arc of Riolan). The
University of Paris (where his father had been Dean of the faculty of
medicine) was an institution seen (in retrospect) as intellectually
conservative. The Riolans father and son were Galenists and staunch
opponents of Harvey's *De Motu Cordis*. On balance, it seems very unlikely
that Riolan intended his thesis to present a controversial view or that he

expected his choice of subject to come as a surprise to the medical faculty that he was about to join. That such a well-connected scholar should choose to begin his teaching career in this way shows that since the dismissive comments made about Paré's monsters just over thirty years earlier, attitudes had changed and they had become an accepted, even a praiseworthy, subject for academic study.

Throughout the seventeenth century, monstrous births featured in doctoral disputations in faculties of theology and philosophy in Protestant universities. From being innovative they descended into something of a safe subject for the unimaginative.[83] As these later authors were not medical men no dissection was involved, and their theses generally consisted of a description of a recent monstrous birth and a brief summary of the literature. The time-honoured questions of the appropriateness of baptism and whether demons could generate monsters were the most popular topics for discussion. In contrast to the volume of early modern literature on monsters that can be assembled today, dissertation writers, despite access to university libraries, generally made scant reference to earlier cases – Laurent Gerlin, for example, who published his thesis in Wittenberg in 1624, was able to identify only three cases of monstrous births in the entire sixteenth century; these he attributed to maternal impressions and discussed according to the theories of Aristotle. Thirty-one years later, Christophor Wallrich took as his subject the highly publicised John-Baptiste and Lazarus Colloredo, the flamboyant Italian and his parasitic twin who toured Europe exhibiting themselves.[84] Monstrous births were a popular subject for study at Wittenberg (Luther himself had written on the subject), and in 1665 Johann Stricer produced a summary of what was known about them[85] in which he defined '[a] natural monster' as 'a natural product with stigmata of deformity of some kind caused by deficient or aberrant development'[86] and categorised plant, animal and human monsters:

DIVISIONS OF MONSTERS

1. Monsters are divided by reason of subject, because some are plants, some animals; by reason of type, because in some their shape is changed whereas in others it remains the same.

2. When their shape is altered they may have a well-formed and perfect shape, but different, for example a mule.

3. When the type stays the same, when they do not differ from a straight and perfect type but nevertheless in another way their shapelessness or deformity set them apart, eg. bicephaly, cyclopia, etc.

4. Those concerning either gender or the arrangement of generative parts, the gender (in this latter case) being preserved.

5. Concerning sex, there are certain forms of doubtful sex or of both, eg. hermaphrodites.

6. Concerning the arrangement of parts there are four groups: i. concerning number, ii. concerning size, iii. concerning unity, iv. concerning shape.

7. There may be defect or excess of number. Monsters with defects have parts absent or deficient, eg. men born without arms, feet, heads, etc. Those with excess have parts added on or increased, eg. men born with two heads, four arms, etc.

8. Regarding the size of monsters, some are deficient and others excessive. In the deficient sort either the entire body is decreased in size, as seen in pygmies, whose whole body is not bigger than a single foot (*pede*), or some men are born with short arms, feet, etc. In the excessive kind either the whole body is affected or one part is conspicuously large, as with giants, megalocephalics, etc.

9. Regarding united monsters, either the parts are fused together, or they are side-by-side but separated, as with newborn children, too large and too many, pressing to be born.

10. Regarding those of a deformed shape, with regard to appearance, position, or in any other way. Now for instance children are born with their eyes in their chests, their noses in their sides and their ears at the back of their heads: others appear which have their faces at the back and their hands towards their scapulae; now appear men who are quadrupeds with faces looking forwards; dogs or wolves, etc.

Some historians unfavourably contrasted the work of universities in the seventeenth century with that of learned societies. The extreme view, articulated by Ornstein, is that outdated scholastic methods and religious intolerance in European universities frustrated learning,[87] until the rise of learned societies formed a true republic of letters, an international community of scholars in which learning could flourish freely. Before turning to accounts of monstrous births published by learned societies it is worth noting that in the late-sixteenth and early-seventeenth centuries universities were the principal source of scholarly accounts of monstrous births, particularly those in which morphological classifications of monsters were developed. The dissection of monstrous bodies took place in universities and, although after the advent of scholarly periodicals most of the information we have on these dissections has come down to us through the work of learned societies, their members were in most cases using the knowledge of anatomy that they had acquired in the medical faculties of universities. Paré did not publish descriptions of the internal anatomy of monsters, despite possessing the preserved bodies of several and opening several more. A century later, learned societies such as the *Collegium Naturae Curiosorum* were made up of university graduates who had not only acquired, through their training in anatomy, the technical skill to undertake difficult dissections of infants whose structure was markedly abnormal but who saw as an end point not the dissection itself but the description of what they found.

Notes

1. O. Wilde, *The Decay of Lying.*
2. G. Peignot, *Manuel du Bibliophile* (Dijon: V. Lagier, 1823).
3. This idea was particularly suggested by Biagioli's thesis that Galileo's astronomical discoveries supplied emblems of the power of his Medici patrons: M. Biagioli, 'Galileo the Emblem Maker', *Isis*, lxxxi (1990), 230–58.
4. Aldrovandi enjoyed the patronage of popes Gregory XIII and Sixtus V, and of Cardinal Barberini (later Urban VIII), who wrote his epitaph.
5. Nothing is known of Obsequens apart from this work, the dating of which rests solely on textual grounds. Livy's prodigies were reports of reports, but he was not unconcerned with accuracy and reliability; see J.P. Davies, *The Articulation of Roman Religion in the Latin Historians Livy, Tacitus and Ammianus Marcellinus* (PhD, University College London, 1999), 54–5.
6. Lycosthenes' Latin text was translated into Italian in 1554 and French the following year: see D. Wilson, *Signs and Portents…* (London: Routledge, 1993), 63–7.
7. This and subsequent quotations are taken from the translation by S. Batman, *The Doome Warning All Men to the Judgement…* (London: R. Nubery, 1581),185.
8. K. Park and L.J. Daston, 'Unnatural Conceptions: The Study of Monsters in Sixteenth and Seventeenth-Century England and France', *Past & Present*, xcii (1981), 20–54.
9. Scholarly writers since Livy have written of the concept of monsters as portents as a historical curiosity – see Davies, *op. cit.* (note 5), 59 – though as a popular belief it has never died out.
10. S. Münster (1488–1552), German cosmographer, mathematician and

Hebrew scholar. He taught at Basel, where, in 1540, the first edition of his *Cosmographia* was published.

11. Wilson, *op. cit.* (note 6), 65.

12. Batman, *op. cit.* (note 7), 339; Appendix, 1545a.

13. *Ibid.*, 356; Appendix, 1551a.

14. Some thirty-four monstrous births from after 1500 are described: see Appendix, 1531a, 1536a, 1538a, b, 1540a, 1541a, 1543a, b, 1544a, b, c, 1545a, b, 1546a, 1547b, 1548a, 1550b, c, 1551a, 1552a, c, 1553a, b, c, 1554a, b, 1555a, 1556a, b, c, d, e, 1557a, b.

15. Appendix, 1538b.

16. C. Rhodiginus, *Antiquarum Lectionum...*(Venice: Aldus, 1516).

17. *NBG*, xlvi (1866), 821.

18. A. Walsham, 'Sermons in the Sky (Celestial Visions Reported Across Early Modern Europe)', *History Today*, li (2001), 56–63.

19. See for example Appendix, 1576a.

20. William Shakespeare, *Othello*, I, iii, 166–70; all were described on a single page.

21. L. Daston and K. Park, *Wonders and the Order of Nature, 1150–1750* (New York: Zone Books, 1998), 360.

22. *O felix culpa, quae talem ac tantum meruit habere Redemptorem*: from the office for Holy Saturday.

23. Batman, *op. cit.* (note 7), 412.

24. *Ibid.*, 401.

25. For example the woodcuts illustrating F.M. Guazzo's *Compendium Maleficarum* (Secaucus: University Books, 1974), first published in 1608. On pictures of devils as a cause of maternal impressions see J. Riolan, *De Monstro Nato Lutetiae Anno Domini 1605: Disputatio Philosophica* (Paris: O. Varennaeum, 1605), fo. 11r.

26. D. Cressy, *Travesties and Transgressions in Tudor and Stuart England: Tales of Discord and Dissension* (Oxford: Oxford University Press, 2000), 47.

27. London, 1615.

28. See Cressy, *op. cit.* (note 26), 40.

29. Appendix, 1580a.

30. See Park and Daston, *op. cit.* (note 8), 30.

31. For a bibliographic history of the work see P. Boaistuau (ed. S. Bamforth), *Histoires Prodigieuses: MS 136 Wellcome Library* (Milan: F.M. Ricci, 2000), 22–3.

32. E. Fenton, *Certaine Secrete Wonders of Nature...* (London: H. Bynneman, 1569), fo. 3v.

33. *Ibid.*, sig. A iv r.

34. Variously Boaistuau, Boiastuau, Boisteau, Boaystuau, Bosteau, Boiestuau, or Baistuau.

35. *NBG*, vi, 282.

36. Fenton, *op. cit.* (note 32), fo. 12v.

37. *Ibid.*, fo. 15r.

38. T. Aquinas, *Summa Theologia*, III (suppl.), q. 86, art. 1, discussed bodily deformity as a punishment for sin, an association made throughout the Middle Ages, when as Eustache Deschamps (*c.*1345–*c.*1406) wrote: 'a man with deformed limbs is misshapen of mind – Full of sins and full of vices'; see J. Huizinga (transl. F. Hopman), *The Waning of the Middle Ages...* (London: Folio Society, 1998), 26.

39. Appendix, 1530b.

40. *Et dit on qu'il auoit esté engendré de quelque femme perdue, qui se prostitoit à tout le monde indifferemmêt.* P. Boaistuau, *Histoires Prodigieuses...* (Paris: V. Sentenas, 1560), fo. 83r.

41. M. Foucault, *The Order of Things* (London: Routledge, 1989), 129–30.

42. In the same year a German translation, *Ein Schon Lustig Trostbuechle...* was published in Zürich by C. Froschover. After Rueff's death, there were further editions of *De Conceptu*, illustrated with improved woodcuts by Jobst Amman.

43. Known as the 'Rosengarten', it was based on Soranus of Ephesus's instructions for midwives 1,400 years earlier. The Rosengarten was widely translated, into English as *The Byrth of Mankynde* in 1540; see O. Hagelin, *The Byrth of Mankynde...* (Stockholm: Svenska Läkaresällskapet, 1990), 12.

44. *Ibid.*, 19.

45. I.S. Cutter and H.R. Viets, *A Short History of Midwifery* (Philadelphia: W.B. Saunders, 1964), 188–90.

46. J. Rueff, *De Conceptu et Generatione Hominis...* (Basel: C. Waldkirch, 1586), I, 383; Appendix, 1547b.

47. It is not the earliest classification – St Albert the Great (*Physics* II, part 3, ch. 3) distinguished four causes of failure of normal foetal development: diminution of matter, abundance of matter, disproportion of matter with regard to the qualities conveyed upon it and deficiency of the container.

48. A. Paré (ed. and transl. J.L. Pallister), *On Monsters and Marvels* (Chicago and London: University of Chicago Press, 1982), xxv.

49. *Ibid.*, 3–4.

50. Park and Daston, *op. cit.* (note 8), 41.

51. For example Appendix, 1536c, 1540b, 1544a.

52. Paré, *op. cit.* (note 48), xxiii.

53. *Ibid.*, xxvi.

54. Park and Daston, *op. cit.* (note 8); R. Hole, 'Incest, Consanguinity and a

Monstrous Birth in Rural England, January 1600', *Social History*, xxv (2000), 183–99, saw a 'new metropolitan orthodoxy' in writers such as Paré and Lemné moving away from the concept of divine punishment towards physical causes of monsters.

55. Paré, *op. cit.* (note 48), 5. Despite his apparent piety, Paré's religious allegiance is unknown.

56. Bauhin defined an hermaphrodite as 'a man [human] whose genitalia are malformed, and in whom, in addition to the proper pudenda, the pudenda of the opposite sex are present': C. Bauhin, *Hermaphroditorum Monstrosorumque...* (Frankfurt: M. Becker, 1600), 22.

57. T. Aquinas, *Summa Theologica*, II, ii, q. 51, art. 4.

58. Bauhin, *op. cit.* (note 56), 58 (facing).

59. A bibliography of the French sources on the life of Liceti is to be found in *NBG*, xxxi, 131–5. A brief account in English is A.W. Bates, 'The *De Monstrorum* of Fortunio Liceti: A Landmark of Descriptive Teratology', *Journal of Medical Biography*, ix (2001), 49–54.

60. Harvey saw his own account of the circulation of the blood as proof of Aristotle's position – see W. Pagel, 'The Reaction to Aristotle in Seventeenth-Century Biological Thought...', in E.A. Underwood (ed), *Science, Medicine and History...* (London: Oxford University Press, 1953), I, 489–509. On opposition to Harvey's theory see R. French, *Medicine Before Science* (Cambridge: Cambridge University Press, 2003), 179–80.

61. *Quaecumque raro contingentia communem rerum sui generis ordinem, ac legem magno excessu cum summa hominum admiratione transgrediuntur; ea, sive in bonorum, sive in malorum serie contineantur, publico sapientum consensu Monstra nuncupare consuevere: sic viri virtutibus heroicis mire praestantes, quasi humanam supergressi naturam prope ad Divinam accesserint, sic ex adverso ferinis vitiis homines turpissime foedati:* F. Liceti, *De Monstrorum Caussis, Natura, & Differentiis* (Padua: P. Frambott, 1634), 3.

62. F. Houssay, *De la Nature, des Causes, des Différences de Monstres d'après Fortunio Liceti* (Paris: Collection Hippocrate, 1937), 11.

63. *...ut propterea eximia haec Physiologiae seges etiamnum inculta, & fere deserta nos ad sui culturam accuratiorem acrioribus dudum stimulis excitaverit. Qua quidem in speculatione licet omnia Monstrorum attributa persequi decreverimus; quia tamen ex rei natura praecipue caussas, originem, & differentias...:* Liceti, *op. cit.* (note 61), 1.

64. French, *op. cit.* (note 60), 78.

65. Liceti, *op. cit.* (note 61), 1, 7. Daston and Park, *op. cit.* (note 21), 200–1 trace the neo-Aristotelian concept of monsters as errors to a lecture published in 1560 by the Florentine philosophical writer Benedetto Varchi.

66. J. Bondeson, *The Two-Headed Boy, And Other Medical Marvels* (Ithaca:

Cornell University Press, 2000), viii–xii, plausibly identifies these with the Colloredo twins (Appendix, 1617) and assumes that the year 1607 given in *De Monstrorum* is in error.

67. Appendix, 1624.
68. *Monstra non indicant future.* Liceti, *op. cit.* (note 61), 6.
69. *Monstra non nisi malorum: ibid.*, 5.
70. Bates, *op. cit.* (note 59), 49–54.
71. 'Uniform monsters are mutilated or deficient, excessive, of two natures, double, unformed, enormous. Multiform monsters are formed of divers parts; different species, but the same genus, or they may have the parts of different genera.'
72. C. Schott, *Physica Curiosa...* (Würtzburg: J. Hertz for J.A. Endter and Wolff, 1662), I, 12.
73. The seven-headed monster appeared in P. Boaistuau's *Histoires Prodigieuses...* (Anvers: Chez G. Ianssens, 1594), IV, 607.
74. An observation first made by G.J. Fisher, 'Diploteratology', *Transactions of the Medical Society of the State of New York* (1866), 207–96: 208: 'The grand objection to a strictly scientific classification of compound monsters is found in the fact that they cannot be continued by natural propagation... yet it cannot be denied that there are certain well determined facts, constant and definite characters, upon which orders, genera, and species may be founded'. Riolan however denied that there were different 'species' of monsters, seeing each as unique: Riolan, *op. cit.* (note 25), fo. 5r
75. Riolan, *op. cit.* (note 25).
76. Wilson, *op. cit.* (note 6), 101–4, stresses Riolan's omission of theological considerations such as 'baptism or even last rites' but this omission can be attributed to Riolan's lack of theological training. Writers with a theological background usually did deal with the question of baptism. The sacrament of 'last rites' is not appropriate to an infant.
77. Appendix, 1605.
78. Riolan, *op. cit.* (note 25), fo. 18r
79. See Wilson, *op. cit.* (note 6), 103–5.
80. Suggesting that he may have been aware of the longstanding belief that twins are mirror images: see for example C. Dareste, 'Recherches Sur les Conditions Organiques des Hétérotaxies', *Comptes Rendus Séances de la Societe de Biologie et de ses Filiales*, series 3, i (1859), 8–11; H.H. Newman, *Twins and Super-Twins...*(London: Hutchinson, 1942), 52–62.
81. C. Coury, 'The Teaching of Medicine in France From the Beginning of the Seventeenth Century', in C.D. O'Malley (ed.), *The History of Medical Education* (Berkeley: University of California Press, 1970), 121–72.
82. French, *op. cit.* (note 60), 115

83. P. Sperling, *Disputatio Philosophica de Monstris* (Wittenberg: C. Tham, 1624); A. Lehmann, *De Monstris* (Wittenberg: G. Müller, 1634); A. Senguerd, *Continens Quaestiones de Monstris* (Utrecht: P.D. Sloot, 1645); C. Posner, *De Monstris* (Jena: S. Steinmanniano, 1652).

84. C. Wallrich, *Disputatio Physica de Monstris quam Deo Juvante* (Wittenberg: J. Borckardt, 1655).

85. J. Stricer, *Disputatio Physica de Monstro* (Wittenberg: J. Röhner, 1665).

86. '*Monstrum est Effectus naturalis cum insigni aliqua deformitate à causa deficiente & aberrante productus.*'

87. M. Ornstein, *The Rôle of Scientific Societies in the Seventeenth Century* (Chicago: University of Chicago Press, 1938).

4

A Farrago of Medical Curiosities

From the latter half of the seventeenth century, scholarly journals become an important source of material on monstrous births. Most journals were linked with learned societies – being published by them, or under their auspices, or at least through the efforts of their members – and communications that would previously have been the subject of correspondence between scholars acquired permanence through inclusion in journals. Though it is perhaps neither possible nor desirable to attempt a rigid definition of a learned society, the particular features that distinguished them from other groups of scholars such as universities or religious orders are worth considering briefly. Learned societies did not usually function as examining or licensing bodies, and membership was not normally dependent upon occupation or formal qualifications. For this reason they were paradoxically more exclusive, since membership was largely dependent upon social connections. The personal recommendation of existing members, necessary to join most learned societies, may have been much more difficult to attain than the passing of an examination.

The theory that the resistance of universities to new methods and fields of intellectual or scientific enquiry encouraged the establishment of learned societies sees their flourishing in the seventeenth century as a response to the deficiencies of universities as centres of learning.[1] Although their members were mostly university men, the learned societies certainly acquired influence on their own account; probably no organization before the Royal Society made itself known internationally in such a way, and it has been said that by the eighteenth century the natural philosophical community was significantly divided into those who were and were not Fellows of the Royal Society (FRS).[2] The high social standing of learned societies added to the authority of material published under their auspices, on the basis that: 'Arts and Sciences, when cultivated by Persons of quality... derive lustre from the rank of their Professors'.[3]

A journal is as difficult to define as a learned society. The three journals examined here – the *Philosophical Transactions* of the Royal Society, *Miscellanea Curiosa* and the *Journal des Savans* – had different backgrounds and aims; one was the mouthpiece of the elite Royal Society, one the organ of a group of German physicians and one an independent forum for news

95

and scholarship in many fields. Did these, and indeed other scholarly journals, have particular qualities that justify treating them as a distinct category? Kronick[4] summarised earlier work by Joachim Kirchner in which seven characteristic features of a periodical were proposed: periodicity, duration, collectivity (that is, multiple authors), availability to all who want to pay for it, continuity (similarity of issues), timeliness and lack of universality (ie. they are aimed at a specific audience). These criteria do not distinguish scholarly journals from newspapers or other periodicals;[5] the former might perhaps contain material that is more complex, though 'complexity' in this situation is difficult to define. An association with a learned society is a defining characteristic of a scholarly journal if present, though some (nowadays most) journals have no such association. I would add that the contents of a scholarly journal are intended to be of more than passing value, and therefore a journal almost invariably has an annual or collected index. The purpose of defining a periodical is not merely semantic, but is relevant to understanding the treatment of the subjects in its pages: in this chapter we will consider why monstrous births were represented in periodicals, and what effect this new forum had on the study of monsters.

Miscellanea Curiosa

Miscellanea Curiosa,[6] the journal of the *Collegium Naturae Curiosorum*,[7] has been called the earliest medical journal. Dr Lorenz Bausch (1605–65), *Stadtphysicus* (municipal physician) of the ancient walled city of Schweinfurt in northwestern Bavaria, had worked in Italy, where he had encountered the *Accademia dei Lincei*.[8] After returning to Germany, Bausch, who kept a museum of 'rarities' and was an enthusiast for Bacon's writings, founded the *Collegium Naturae Curiosorum* in 1652, along with three other physicians. Their stated aims were 'the advancement of medicine and pharmacy through observation; by presenting observations in monographs, and communicating them to members for correction and further elaboration.'[9] The president assigned a topic to each member (which was printed after his name in publications), and members were required to demonstrate the 'truth' of any communications to the society. In practice, this meant that eyewitness accounts from members themselves or from professional colleagues were expected; physicians were to be self-appointed expert witnesses, whose testimony was reliable not only because of their social status, but because they were possessors of specialist knowledge. As physicians, they would have been used to treating every case on its merits rather than making generalisations, and each published observation was treated as a separate contribution to knowledge, a format that encouraged reporting monstrosities, which were notable for their singularity.

By 1662, the *Collegium* had twenty-five members; membership was open to 'doctors, licentiates, or those approximating them in learning', but initially the society remained largely for German medical men (there were four foreign members by 1693). In 1687 the *Collegium* (like the Royal Society) acquired a royal patron and became the *Sacri Romani Imperii Academia Caesareo-Leopoldina Naturae Curiosorum*, having come under the nominal protection of the Holy Roman Emperor, Leopold I. Once under his patronage, it had the same privileges as a university, including a license to print books.[10] The badge of the *Collegium* was the ship *Argo*, the Golden Fleece representing scientific truth. The fleece, like the truth, was perceived as valuable and difficult to obtain (like the Order of the Golden Fleece, of which Leopold had been created a knight in 1654, the insignia of which were shown in the frontispiece of *Miscellanea Curiosum*), and there was also, in my view, more than a suggestion of a quest for something hidden, of the natural philosopher as the discoverer of occult meaning.[11] On 13 December 1664, Dr Johann Daniel Major (1634–93), physician in ordinary to the City of Hamburg and a newly-appointed member of the *Collegium*, wrote to Henry Oldenburg (a German by birth, who, as secretary of the Royal Society, corresponded with many European learned societies) informing him of the work of the *Collegium*, whose members were, he reported: 'scattered through certain of the more cultured German cities and provinces'.[12] Oldenburg graciously replied '[w]e do not doubt that Germany, ever fertile in learned men, will greatly add to the store of knowledge',[13] and agreed an exchange of information with the Royal Society.

After a re-organisation in 1670, undertaken by Dr Philipp Jakob Sachs von Lewenhaimb (1627–72), who had joined in 1658, new regulations stated that the *Collegium* would publish its collected observations every year, and that each member would be required to submit an account of his special subject for publication. It was also open to non-members to make contributions to the society's journal,[14] and those who did so included distinguished foreigners such as Thomas Bartholin the Elder (1616–80).[15] In the first ten years of publication, ninety-eight contributors to the journal were members and 198 were not; early editors were called 'collectors', the first of these being Sachs. Most members of the *Collegium* and, arguably, most readers of *Miscellanea Curiosa* were physicians; its content is therefore an indication of the broad range of interests of physicians at the time. Each volume contained more than a hundred communications, and there was usually a longer treatise printed as an appendix, the whole amounting to some five hundred pages. Topics included anatomy, monsters, zoology and botany, with an emphasis on the unusual.[16] Many of the communications were very brief; some were historical reviews, but most were reports of new cases. Production standards were usually high, and accounts of human monsters often included detailed autopsy findings and engravings of dissections and skeletal preparations. Most of the engravings of monstrous births show recognisable types, from which I infer that they were realistic representations that appear to have been made from the actual specimens, though some artists, for example the illustrator of Carol Patini's 'Monstrum biceps masculinum',[17] continued the tradition of showing monsters alive and standing in a landscape, as they had been depicted in the wonder book and broadside literature of the previous century.

These observations of monstrous births resemble modern case reports, and the detailed texts and engravings place the emphasis on a high standard of anatomical description. The current trend to regard observational disciplines such as anatomy and taxonomy as intellectually inferior to experimentation is probably responsible for the comparative obscurity into which *Miscellanea Curiosa* has fallen compared with the journals of learned societies that adopted a more experimentalist approach.[18] Ornstein argued that '[s]cience seems somewhat more backward in Germany than in the other countries'[19] and declared that the *Collegium* 'hardly deserves to be classed as a learned society',[20] largely because it did not hold meetings or sponsor experimentation. However the *Collegium* was never intended to operate on the same lines as the Royal Society – one of its main functions was the recording of notable cases in *Miscellanea Curiosa*. Even the more experimentally inclined Royal Society did not adopt an experimental approach to monstrous births. Although experimentation on human foetuses was perhaps neither practical nor acceptable, animal studies would have been a real possibility; at a time when maternal impressions (the idea that the foetus resembled something seen by the mother at conception or during early pregnancy) were generally accepted as a cause of monstrous births it would have been quite straightforward to test the theory on animals; there was even the biblical story of Laban's sheep to point the way.[21] That no such experiments were tried suggests that the causes of monsters were not the key to their significance. In *Miscellanea Curiosa*, the causes assigned to them were peripheral to the observations themselves, and investigation was usually limited to enquiring of the parents whether there were any special circumstances surrounding the pregnancy. The lack of attention given to causes is in contrast to the increased emphasis on description. The detailed descriptions and engravings offered access to information, a form of 'virtual witnessing' for physicians who were unable to see a case for themselves.[22] The initial circulation numbered only a few hundreds, but *Miscellanea Curiosa* also functioned as an archive of information for future readers. While all publications could potentially be archived, scholarly journals were unique in that they were intended to be cumulative in this way (there was a yearly index, with a collected index after the first twenty years), and their editors were, like the curators of museums, engaged in the process of 'collecting nature'.[23] As the accumulation of data, as Oldenburg put it, to 'add to the store of knowledge' was their stated objective, they have perhaps been unfairly criticised in retrospect for achieving what they set out to do.

The *Philosophical Transactions* of the Royal Society

The Society was originally founded in 1660,[24] and in 1662 Charles II – who had been sufficiently interested in their work to send them 'rarities' – granted a Royal Charter to 'The Royal Society of London for Improving Natural Knowledge'.[25] The Royal Society is usually seen as the foremost learned society of the seventeenth century and its roll of presidents was certainly unequalled – Christopher Wren, Samuel Pepys and Isaac Newton all within the first forty-five years. Medical practitioners were, however, the largest and most active single group (about a fifth) of the early fellows and this was reflected in the papers published in the Society's proceedings. The *Philosophical Transactions* were not published by the Society itself, but were the private venture of its secretary, Henry Oldenburg (*c.*1618–77), whose correspondence[26] is an invaluable historical record of the Society's early activities. Oldenburg remained in London during the plague and the Great Fire, only to be imprisoned in the Tower in 1667 for obscure reasons most probably related to his suspiciously large foreign correspondence (information was Oldenburg's business and although at times he collected European intelligence for the English government the flow was not necessarily all one way) at a time when England was at war with both France and Holland.[27] His concerns over the status of the authors of correspondence to the Royal Society are very much apparent in his letters:

> I am sorry, the Dissector of the Doublechild did not putt his name to the Account, he gave of the operation; and we must contrive some way or another, to have it yet done, for the more authentickness of the relation, now it is to be recorded by a Royall Society of severe Philosophers.[28]

Notwithstanding the bantering tone of Oldenburg's remarks, he was evidently disappointed not to have an author's name to append to the description of the doublechild and he added that the Society 'would be very glad to have that double attestation of the 2. Physitians among their records.' The status of the witnesses was detailed by his correspondent, Robert Boyle (1627–91, whose agent Oldenburg was, and to whom he dedicated volume 5 of the *Philosophical Transactions*): one, Dr Turbervill, 'an Excellent Oculist', was 'deservedly famous in those parts', and the other was a physician 'late of this University [Oxford]', who, having seen the child alive, was looking forward to dissecting it.[29] This anxiety over suitably qualified witnesses related to a case seen by over a thousand people.

The medical witnesses compared the case to a double monster born in Oxford over a century earlier,[30] and Oldenburg himself ('Having Rueffus among my books') made the same comparison. Boyle described the scene:

> On Tuesday night last [letter dated 27 November 1664], there was borne in Fisherton adjoyning to our towne of Salisbury a Monstrous Issue in part, the Woman has three Children Girles, ye one very well formed & fatt, the other two as you may call them hath but one Body, continued hansomely to their shoulders, from whence groweth foure Armes compleatly made, two Necks & two heads very well featur'd, wth all ye parts...they were at writing hereof very lusty, & doe take their food, sugar & water, looke abroade & wagg all parts; the one is more sleepy than ye other, both very pretty, I saw them this Evening (being Thursday) there hath been a thousand to see them.[31]

The girls died at the age of three days, one fifteen minutes after the other. A letter, now lost,[32] giving an account of their death and dissection, was read to the Society on 9 November 1664: 'they were found to have their parts double... except that the guts... met in a common channel; as also the matrix [uterus].'[33] This was the first monstrous birth published in a journal, as an anonymous letter to the *Journal des Savans*.

Of the few monstrous births mentioned in the Oldenburg correspondence, the most detailed account, in correspondence from the Reverend Nathaniel Fairfax (1637–90), concerned another double monster. Fairfax was a Cambridge graduate who obtained an MD from Leiden and practised medicine in Suffolk. In a letter dated 28 September 1667 he told of a Mrs Burroughs of Woodbridge who, aged 23, conceived for the third time by her husband and delivered, at 4pm on 23 October 1661, 'a twobodyed one headed daughter or daughters', which were stillborn at around the twenty-eighth week of gestation: 'being drowned in the waters (as the good wives thought)'. As the midwives suggested that death occurred during labour the twins were presumably delivered vaginally, and one might speculate that their death resulted from prolonged labour due to their malformation. They had a single face, but 'some of the Wives sd. the head was bigger th[a]n for the body'. Fairfax, wondering if a second conception could account for the twinning, accordingly spoke to the mother, whose husband was by then dead:

> [U]nderstanding th[a]t nothing immodest was driven at, nor should any light or unseemly use be made of it, she told me th[a]t (according as I gheest,) she did think (too) th[a]t she might conceive it at twice. for w[he]n

she was 9 or 10 weeks gone she had a most strang restless longing w[hi]ch she kept to her self some days & weeks but at length fearing a miscarryage she let her husband know it, w[hi]ch was this, viz. Th[a]t she would yeild to be the under sheet, whilst they should joyne [i]n [th]e deeds of nature. this was done about the 14th week. now since she understood the bodyes came from her in the armes of each other, she has been often ready in her thoughts to drive it up to th[a]t, more longd for, th[a]n kindly embrace.[34]

Mrs Burroughs, who had had six years to ruminate on the cause of her monstrous birth, may have harboured feelings of guilt; did the conjoined twins, embracing one another,[35] mimic her embrace of her husband during pregnancy and was this therefore an example of a maternal impression?[36] Fairfax speculated that two children conceived on different occasions, 'a conception upon a conception', had somehow become fused: 'one whole soul may snug to, or ly hid in another....' By asking 'whither nature aymd at a single birth or a twinne', he was implicitly accepting Aristotle's (and Liceti's) view of the monster as a mistake. He also considered whether the monster could be regarded not only as a result of the mother's lustful thoughts but also as a punishment for them:

Methinkd tis easyer to rais a great many questions about this Case th[a]n to answer a few, as Whither the two-bodied burden in the womans womb put her upon the longing after an hugg th[a]t should bear some resemblance to it, or, w[hi]ch is more likely, this unsatiable desire of hers, should stamp such an image upon th[a]t w[i]th in her... whither there is more in it of morall th[a]n of naturall, as th[a]t were a punishment of an unkind list. (as the woman her self ghesses). I would be loth to be a lessener of sins, but I think the thing in itself is not so much abhorrent from the nature of mankind th[a]t comparing it w[i]th wh[a]t god does in the world in the like cases...but w[he]n I consider it as the child of a longing... for I am so much a friend to the pasionte bout in a woman w[hi]ch springs more from the hurry of materiall particles th[a]n from the rationall soul, th[a]t I scruple whither longings shall be layd to the rule of a law, at domesday.[37]

In a second letter of 26 September 1667 he returned to the idea of maternal impressions: 'the breeders unwonted longing (w[hi]ch th[a]t posture onely could fulfill) had some way or other to doe with the shaping of the burthen.'[38] There are no theories here (maternal impressions, punishment of sins, unacceptable sexual behaviour) that were not current a century or more before, though Fairfax was the first to describe an attempt to establish the background to a monstrous birth by questioning the mother.

The *Philosophical Transactions* was one means for the Royal Society to become – on Baconian principles – part of the 'economy of knowledge' by serving as a 'channel of transmission' for the exchange of information,[39] at the same time enhancing its own reputation by publicly identifying itself with philosophical advancement. It had a far broader scope than *Miscellanea Curiosa*, including mathematics, optics, astronomy, geography, architecture, painting, music, mineralogy, botany, zoology, grammar and history, as well as medicine and (as they would now be called) the medical sciences, and the eight accounts of human monsters in the first thirty-five years of publication represent little more than a footnote to the medical content. European scholars 'clamoured' for a Latin reprint of the *Philosophical Transactions* which was, however, not forthcoming.[40] During these early years, the Fellows of the Royal Society introduced no new insights into monstrous births, explaining them in conventional terms of maternal impressions that the parents of monsters, such as Mrs Burroughs, readily accepted.[41] The Fairfax correspondence however suggests that, despite the descriptive emphasis of accounts of monstrous births offered for publication, a more traditional debate on their meaning in moral terms may have been taking place privately.

The *Journal des Savans*

First published five years before the *Philosophical Transactions*, the *Journal des Savans* (or *Sçavans*) was claimed by Voltaire as 'the father of all the publications of this genre which today fill Europe.'[42] Its originator was Denys de Sallo (1626–69), *conseiller* to the Court of Parliament and part of the coterie of the powerful Jean-Baptiste Colbert (1651–90, Marquis de Seignelay), *contrôleur général* (minister of finance) to Louis XIV and a founder of the Academy of Sciences, the Academy of Inscriptions and Medals, and the Paris Observatory. In 1664, Sallo was granted a *privilège* for the printing of a journal, and the first issue appeared on 5 January 1665; it was published by the Parisian printer Jean Cusson, and sold for five sous. In an introductory note to the reader, Sallo (under the *nom de plume* Sieur de Hedouville) outlined his five-fold purpose for the publication:

1. To provide a catalogue and brief description of the principal books printed in Europe.
2. To print obituaries of famous men.
3. To publish findings from experiments in physics and chemistry, new discoveries in the arts and sciences such as machines and useful or curious inventions of mathematicians, celestial and meteorological observations, and new anatomical findings made on animals.
4. To document the findings of secular and ecclesiastical tribunals as well as universities in France and the rest of Europe.
5. To report items of news that might be of interest to men of letters.[43]

He also stated that the journal would contain differing points of view and that the editor would be impartial.[44] The first issue had ten articles on such diverse topics as a monstrous birth, Giuseppe Campani's new telescopes and lenses, a new edition of Descartes's *De l'Homme*, and the history of the African church.

The *Journal des Savans* was suppressed following the thirteenth weekly issue on 30 March 1665, the reason given being that Sallo was not submitting his proofs for official approval before publication. Sallo had undertaken the editorship out of interest (the profits went to the printer) and relinquished it rather than lose his independence.[45] After a hiatus of several months, the journal returned on 4 January 1666, under the editorship of the Abbé Jean Gallois (or Galloys, 1632–1707), who edited the next forty-two issues.[46] The *Journal* continued to appear on a weekly basis, under various clerical editors, until 1724 when it became a monthly issue.[47] It was not linked to a particular learned society but reports from the French Academy, the Academy of Sciences, and the Academy of Inscriptions and Belles-Lettres (Petite Académie), along with reports from the Royal Society and other foreign societies all found their way in.[48] Among the authors of contributions from the first two years of publication were Bausch and Sachs of the *Collegium Naturae Curiosorum*,[49] and Henry Oldenburg, whom Sallo had consulted before the inception of the *Journal*, and who supplied an account of the conjoined twins from Oxford.[50] Although they were included from the journal's inception, monstrous births were only a minor part of the total content.

The existence of holy things

Thomas Shadwell's *The Virtuoso* (1676) included a parody of the gentleman natural philosopher in the person of Sir Formal Trifle (presumably FRS), a somewhat pompous and effete character who studied swimming in theory, without entering the water, and who was of the opinion that 'To study for use is base and mercenary, below the serene and quiet temper of a sedate Philosopher.' The point of the satire was not that learned societies had a less utilitarian attitude to knowledge than, say, the universities, but that they studied practical things in a theoretical way; Shadwell's message was that not everything amenable to scholarly study is necessarily worthy of it. The view that monstrous births are unworthy of study – which as we have seen was one response to Paré's work – coupled with a perception that experimentation is inherently more valuable than observation may explain why until recently reports of monsters in early journals received little attention from historians of science, and those in the *Philosophical Transactions* of the Royal Society could be dismissed as 'a farrago of medical curiosities… evidence of triviality and misguided enthusiasm among English medical practitioners',[51] who it was felt, in following the example of Francis Bacon, had tended to 'linger too long over "prodigies" and "marvels"'.[52]

Despite the greater anatomical detail, descriptions of monsters in journals resembled those in broadsides with their 'picture, description, interpretation' format, and they can thus be seen as an example of the 'surfacing into [scholarly] visibility'[53] of vernacular knowledge that occurred during the Scientific Revolution. The furore surrounding monstrous births would have drawn the attention of local physicians to them, even if they were not actually consulted by the parents. The large crowds through which they often had to make their way to examine monstrous births indicated their continued appeal to the general audience; their entry to the journal literature reflected the interest of scholars who took advantage of this new means of publishing their observations and in so doing brought university-acquired skills in anatomy to the pre-existing framework within which monsters were described.

For publishers of popular literature, monsters were a subject likely to sell both because of the general interest in them and because they were suitable emblems for theological and moral discussion. The inclusion of monsters in wonder books and obstetrical works may have served to broaden their potential readership; the market for vernacular translations of such works indicates general as well as academic interest, and as book production was costly it was shrewd business to cater for both. Periodicals, although not intentionally loss-making, were less directly driven by financial gain than books or ballads as they were probably purchased not for a specific item of content but because of their overall reputation, which was bound up with the reputation of the learned society with which they were associated. Journals enabled material from a wider range of authors to find its way into print, and men who lacked the funds, time, material or reputation to write a book could now make, and be seen to make, a contribution, however small, to knowledge. It was easier than ever to publish, and editors faced the problem of filling the available space; as Kronick[54] remarked: 'One of the problems of regularity of issue [of journals] was that of finding an adequate pay-load for the vehicle.'

The empiricist motto of the Royal Society, *Nullius in Verba* (meaning 'take no-one's word for it') seems inconsistent with the many observations in the *Philosophical Transactions* that the reader was expected to believe 'on trust'. Those who contributed to the *Philosophical Transactions* did so as amateurs, content to write as an interest or to enhance their reputation; indeed, although it was possible to make a living as a freelance writer and translator if one could successfully combine this with publishing and administration, as Oldenburg did, it was not possible to make a living from natural philosophical writing in the seventeenth century. From the start, the Society had been anxious to emphasise the social status of its members (for example by appointing several high-ranking but intellectually undistinguished presidents and fostering Royal connections), which, as we saw from Oldenburg's remarks on the 'doublechild', was seen as guaranteeing their intellectual probity,[55] partly because they were perceived as being intellectually 'free and unconfined'.[56] A gentleman's word was accepted as honest, and he was considered intellectually capable of producing an accurate account; furthermore, unlike the writers of broadsides and newspapers, he had no direct financial incentive to write. Perhaps 'don't take just anyone's word for it' was closer to the society's ethos.

The intended readers were also professional men and gentlemen amateurs, many, perhaps most, of whom were members, or would-be members, of the sponsoring society, and some of whom would have had the added incentive of seeing their own work in print from time to time. In his preface to the abridged version of the *Philosophical Transactions*, Lowthorp[57] identified two classes of reader: 'those who make use of Books for their private Instruction or Entertainment, and those who consult them in order to publish something of their own.' By the fifth edition the Latin papers were, for the first time, translated into English; the preponderance of contributions in the English and French languages may have helped the popularity of the *Philosophical Transactions* and *Journal des Savans* over the all-Latin *Miscellanea Curiosa*, although it limited their geographical range. Journals were a suitable forum for material that was short, self-contained, and topical. Though the readership of early journals may have been numerically less than that of broadsides, which could be produced more quickly and cheaply and sold locally while the birth of a monster was still fresh in everyone's minds, journals had two advantages to the scholarly author: they were targeted at other scholars and they were intended to be permanent. *Miscellanea Curiosa*, the *Philosophical Transactions* and the *Journal des Savans* were indexed, so each contribution was a unit of knowledge that would remain available for the conceivable future.

Reports of monstrous births contained an element of surprise that they shared with popular accounts of monsters and museum specimens: almost by definition, they were not what the reader or viewer expected to see. Reports of monstrous births from before 1700 often made no mention of earlier cases, and even relatively frequent types, such as foetuses without a head, were treated as a surprising novelty. In terms of modern scientific theory the case report is striking because it runs counter to an accepted hypothesis, even though that hypothesis may not have been explicitly

Figure 4.1
A macerated child with a large encephalocoele and bilateral cleft lip, and a locust's wing bearing a Hebrew inscription. Miscellanea Curiosa, 1690.

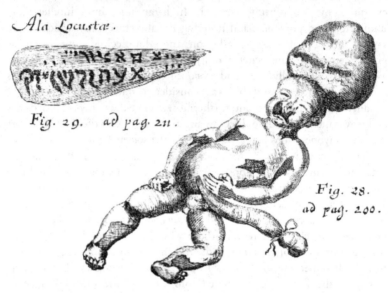

stated;[58] one could claim, for example, that conjoined twins disprove a null hypothesis that human individuality is dependent upon independent bodily existence. Such reports can be seen as essentially subversive, their function being to highlight exceptions to the perceived natural order. The use of exceptions to shed light on normal development – the theory that the edge shows us what the middle is like[59] – provided a fresh motive for the study of the unusual, and by the end of the seventeenth century a new role for the monster as a natural experiment was beginning to emerge. A child born without nostrils was used as evidence to support the theory that the foetus *in utero* breathes through its mouth,[60] and an anencephalic child posed a question for Cartesians: how did it move its limbs if the pineal gland, the seat of the soul, was lacking?[61]

Before 1700, such interpretations were a minority; monsters still spoke of the order of creation. Many of the contributions to *Miscellanea Curiosa* noted resemblances between the natural world and Christian images: a root shaped like a crucifix, or the image of the Virgin Mary in a rock formation. Johann Musche de Moschau translated a message in Hebrew that had been found in the pattern of the wing of a locust.[62] These do not qualify as emblems in the traditional sense – the reader is told what they represent rather than left to work it out – but they do suggest that the natural world was seen as a kind of emblem book in which God had concealed messages that men could discover. Coincidentally, but significantly, the image of a stillborn infant with multiple congenital malformations was placed under that of the locust's wing (Figure 4.1). A description of a monstrous birth ended with the words 'Benedictus sit Deus in omnibus Operibus suis',[63] ['Blessed be God in all His works.'] and, commenting on another monstrous foetus, the editor wrote 'Whatever, therefore, one thinks, these selfsame monsters cry out: IN ME YOU CAN SEE THE EXISTENCE OF HOLY THINGS: BE THANKFUL UNTO GOD.'[64]

Notes

1. M. Ornstein strongly advocated this view in *The Role of Scientific Societies in the Seventeenth Century* (Chicago: University of Chicago Press, 1938); entries under 'universities' in the book's index included 'opposition to freedom of thought', 'fundamental reforms needed', 'flood of criticism against' and 'contributed little to the advancement of knowledge'.

2. J.E. McClellan, *The International Organization of Science and Learned Societies in the Eighteenth Century* (PhD, Princeton University, 1975), 17; published as *Science Reorganized: Scientific Societies in the Eighteenth Century* (New York: Columbia University Press, 1985).

3. T. Renaudot, *A General Collection of Discourses of the Virtuosi of France...* (London: T. Dring and J. Starkey, 1664), 3.

4. D.A. Kronick, *A History of Scientific and Technical Periodicals...* (New York: The Scarecrow Press, 1962), 30–1.

5. Newspapers appeared in Antwerp in 1605, Augsburg in 1609, Hamburg in 1616, Vienna in 1623 and England in 1641: see E.W. Allen, 'International Origins of the Newspaper: The Establishment of Periodicity in Print', *Journalism Quarterly*, vii (1930), 307–19.

6. Sometimes known as the *Ephemerides*, or other variants of its alternative title *Ephemeridum Medico-Physicarum Germanicarum Academiae Imperialis Leopoldinae Naturae Curiosorum.*

7. On the early history of the *Collegium* see R. Toellner, 'Im Hain des Akademos auf die Natur Wißbegierig sein: Vier Ärzte der Freien Reichsstadt Schweinfurt gründen die *Academia Naturae Curiosorum*', in B. Parthier and D. von Engelhardt (eds), *350 Jahre Leopoldina – Anspruch und Wirklichkeit: Festschrift der Deutschen Akademie der Naturforscher Leopoldina, 1652–2002* (Halle: Deutsche Akademie der Naturforscher Leopoldina, 2002), 15–43; and on its early presidents, U. Müller, 'Die Leopoldina unter den Präsidenten Bausch, Fehr und Volckamer (1652–1693)', *ibid.*, 45–93.

8. The Academy of Lynxes operated from 1600 until 1630. The lynx, an animal proverbial for its acute observation, was shown in the badge of the

society engaged in a symbolic struggle with ignorance: Ornstein, *op. cit.* (note 1), 74.

9. *Ibid.*, 170.

10. The name of Leopold has remained in the title of the society, currently the *Deutsche Akademie der Naturforscher Leopoldina.*

11. On the occult connections of learned societies see F. Yates, *The Rosicrucian Enlightenment* (London: Routledge and Kegan Paul, 1972).

12. A.R. Hall and M.B. Hall (eds and transl.), *The Correspondence of Henry Oldenburg* (Madison: University of Wisconsin Press, 1965–77), II, 337.

13. Quoted in Ornstein, *op. cit.* (note 1), 172.

14. W. Röpke, 'Die Veroffentlichungen der K. Leopoldinische Deutsche Akademie der Naturforscher', *Leopoldina*, i (1926), 151.

15. Bartholin presumably approved of the emphasis given to maternal impressions: see J. Bondeson, *A Cabinet of Medical Curiosities* (London: I B Tauris, 1997), 148–9. He contributed a teratological case, 'De sirene Danica' [the Danish siren], *Miscellanea Curiosa*, i (1670), 73–7, which, with its human face and bifid tail, is very reminiscent of later fakes; see J. Bondeson, *The Feejee Mermaid and Other Essays in Natural and Unnatural History* (Itheca: Cornell University Press, 1999), 36–63. At the time Bartholin was working at the University of Copenhagen, a post acquired through the influence of Ole Worm, who was married to Bartholin's aunt.

16. In some cases the very unusual: 'Flatus per penem emissi' and 'De cati ex ore mulieris nativitate' are two of the more bizarre cases.

17. Appendix, 1691a.

18. See Bondeson, *A Cabinet of Medical Curiosities*, 38.

19. *Op. cit.* (note 1), 165.

20. *Ibid.*, 175.

21. Genesis 30:35–43.

22. For example the detailed osteological illustrations in M. Hofmann, 'Anatome Partus Cerebro Carentis', *Miscellanea Curiosa*, series 1, ii (1671), 60–4.

23. Some of the material remains of interest to developmental pathologists today; there is, for example, arguably the earliest description of Roberts syndrome (Appendix, 1672) and the first successful surgical separation of conjoined twins (Appendix, *c.*1689).

24. The connections between the Royal Society and earlier groups such as the Invisible College are tenuous but it is possible to interpret the Royal Society as a development of a more arcane tradition, a thesis advanced by Yates, *op. cit.* (note 11).

25. For accounts of the early history of the Royal Society see Ornstein, *op. cit.* (note 1), ch. 4; H. Hartley (ed.), *The Royal Society, Its Origins and Founders* (London: The Royal Society, 1960); C. Webster, *The Great Instauration:*

Science, Medicine, and Reform, 1626–1660 (London: Duckworth, 1975).

26. Published in thirteen volumes: Hall and Hall, *op. cit.* (note 12).

27. D. McKie, 'The Arrest and Imprisonment of Henry Oldenburg', *Notes and Records*, vi (1948), 28–47; Hall and Hall, *op. cit.* (note 12), III, xxviii.

28. Hall and Hall, *op. cit.* (note 12), II, 309.

29. See Appendix, 1664b.

30. Appendix, 1552a.

31. Hall and Hall, *op. cit.* (note 12), II, 277.

32. *Ibid.*, 294.

33. T. Birch, *The History of the Royal Society of London...* (London: for A. Millar, 1756), I, 485.

34. Hall and Hall, *op. cit.* (note 12), III, 496.

35. A conventional way of depicting such twins; see Fig. 2.1.

36. J.M. Hoffmann, 'De Monstro Gemello', *Miscellanea Curiosa*, series 2, iv (1685), 288–90, also put forward this explanation for double monsters.

37. Hall and Hall, *op. cit.* (note 12), III, 496.

38. The implication is that the twins were joined owing to the mother having sexual relations with her husband while already pregnant. This not only laid her open to a charge of concupiscence, but also suggested the operation of maternal impressions, the embrace of the twins resembling that of husband and wife. Fairfax adds in a footnote – Hall and Hall, *op. cit.* (note 12), III, 497 – that 'the nature of the thing [the relations between the woman and her husband] is such as to bespeak a Cover', which will harm his trustworthiness if the details are made known.

39. R. Porter, 'The Early Royal Society and the Spread of Medical Knowledge', in R. French and A. Wear (eds), *The Medical Revolution of the Seventeenth Century* (Cambridge: Cambridge University Press, 1989), 272–93.

40. See Hall and Hall, *op. cit.* (note 12), III, xxiv.

41. For example in the case of a child resembling an ape with 'a Mass of Flesh that came from the hinder part of the head... the Woman which brought it forth had seen on the Stage an Ape so clothed': Anon., 'Extract of a Letter, Written from Paris, Containing an Account of Some Effects of the Transfusion of Bloud; and of Two Monstrous Births, &c.', *Philosophical Transactions*, ii (1667), 479–80.

42. Quoted in B.T. Morgan, *Histoire du Journal des Scavants Depuis 1665 Jusqu'en 1701* (Paris: Presses Universitaires, 1929), 17.

43. Ornstein, *op. cit.* (note 1), 200.

44. H. Brown, 'History and the Learned Journal', *Journal of the History of Ideas*, xxxiii (1972), 365–78.

45. *Ibid.*

46. Gallois was a *conseiller* and an active member of the French Academy: *NBG*, xv, 257–8.

47. See Morgan, *op. cit.* (note 42). In 1903 the Journal came under the auspices of the *Académie des Inscriptions et Belles-Lettres*.

48. The French Academy of Sciences, founded in 1666 and made a royal institution by Louis XIV in 1699 had its own journal from 1700, and the *Mémoires de l'Académie Royale des Sciences* for 1666–99 were published retrospectively in ten volumes between 1729 and 1734. Both contain accounts of monstrous births.

49. Ornstein, *op. cit.* (note 1), 201.

50. It was published anonymously: 'Extrait d'une Lettre Escrite d'Oxfort, le 12. Novembre 1664', *Journal de Savans* (1665), 11–12.

51. A.R. Hall, 'Medicine in the Early Royal Society', in A.G. Debus (ed.), *Medicine in Seventeenth-Century England* (Berkeley: University of California Press, 1974), 421–52. Porter, *op. cit.* (note 39), 285, saw this distinction from as too sharply drawn, as well as being the antithesis of the Baconian theory of learning through observation.

52. E. Cameron (ed.), *Early Modern Europe* (Oxford: Oxford University Press, 2001), xxiv.

53. P. Burke, *A Social History of Knowledge: From Gutenberg to Diderot* (Oxford: Polity, 2000), 14.

54. Kronick, *op. cit.* (note 4).

55. S. Shapin, *A Social History of Truth* (Chicago: University of Chicago Press, 1994).

56. As the Society's historian Thomas Sprat (1636–1713) optimistically stated; see Burke, *op. cit.* (note 53), 26.

57. J. Lowthorp (ed.), *The Philosophical Transactions and Collections, To the End of the Year MDCC, Abridged and Disposed under General Heads* (London: W. Innys *et al.*, 1749), I, xiii.

58. J.P. Vandenbroucke, 'Case Reports in an Evidence-Based World', *Journal of the Royal Society of Medicine*, xcii (1999), 159–63.

59. See Aristotle, *On the Heavens*, 2 293a.

60. Vander Wiel, 'Extrait des Nouv. de la Rep. des Lettres', *Journal des Savans* (1686), 263–4.

61. Anon., *op. cit.* (note 41).

62. J.I. Musche de Moschau, 'Ala Locustae Literis Hebraicis Decorata', *Miscellanea Curiosa*, series 2, ix (1690), 204–11.

63. J.J. Wepfer, 'De Puella Sine Cerebro Nata, Historia', *Miscellanea Curiosa*, series 1, iii (1672), 175–203.

64. *'Quivis ergo ab ejusmodi monstris sese inclamari putet: IN ME INTUENS
    PIUS ESTO: DEO GRATUS ESTO!*: H. Volgnad, 'De Monstroso Foetu',
    Miscellanea Curiosa, series 1, iii (1672), 446–7.

5

Finding Fault with Nature:
Some Causes of Monstrous Births

> We ought not to set them aside with idle thoughts or idle words about
> 'curiosities' or 'chances'. Not one of them is without meaning; not one that
> might not become the beginning of excellent knowledge, if only we could
> answer the question – why is it rare? Or being rare, why did it in this instance
> happen?[1]

The distinction between monsters and prodigies was first established in the
sixteenth century: neither classical embryology nor its mediaeval
interpretation required it to be made. In mediaeval times monsters were
peccata naturae (slips of nature)[2] and in common with other rare or unusual
happenings they were 'unnatural': to the mediaeval mind expressions such as
praeter ut in pluribus (outside that which occurs frequently) and *praeter
naturam* (beyond the range of nature) were interchangeable.[3] The concept of
nature making a mistake (*peccata naturae* were also sins of nature) entailed
the assumption that, as Aristotle had written in the second book of his
Physics, Nature had particular aims.[4] Aquinas developed this further,
concluding that it was legitimate to find fault with nature:

> Actions are open to criticism only so far as they are taken to be done as means
> to some end. It is not imputed as a fault to any one, if he fails in effecting
> that for which his work is not intended. A physician is found fault with if he
> fails in healing, but not a builder or a grammarian. We find fault in points
> of art, as when a grammarian does not speak correctly; and also in points of
> nature, as in monstrous births.[5]

According to St Augustine, God would correct these mistakes of nature
on the last day:

> We are not justified in affirming even of monstrosities, which are born and
> live, however quickly they may die, that they shall not rise again, nor that
> they shall rise again in their deformity, and not rather with an amended and
> perfected body. God forbid that the double limbed man who was lately born
> in the East, of whom an account was brought by most trustworthy brethren
> who had seen him, – an account which the presbyter Jerome, of blessed
> memory, left in writing; – God forbid, I say, that we should think that at the

resurrection there shall be one man with double limbs, and not two distinct men, as would have been the case had twins been born. And so other births, which, because they have either a superfluity or a defect, or because they are very much deformed, are called monstrosities, shall at the resurrection be restored to the normal shape of man; and so each single soul shall possess its own body; and no bodies shall cohere together even though they were born in cohesion, but each separately shall possess all the members which constitute a complete human body.[6]

In the sixteenth century, when theological and moralising interpretations placed the emphasis on monstrous births as evidence of providence, the concept of the monster as a mistake came under attack: nothing that was created by God could be in error. Liceti, who, as we have seen, was an authority on Aristotle's writings, to some extent reconciled the divine origin of monsters with their deformity, by rejecting the 'vulgar' opinion that monsters were 'errors' or 'failures' on the part of nature and proposing instead that they were part of a secondary plan, the results of nature doing its best with the flawed materials available:[7] 'Nature intendeth perfection, but being hindered doth what he can.'[8] This view of the monster as a mistake remained generally accepted by scholars in the seventeenth century.[9] We can thus distinguish two theoretical bases for the interpretation of monstrous births: the first, as 'slips of nature', having classical roots and revived in the work of Liceti and later scholars, and the second, as divinely-mediated signs, often related to the transgression of natural or moral 'laws', expressed most notably in the popular literature of the sixteenth century. Although monsters remained outside the usual course of nature they were, for early modern observers, possible in nature, and unlike prodigies could be explained without recourse to the supernatural. This chapter examines a common theme in early modern explanations of monstrous births – all were thought to be generated from human seed.

Unnatural conceptions

The modern view of birth 'defects' is inseparable from the idea that something has gone wrong during intrauterine development. Most people, even those with little scientific knowledge, believe that the foetus increases in complexity as it develops and that either internal (genetic) or external (environmental) factors can disrupt normal development. The comparable widely held view of foetal development in the early modern period was based on Aristotle's *Generation of Animals*. According to Aristotle, the growth of the foetus was not a stepwise process of development (such as Galen envisaged), but a 'mingling' of seed (male and female) from which the foetus was concocted by a subtle transformation – rather like baking a cake or, as

Aristotle suggested, the setting of cheese from milk. The male's contribution was semen and the female's menstrual blood; the semen imparted form then evaporated and the menstrual blood provided the substance of the embryo. Both had generative capacity (on its own the female chicken could produce an infertile egg), but that of the male was greater.[10]

We cannot suppose that all writers or readers of accounts of monstrous births had a thorough understanding of Aristotle, but by the latter part of the seventeenth century it was considered important for those involved in childbirth to have some idea of foetal development, which they acquired from succinct accounts such as that in Jane Sharp's *Midwives Book:*

> Conception is the proper action of the womb after fruitful seed cast in by both sexes... the mixture of both seeds is called conception, when the heat of the womb fastens them; if the woman conceives not, the seed will fall out of the womb in seven daies, and abortion and conception are reckoned upon the same time.

> The seeds of both must be perfectly mixed, and when that is done, the Matrix contracts it self and so closely embraceth it, being greedy to perfect this work, that by succession of time she stirs up the formative faculty which lieth hid in the seed and brings it into act...[11]

She went on to consider how this process differed when monsters were formed:

> The matter is the seed, which may fail three several ways, either when it is too much, and then the members are larger, or more than they should be, or too little, and then there will be some part or the whole too little, or else the seed of both sexes is ill mixed, as of men or women with beasts; & certainly it is likely that no such creatures are born but by unnatural mixtures, yet God can punish the world with such grievous punishments, and that justly for our sins.... But the efficient cause of Monsters, is either from the forming faculty in the Seed, or else the strength of imagination joyned with it; add to these the menstruous blood and the disposition of the Matrix.... The second cause is the heat or place of conception, which molds the matter quickly into sundry forms. But imagination holds the first place, and there it is that children are so like their parents.[12]

Understanding of the development of monsters was also based on Aristotle, whose account of their formation from excess of seed ('[t]he reason why the parts may be multipled contrary to nature is the same as the cause of the birth of twins – excess of material')[13] had been accepted by European scholars since mediaeval times.[14] St Albert the Great (1193–1280) wrote that twins resulted from abundance (*superfluitas*) and division (*divisio*) of semen.[15] Incomplete division caused a double monster; hence John of Jandun (*c.*1285–1328) wrote: 'it is dangerous that the female moves during sexual intercourse in the way prostitutes are reputed to do, because if at such a moment they would conceive, they could generate an awful two-headed monster.'[16] Sixteenth-century commentators also accepted excess of seed as a cause of monstrous births,[17] a theory that derived support from many classical sources: '*Empedocleus* and *Dephilus* do attribute [monsters] to come of the superabundance or defaulte and corruption of the seede'.[18] Lack of seed resulted in missing parts: '[i]f the quantity of seed (as we said prior to this) is deficient, similarly one or more members will be lacking.'[19] It was thought to be the female that provided the substance for the embryo, but references to excess or deficiency of seed also applied to the male, since although the male semen did not contribute to the matter of the embryo, the magnitude of its 'spirit', rather than its physical quantity, was significant. Lodovico Maria Sinistrari (1622–1701) wrote in *De Daemonialitate* (completed around 1700 but not published until 1875): 'Medical men are well aware that the size of the foetus depends, not indeed on the quantity of matter, but on the quantity of virtue, that is to say of spirits held by the sperm; therein lies the whole secret of generation'.[20]

A word is needed concerning the preformation versus epigenesis controversy that is such a well-known component of eighteenth-century embryology. The opposing views were that either the form of the embryo existed in the semen (preformation) or it developed gradually *in utero* (epigenesis). At first sight the existence of monsters rules out preformation (unless monsters are preformed too, in which case they could not be caused by, for example, maternal impressions), a point apparently first made by Johann Conrad von Brunner (1653–1727) in 1683.[21] However, although it is no longer believed that the structure of the embryo is preformed in the sense that there are homunculi hidden in sperm, preformation is in some respects still a powerful argument, and with the discovery of the role of genes and of regional variations in the cytoplasmic composition of the unfertilised egg in development it has acquired a new lease of life. Epigenesis is a key concept in the history of embryology, but it does not necessarily mean that form develops out of nothing, as some epigeneticists implied. In retrospect we can see analogies between the 'higher' causes of monsters, such as the 'will' of God or the 'plan' of Nature and preformation and between the 'lower' causes, such as the 'virtue' of the seed and epigenesis; but to imply that there was held to be a dichotomy between them in accounts of monstrous births is anachronistic.

Most of the suggested causes of monsters were external to the foetus; for example, a widely accepted cause of misshapen limbs was physical constraint within the uterus. Paré attributed a child's deformed hands and feet to its having been 'pressed against the mother's body'. To him the cause was self-evident, but Fenton characteristically supported the association between 'narrowness of the womb' and deformities with an appeal to antiquity:

> Hippocrates witnesseth in his booke *De Genitura*, wher he sheweth by the similitude of trees, how these children issue from the bellie of theyr mother monstrous and deformed, saying thus: that of force those bodies which cannot move by reason of the straightnesse [narrowness] of the place, must become the rather mishapen and deformed: like as trees before they issue out of the earth, if they have not libertie and scope to spring, but be with holden by some let or hindrance, grow crooked... he sheweth other reasons, by the which children be made monstrous and deformed, as by the natural diseases of the parents: for if the foure kindes of humors, whereof the seede is made, be not wholly contributorie to ye secrete partes, there shall be then some partie wanting. Besides this, he addeth further other reasons... as when the mother receiveth some blow or hurt, or that the childe fortunes to be sicke in the bellie of hys mother, either that the nourishment wherewith he ought to be relieved, happen to slippe out of the wombe: al which things be sufficient to make them hideous, wanting or deformed.[22]

A double monster could also be formed by crowding of seed or pressing together of twins within the uterus,[23] and it was thought that this could occur even if twins were conceived on separate occasions.[24]

Sixteenth-century observers expected children to resemble their parents ('like is born from like')[25] and those that did not were monstrous: '[t]hus Aristotle calls a woman a Monster, and a fault of Nature, which always designs the making of a Male as the more perfect.... And for the same reason he calls a Child, which doth not resemble its Father, a Monster, because the Father design'd to beget a Man like himself.'[26] It was axiomatic that abnormal parents gave birth to abnormal children, and in his account of hereditary diseases, Paré wrote of dwarfs and cripples who resembled their parents: 'Now these kinds of people are far from unusual, which is a thing that anyone can observe and know by his own eye the truth of what I am saying, wherefore I see no reason to continue talking further about it.'[27] Because heredity was an accepted cause of malformations (it was one of the three causes identified by Ballantyne in the Hippocratic writings, the others being trauma and narrowness of the womb[28]), it was noteworthy if the parents of a monstrous birth had had normal children before: 'The father thereof is one Vyncent, a butcher; bothe he and hys wyfe being of honest and quiet

117

conversation, they having had chyldren before in natural proportion, and went with this her full tyme.'[29] Another ballad appears to suggest that the generation of a monster might have involved a hereditary component from both parents: 'The aforesayde Anthony Smyte of Much Horkesley, husbandman, and his wyfe, were both maryed to others before, and have dyvers chyldren, but this defomed childe is the fyrst that the sayd Anthony and his wyfe had betweene them two.'[30]

Offspring that did not resemble their parents, especially those that resembled animals, called for an explanation, and one possibility was that an unnatural appearance was the result of unnatural parentage. Aristotle had written that different gestational periods prevented cross-species unions from being fertile, and although stories of fertile human–animal unions have an honoured place in mythology the existence of actual hybrids has always been tenuous and examples few. There is a well-known story in which St Albert the Great saved the life of a herdsman who, when one of his cows gave birth to a human-like monster, was accused of bestiality, by arguing that the birth was the result of astrological influences. Although this episode of hagiography was probably not intended as a literal account of events, it required the hearer to believe that the monstrous birth was not the result of bestiality, as it was intended to show Albert's cleverness in saving an innocent man by discovering the true cause of the monster, not his skill at excusing the guilty. Thijssen remarks that the modern tendency to describe the use of monsters as evidence of bestiality as 'mediaeval' is misleading,[31] as mediaeval laws did not accept the possibility of human–animal hybrids. Tales such as that of Albert saving the herdsman do however suggest that a link between monstrous births and bestiality was part of popular legend in the Middle Ages, even if people were reluctant to believe the truth of it. Vincent de Beauvais (*c*.1190–1264) presented a hybrid theory of animal monstrous births in his *Speculum Naturale* without specifically applying it to humans: '[t]his type of [hybrid] monstrosity sometimes occurs in this way, that is by means of coitus between two different species'[32] and Gerald of Wales reported the birth of an animal–human hybrid, writing in his *History and Topography of Ireland* of a human-cow:

> From the joinings of the hand with the arms and the feet with the legs, he
> had hooves the same as an ox. He had no hair on his head... his eyes were
> huge and like those of an ox both in colour, and in being round. His face was
> flat as far as his mouth. Instead of a nose he had two holes to act as nostrils,
> but no protuberance. He could not speak at all; he could only low.[33]

By the sixteenth century most writers were prepared to credit such stories. Paré stated that hybrid offspring were produced 'if animals of diverse types cohabit with one another', and as far as humans were concerned: 'it is, when it is done, a very unfortunate and abominable thing, and a great horror for a man or a woman to mix with or copulate with brute animals; and as a result, some are born half-men and half-animals.'[34]

He related the story of a child conceived in 1493 of a woman and a dog: 'having, from the navel up, upper parts similar in form and shape to the mother, and it was very complete, without Nature's having omitted anything; and, from the navel down, all its lower parts were similar in form and shape to the animal, that was the father'.[35] The number of examples of supposed human–animal hybrids described in sixteenth and seventeenth century literature is however small and those mentioned in accusations of bestiality were usually animal abortuses, for example:

> At Birdham near Chichester in Sussex, about twenty-three years ago, there was a monster found upon the common, having the form and figure of a man in the fore-part, having two arms and hands, and a human visage, with only one eye in the middle of his forehead: the hinder part was like a lamb. A young man in the neighbourhood was supposed to have generated the monster by bestial copulation, and that the rather, because he was afterwards found in the like beastly act with a mare; upon discovery whereof, he fled out of the country. This young monster was nailed up in the church porch of the said parish, and exposed to public view a long time, as a monument of divine judgement.[36]

Liceti was even prepared to disagree with Aristotle in order to affirm the existence of true animal–human hybrids, but by the end of the seventeenth century, scholarly opinion was turning against the possibility, though the argument was not yet over: in 1699, Edward Tyson wrote to the Royal Society to disprove the claim that a man-pig could originate from bestiality.[37]

Rare though actual accounts of such hybrids were, it was common to present monstrous births as human–animal intermediates by the use of animal similarities to describe their appearance. In the great majority of cases such descriptions did not imply that the monsters were thought to result from the mixture of animal and human semen. When a child was born with a 'leopard's mouth' there was clearly no question of the mother having encountered a real leopard during her pregnancy: it probably had a cleft lip and palate, a condition still called by its animal resemblance – hare-lip.[38] The use of such human–animal comparisons for descriptive purposes continues in modern teratology: lobster-claw deformity, *cri du chat*, bird-headed dwarfism, and many more. Liceti discussed several explanations for human–animal intermediates but attributed most to association; the resemblance between human and animal was nothing more than that (though the doctrine of signatures shows how important such resemblances could be).[39]

Spontaneous degeneration

Liceti ascribed the birth of other animal-like offspring to human parents to 'degeneration' of the seed:

> If, therefore, the male semen in the female uterus were to degenerate from its original nature through whatever cause, its vital principle becomes transformed to another kind; if the whole of the semen were fully changed in this way, whole creatures of diverse kinds are formed; not monsters, but like monsters.[40]

These births were considered to *be* animals rather than to resemble them, and for this reason Liceti and later commentators such as Bayle wrote that they were not monsters, as they were not human. Among late seventeenth century scholars, degeneration of the seed was an accepted explanation for the births of animals to human mothers, and it was claimed that even after six months gestation a human foetus could still degenerate (*degenere*) into a monkey.[41] The possibility of degeneration may perhaps have been suggested by the resemblance of early human abortuses to animals,[42] and to a modern reader it is reminiscent of the later belief that the human embryo passes through stages of resemblance to lower animals before achieving its definitive form ('ontogeny recapitulates phylogeny'), although there was no such concept of embryonic development in the early modern period.

Because the formation of the human foetus was usually seen in Aristotelian terms as a rather mysterious process of 'setting' rather than as a Galenic sequence of events tending towards greater complexity, there was no widely agreed time at which it was fully formed. Some writers, for example Paré, adopted the timings derived from Hippocrates and Pliny the Elder and stated that the formation of the male foetus took thirty days and the female forty-five, but these were not universally accepted and the exact time at which it formed remained nebulous.[43] There was no lower age limit below which a foetus was presumed to have been born dead: the French man-midwife Guillaume Mauquest de la Motte (1655–1737) baptised one infant 'of the bigness of a cockshafer' so tiny that it was lost in the folds of the bed linen and then accidentally trodden on[44] and wrote of another even smaller, the size of a 'small bee.... I believe this little embryo was alive, but in spite of all my care I could not discover it.'[45]

Uncertainties over when the form of the foetus became established are apparent in accounts of monstrous births due to maternal impressions,[46] the enduringly popular theory that a strong emotional or visual experience during pregnancy could impress itself on the foetus:

> The auncient Philosophers amongst others, which have serched the secrets of Nature, have declared other greate causes of this wonderfull and monstrous childbearing, which Aristotle, Hypocrates, Empedocles, Galene, and Plinie, have referred to an ardent and obstinate imagination, which the Woman hath, whylest she conceives the childe, whiche hath such power over the fruite, that the beames and Charrecters, continue upon the rocke of the infante, whereupon they finde an infinite number of examples to prove the same.[47]

The theory was based on the classical idea that every child is conceived in the likeness of the person or thing seen, or imagined, by the mother at the time of conception. In most cases this was expected to be the child's father, although some embarrassing exceptions could be explained away by claims that the mother's gaze, or imagination, had wandered at the crucial moment:

> Hippocrates saved a princesse accused of adulteries, for that she was delivered of a childe blacke lyke an Ethiopian, hir husbande being of a faire and white complexion, which by the persuasion of Hippocrates, was absolved and pardoned, for that the childe was like unto a Moore, accustomably tied at her bed.[48]

The same explanation could be applied to monstrous births; Remy quoted the story told by Marcus Damascene of a woman whose child was covered with hair because she had gazed at a picture of St John the Baptist (after which Pope Nicholas III is said to have ordered the removal of all such pictures from Rome),[49] and when a woman in early sixteenth-century France gave birth to a child with a head like that of a frog the father suggested that this was because she had been holding a live frog (a cure for fever) at the time of conception.[50]

In the early modern period maternal impressions were thought to affect not just conception but established pregnancy. Although according to the classical tradition it ought not to have mattered once the foetus was fully formed after the first thirty to forty days (and the foetal movements felt), throughout the early modern period and afterwards most pregnant women, at whatever stage, avoided monsters. Unwholesome desires during later pregnancy, such as those of the mother for 'filthie unsavorie meates, as burning coals, mannes flesh, and other like things' which were 'contagious and hurtfull to their fruite',[51] could also engender monsters, as could unpleasant experiences; a woman who had seen the bloated carcass of a horse whilst pregnant gave birth to a child with a swollen abdomen covered only by a thin membrane.[52] In the late seventeenth century it was thought that such experiences could alter not only the shape of the foetus but also its nature: '[m]any apprehensions seize on the pregnant woman and the foetus changes its whole shape, indeed, it changes its nature, from human to that of a beast'.[53] Maternal impression is probably the most durable of all explanations for monstrous births; countless examples have been (and are being) produced and the theory can only be refuted by appeals to the lack of any demonstrable mechanism by which the maternal imagination could materially affect the foetus. Prior to the eighteenth century most observers were convinced by the weight of examples; as Remy wrote: 'In view of the above examples of the power of imagination, what should hinder us from confidently ascribing to the influence of sight those hideous births accomplished by Nature?'[54] Debate began in earnest in the eighteenth century,[55] but in the late-seventeenth century, learned societies continued to publish fresh examples.

One explanation for the popularity of the theory is that questioning relatives to find a cause for monstrous births – whether, as in Remy's case, for forensic reasons or, as the learned societies did, from scholarly curiosity – may have helped to turn superstition into a self-perpetuating truth as mothers who believed in the power of the imagination on the foetus invested minor incidents that had occurred during their pregnancy, such as the loss of a cow, with a significance born of hindsight.[56] These explanations were also relatively acceptable to all concerned; to the moralising writer they offered an opportunity to warn against allowing one's imagination to dwell on lurid subjects, whereas from the parents' point of view, it was better to be accused of a wandering imagination than adultery or witchcraft.

In *De Monstrorum*, Liceti shows that he and his readers were familiar with several explanations for human–animal monsters including co-incidental resemblance, degeneration of the seed and maternal impressions; yet having considered these alternatives he still accepted some as genuine hybrids, as had Paré, and was prepared to contradict Aristotle in order to do so. The increasing acceptance in the late-sixteenth and early seventeenth centuries of the possibility of human–animal hybrids may have been a reflection of increasing unease over the distinction between men and animals, and it enabled monsters to be used as a warning against the transgression of sexual norms.[57] In Salisbury's study of the changing relationships between humans and animals in the Middle Ages *The Beast Within*,[58] she argues that blurring of the once-absolute theologically based distinction between humans and animals led to increasing efforts to maintain the special nature of humankind. Humanity was seen as something that could be lost or degraded unless efforts were made to preserve it, and bestiality therefore attracted increasingly severe religious and legal penalties. The laws against bestiality, a sin treated by mediaeval penitentials as equivalent to masturbation, had been strengthened in most European states until by the sixteenth century it was generally a capital offence. Prohibitions against animal behaviour extended from copulation with animals to copulation like animals;[59] the latter including not only dorsal intercourse but excessive lust and uncontrolled sexuality, characteristics with which, however unjustly, animals were associated.[60] These laws were the consequence of 'a new fear about the status of humanity', at a time when the once seemingly certain uniqueness of mankind was increasingly open to question.[61]

It does not seem plausible that the association of monstrous births with criminal acts was intended as a deterrent, as the threat of a monstrous birth would hardly have done much to prevent bestiality, or for that matter witchcraft, which were already capital offences. A more likely explanation for the early modern preoccupation with human–animal monsters is that the link between bestiality and monstrous births was an attempt to make human law part of the wider natural world rather than just an arbitrary system. Monsters were 'against nature' and their birth was evidence that their parents had transgressed natural, as well as human, laws. Mediaeval writers had recognised that animals differed from humans in that they were 'governed by their own wishes' and so unlike men they did not have social or legal obligations; yet in the sixteenth and seventeenth centuries animals were prosecuted, and in increasing numbers, in an attempt to apply human laws to the whole of nature.[62] These animal trials cannot be explained on the basis of Christian concepts of the dominion of man over animals, for,

> if the pivotal fact in explaining the disappearance of animal trials was the rise of science and the secularization of religion, then why did the trials peak between 1600 and 1700, at the very moment when the movement in science was at its height, and why did they continue, albeit sporadically, well into the nineteenth century?[63]

This peak coincided with the period of greatest interest in human–animal monsters and of concern over 'degeneration' of humans into animals.

Accounts of humans giving birth to animals occur throughout the early modern period. A case from Elizabethan England that has been the subject of recent study is that of Agnes Bowker who, on 16 January 1569, claimed to have given birth to a cat, the macerated, or flayed, body of which she produced for inspection.[64] None of the six women, including her mother, who helped at the delivery admitted to having actually seen the cat emerge. Dissection of it revealed nothing of significance, but it was noticed that a neighbour's cat had gone missing. The commissary of the court of the

Archdeacon of Lichfield, a clergyman named Anthony Anderson, who was responsible for investigating the case, caused another cat to be killed, flayed and boiled, after which it resembled Agnes Bowker's creature. Anderson was satisfied that it was a cat, but found it hard to accept that Agnes had given birth to it. Only Agnes and her midwives knew the truth, and it may have been a deception, in the manner of the later and more celebrated 'rabbit breeder', Mary Toft,[65] designed to produce notoriety. Agnes variously confessed to having had commerce with a cat and with a man named Hugh Brady, a schoolmaster and alleged witch by whom she appears to have become pregnant. Her free confession to these actions, which implied that she was a party to witchcraft, suggests that either she prepared to risk prosecution to achieve prominence, or that she was attempting to conceal the more serious crime of infanticide, the women hoping that a flayed and boiled cat might pass for a macerated foetus. If her story was an attempt to conceal the truth, it was successful: none of the people involved in this bizarre case was punished. One significant aspect of Agnes's story is the reluctance on the part of the authorities to credit either that she had given birth to an animal or that the birth was evidence of witchcraft.

There was, however, a popular tradition that demons could beget monstrous children and the possibility was much debated by those involved in witchcraft trials and later by academic theologians.[66] The consensus amongst scholars throughout the early modern period was that such conceptions were theoretically possible only if it used semen extracted from a man, as the demon could not contribute of itself the physical matter necessary for conception. The term *demons* referred to 'spirits' in general ('spirits' is the appropriate translation of the Latin *daemones* used in legal textbooks of the time); the evil spirits presently thought of as 'demons' were *cacadaemones* or, in English, devils.[67] In essence, demons were creatures of a higher order of nature than men, but lower than angels; like a man, a demon possessed a soul that required salvation. Some writers envisaged demons as purely spiritual creatures, while others, notably Sinistrari, considered them to possess physical, though praeternatural, bodies.[68] In his *Demonolatry*, first published in 1595, Nicholas Remy (1530–1615), Public Advocate to the Duchy of Lorraine, who presided over more than nine hundred capital trials for witchcraft and was familiar with popular opinion on the subject, considered the significance of monstrous births in accusations of witchcraft:

> …to this day nearly all men show by their speech and their thoughts that they truly and firmly believe in the procreation of men by Demons; and they think that their strongest and most unassailable proof lies in the fact that they can point to certain women who have lain with Demons and have given birth to deformed and portentous monsters, such as have been noted by

Cardan (*De Rerum Varietate*, XVI. 39) in Scotland, by Levin Lemne (*De Miraculis Occultis Naturae*, I, 8) in Belgium, and more than once by ourselves in Lorraine during our examinations of witches. But this argument can easily be refuted by anyone who cares to probe and delve more deeply into the whole matter. For, as Ulpian says… phenomena of this sort are against nature; and I take him to mean by this that they are disaccordant with the common laws of nature.[69]

Remy then considered several cases that he had read of, including: a child with 'two mouths, two sets of teeth, a long beard, and four eyes' born at Daphne near Antioch; 'that shapeless mass like a palpitating sponge or marine zoophyte with every evidence of life, which Levin Lemne says [*De Miraculis Occultis Naturae*, I, 8] an island woman brought to birth not long since in Lower Germany', and the Monster of Ravenna.[70] Summing up, he concluded:

> [N]obody, who is amenable to the processes of reasoning which always carry the most weight in this kind of argument, will fail to agree readily that all these creatures, in respect of the formation of their animal bodies, owe their inception to the same causes which actuate Nature in her undertaking of other matters.[71]

Of the 'palpitating sponge'[72] described by Lemne, he wrote:

> Not even among physicians is there any doubt that this was begotten in the natural manner: they only differ in their opinion of the cause of its deformity. For some ascribe it to a malformation of the womb; some to unclean and evilly infected semen; some to the influence of the stars and the heavens, and especially to that silent quarter of the moon which Varro calls intermenstrual.[73]

In effect, Remy assigned all deformed births to the category of 'monsters' and denied that supernatural intervention occurred at all, quoting from Euripides' *Electra*: 'There is no birth but Nature is its mother'. He also indicated that although physicians did not doubt that monstrous births were 'natural' (that is, not supernatural) they did not fully understand their causes. Remy was well aware of the difference between popular and learned thinking:

> Whatever may be the truth of it, I have never yet heard any suggestion made that a foetus of this sort originates from nature, and not from Demons. For even honest matrons, far from the least suspicion of such execrable copulation, have often been known to give birth to such a child. And, on the other hand, witches who are said to have daily carnal relations with Demons

often bear children complete with every natural attribute and absolutely perfect.[74]

Man and demon were: 'so utterly opposite by nature as are the mortal and the immortal, the corporeal and the incorporeal, the sentient and the insentient', he wrote. 'How such incompatibles can mingle and copulate together passes my understanding.'[75] The union, if it occurred at all, was 'Cold, Joyless, Vain and Barren'.[76] In *Demonolatry*, Remy was concerned with whether giving birth to a monstrous child could be regarded as legal evidence of intercourse with demons, and he concluded that it was not, both for the practical reason that witches did not, in his experience, give birth to monsters, and for the theoretical reason that all monstrous births had natural, rather than supernatural, causes. While this was the official view, however, he accepted that the general population did not share it.[77]

Paré, writing some twenty-two years before Remy, had taken a similarly practical approach, denying either that demons could use human semen to conceive (as it would lose its efficacy in transportation) or conceive themselves (since they were incorporeal), and remarking pragmatically that if such things were possible the world would contain large numbers of demons.[78] Even Liceti, who apparently accepted the *possibility* of animal-demon hybrids and included at the end of his classification of monsters of non-uniform type four short chapters on monsters resulting from the actions of demons, did not seem to regard them as a serious consideration. He may have included every proposed cause of monsters, however implausible, out of scholarly completeness, in order to present a complete picture of the subject, as his near-contemporary Aldrovandi did in his natural history, but the engraving of purported demons in *De Monstrorum* appears deliberately to subvert the text. The original of this illustration had accompanied Lycosthenes' description of a child born to 'honest and noble' parents,[79] but in *De Monstrorum* it appears as a fantastic demon, festooned with cobwebs, a museum piece more likely to have provoked amusement than horror amongst the scholars of Padua (Figure 5.1).[80]

The sooterkin dissected

'Mingling of seed',[81] encompassed more than just what would now be called cross-fertilization; conception during menstruation ('women perfourming the desire of the fleshe being in their Sanguine menstruali, bring forth these monsters')[82] was also regarded as mingling of seed and could lead to something even stranger than a monstrous birth – the sooterkin. This creature, also spelled *sooterkijn* and known as *de Suyger*, was a type of parasitic animal thought to afflict pregnant women, especially in Holland, and was particularly prominent in the literature towards the end of the

Figure 5.1
Daemones*: In the centre, a monster born at Krakow (Appendix, 1547b).
To the right is Melanchthon's 'popish ass' and to the left a child
with the head of a rabbit.* Liceti, De Monstrorum *(1634)
adapted from an illustration in Lycosthenes'* Prodigiorum.

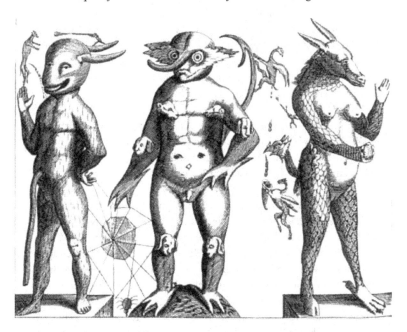

seventeenth century. It accompanied the birth of a normal child and was usually expelled with the afterbirth, to the surprise of those present. It became notorious in England following the publication in 1724 of *The Female Physician* by the man-midwife John Maubray (or Mowbray, 1700–32), who claimed to have seen the sooterkin:

> That these BIRTHS in those *Parts*, are often attended and accompany'd with a *Monstrous* little *Animal*, the likest of any thing in Shape and Size to a MOODIWARP; having a *hooked snout, fiery sparkling Eyes*, a long *round Neck*, and an acuminated *Short Tail*, of an extraordinary *Agility* of FEET. At first *sight* of the World's Light, it commonly *Yells* and *Shrieks* fearfully; and seeking for a *lurking Hole*, runs up and down like a little *Daemon*, which indeed I took it for, the first time I saw it, and *that* for none of the better sort....

[N]ot many Years ago, in coming from Germany over East and West *Friesland*, to *Holland*, I took passage in the ordinary Fare-Vessel, from the City of Harlingen for Amsterdam....

Amongst the better Sort of the Passengers, who posses'd the Cabine, there happen'd to be a *Woman big with Child*, of a very creditable Aspect, who... was taken all at once, aboard the *Ship*, with a sudden and surprising LABOUR: upon which occasion, in short I immediately lent her a helping *Hand*, and upon the *Membran's* giving way, this forementioned ANIMAL made its wonderful *Egress*; filling my Ears with dismal SHRIEKS, and my *Mind* with greater CONSTERNATION....

I heard some of our *Accidental Company* call it *de Suyger*, as they went about to kill it: upon which I immediately laid [delivered] the *Woman* of a pretty *plump* GIRL; who, notwithstanding all this, had no *Deformity* upon it, save only many *dark*, *livid* SPOTS all over its Body....

AFTERWARDS I had occasion to talk with some of the most learned Men, of the several famous Universities in these *Provinces* upon this Head; who ingenuously told me, that it was so common a Thing, among the *sea-faring*, and *meaner sort* of *People*, that scarce ONE of these *Women* in *Three* escaped this kind of strange BIRTH; which my own small Practice among them afterwards also confirmed: Insomuch, that I always as much expected the Thing *de Suyger*, as the CHILD it self: And besides the Women in like manner, make a respective suitable *Preparation*, to receive it warmly, and throw it into the Fire; holding Sheets before the *Chimney*, that it may not get off; as it always endeavours to save it self, by getting into some dark *Hole* or *Corner*, They properly call it *de Suyger*, which is (in our Language) the SUCKER, because, like a *Leech*, it sucks up the INFANT'S *Blood* and *Aliment*.[83]

Maubray's claim was ridiculed by the surgeon James Douglas (1675–1742) in a pamphlet entitled *The Sooterkin Dissected*,[84] written under the pseudonym of Philalethes or 'a lover of truth and learning'. Dutch mothers, Douglas observed, called their children 'sooterkints', or sweet children, but there was no creature called *de Suyger*, and he offered readers a guinea for every sooterkin brought from Holland. This sort of satire made an impression, and Maubray became popularly known as 'the sooterkin doctor'.[85]

Sooterkin-like creatures had a long history and had been likened to various animals. They were not considered to be progeny in the way that monstrous births were, and were sometimes compared to spontaneous

128

generations, but were thought to arise from human semen. According to Aristotle's *Problems*:

[A]nything else which is produced from the semen, as for instance, a worm, or the so-called monstrosities, when there is corruption in the womb, are not to be reckoned as offspring. In a word, anything which is produced from corruption is no longer produced from that which is our own but from that which is alien to us, like that which is generated from excretions such as ordure.[86]

The Northern Italian physician Michele Savonarola (1385–*c*.1468) wrote of women giving birth to a thing called a *fera* ('a piece of flesh bearing the form of a living animal') that he attributed to superfecundation.[87] In early sixteenth-century Augsburg in Germany 'a woman gave birth first to a human head wrapped in membranes, second to a two-footed serpent, which had the head of a pike, the body and feet of a frog and the tail of a lizard, and thirdly a pig with all its parts complete.'[88] Batman gave an early description of an English sooterkin in 1581:

The same day of the tempest, was delivered an aged woman, who hadde to name Alice Perrin of the yeres of 60, being the day before in great pain, of a strange monster: whose head was like to a sallet or head piece, the face somewhat formall, onely the mouth long as a Rat, the fore parte of the body like unto a man, having eight legges, and the one not like the other, a taile in length halfe a yard, like to the tayle of a Rat. A strange sicknesse followed.[89]

Creatures resembling amphibians also appeared; Lycosthenes related that: 'In a farme of Thuring by Unster a woman brought forth a toade with a tayle long and strange to behold',[90] and in 1558 Giovanni Battista della Porta (1535–1615) remarked that 'neither is it hard to generate Toades of women... for women do breed this kind of cattel, together with their children',[91] adding that the women of Salerno 'were wont to use the juice of parsley and leeks, at the beginning of their conception... to destroy this kind of vermin.'[92] Similar stories continued throughout the next century; on 8 May 1646 the Reverend Ralph Josselin heard of 'a monster borne about Colchester, first a child, th[e]n a serpent, th[e]n a toad which lapped',[93] and a few years later Edward Topsell wrote that these creatures were co-conceptions with a normal child: 'Women conceiving with childe have likewise conceived at the same time a Frog, or a Toad, or a Lizard.'[94] There is no early modern Dutch literature on the sooterkin but it was a convenient insult and during the first Anglo-Dutch war John Cleveland (1613–58) wrote: 'There goes a report of the Holland Women, that together with their Children, they are delivered of a Sooterkin, not unlike to a Rat, which some imagine to be the Offspring of the Stoves.'[95] There were tales of Dutch women giving birth to 'a living Creature besides the Child… likest a *Batt* of any other Creature; which the midwifes throw into the fire.'[96] Sharp's *Midwives Book* described sooterkins along with different animals generated in the wombs of women from various places:

> As for monsters of all sorts to be formed in the womb all nations can bring some examples; Worms, Toades, Mice, Serpents, Gordonius saith, are common in Lumbardy, and so are those they call Soole kints in the Low Countries, which are certainly caused by the heat of their stoves and menstrual blood to work upon in women that have had company with men; and there are sometimes alive with the infant, and when the Child is brought forth these stay behind, and the woman is sometimes thought to be with Child again; as I knew one there my self, which was after her child-birth delivered of two like Serpents, and both run away into the Burg wall as the woman supposed, but it was at least three months after she was delivered of a Child, and they came forth without any loss of blood, for there was no after burden.[97]

Broadsides, meanwhile, continued to turn out similar (or different versions of the same) tales, for example this one in which one of the monsters was a serpent that partially devoured the child:

> The first monster which came to sight,
> Was a live toad, which did them fright,
> It sprauled and creeped all about,
> Which put the women all in doubt.
>
> It had four legs as it is told,
> A loathsome creature to behold,
> In ugly shape it did appear,
> The like no woman e're did bare.
>
> The next that came unto their view,
> As for certain it is just and true,
> It was a serpent and a dead child,
> Whose life the serpent did beguile.
>
> For why some of it's face and head,
> By this monster was devoured,
> And it's body injured full sore,
> The like was never seen before.

The serpent had ears like a Pig,
Which was considerable big,
It had a great long tail likewise,
With a pair of wings, and eke two eyes.

This monster joyn'd to the childs side,
Which they endeavour'd to divide,
But before they could bring it to pass,
The Midwife sunk down in the place.

But other Woman in the town,
Who having stouter hearts than some,
Without delay they did contrive,
To burn these two Monsters alive.[98]

The stout-hearted women made a distinction between the 'monsters' and the child, as another ballad relates: 'the two foul ugly creatures was burned, but the child descently [sic] buried'.[99] The sooterkin was distinct from normal and monstrous births as it was a non-human generation, a product of the corrupted womb, which accompanied a normal child as a kind of afterbirth and as such did not merit the humane treatment usually given to monstrous children.

Gélis has attempted to explain the phenomenon of the sooterkin through retrospective diagnosis as a misinterpretation of hydatidiform moles: 'Its [the mole's] irregular shape gave rise to the weirdest interpretations on behalf of the women who had witnessed the event. Some would have 'seen' the woman give birth to a dead animal, rat, mole, or tortoise; others saw a living four-footed animal, armed with claws and hooked nails'.[100] In my view there are several problems with this theory; firstly, hydatidiform mole, known simply as *mola*, a mass, was well known in the seventeenth century; Mauquest de la Motte described it as 'a false Conception' and 'a Shapeless mass', and 'The Countess of –', two months pregnant, told la Motte 'that it was a Mole', a diagnosis subsequently confirmed at delivery.[101] Secondly, the misinterpretations proposed by Gélis are not likely – a mole looks nothing like any of them. When molar pregnancies were described it was as a 'palpitating marine zoophyte'[102] or Countess Margaret's 365 children, each, presumably, in its own gestational sac. Thirdly, the sooterkin was said to emerge after the birth of a baby, a kind of monstrous afterbirth: one of the characteristics of a complete hydatidiform mole is that there is no associated foetus (except for the extremely rare possibility that one of dizygotic twins is a mole). An alternative explanation for some sooterkins is that they were the abnormal stillborn twin in a twin pregnancy; a *fetus papyracious*, or an acardiac monster. The supposedly liveborn sooterkins may have been imaginative explanations of the origin of these abnormalities devised by midwives or mothers who wanted a story to tell when they exhibited the remains of an almost unrecognisable foetus.

Paracelsus saw 'putrefaction' as the first step of all generation[103] and the sooterkin's unpleasant and verminous appearance had some similarities with other animals such as worms and mice that were thought to be formed by spontaneous generation. Were they, therefore, an example of spontaneous generation in humans?[104] Rueff rejected the possibility of spontaneous human generation even for false conceptions – they arose not from corruption alone but required semen, however defective:

> Averrois and Paulus Aegineta doe declare that this deformed lump of flesh is ingendered of the weaknesse and debility of both the seedes, that is to say, of the mans and womans, or else of the corruption of good seedes, which happeneth about the first time of conception. But others doe say, that it is engendered of the abundance of the flowers or Terms, because through the great heat of the Matrix they are sometimes congealed and clotted together, and brought into a misshapen masse or lump of flesh; but they which doe more narrowly pry and search into the Natures of things, doe attribute this to the more copious and abundant seed of the woman, especially in those women who are somewhat more lascivious than others are, which conceiving little seed from their husbands, dry by nature, by the desire of the Matrix [the first function of which, according to *The Expert Midwife*, was to 'attract' the seed], doe stirre up copious seed of their owne, which augmented with the flowers, by the heat of the Matrix, is congealed together, and by the defect and want of mans seed, the proper worke-man and contriver of it, doth grow together in such a lump: For nothing can be ingendered without the seed of man; as neither any can be ingendered of the seed of women only.[105]

Sooterkins were a separate tradition to monstrous births in early modern writing; they were not monstrous births in the sense in which the other conditions described in this book were; they were not human, nor were they intermediates between humans and animals; their relation to the mother was that of a parasite. The sooterkin was something other than human; it scuttled away, or was killed. However, even their conception still required human semen, albeit imperfect and capable only of giving rise to an animal. Bizarre though the range of creatures to which early modern mothers gave birth seems to the modern reader, all were explicable by, and even predicted by, Aristotelian theories of generation. Nothing born to a human mother, whether an animal, a sooterkin or a monstrous birth, was conceived without human seed.

Notes

1. J. Paget, 'Some Rare and New Diseases', *Lancet*, ii (1882), 1017–21.
2. J.M. Thijssen, 'Twins as Monsters: Albertus Magnus's Theory of the Generation of Twins and its Philosophical Context', *Bulletin of the History of Medicine*, lxi (1987), 237–46.
3. *Ibid.*
4. Physics, book II, pt 8.
5. T. Aquinas, *Summa Contra Gentiles*, book III, ch. 2, 'that every agent acts to some end'.
6. Augustine, Bishop of Hippo, *Enchiridion*, ch. 87, 'the case of monstrous births'.
7. L. Daston and K. Park, *Wonders and the Order of Nature, 1150–1750* (New York: Zone Books, 1998), 200.
8. T. B[edford], *A True and Certain Relation of a Strange Birth...* (London: A. Griffin, 1635), 14.
9. G. Havers (transl.) *A General Collection of Discourses of the Virtuosi of France...* (London: T. Dring and J. Starkey, 1664), 64.
10. D.M. Balme, '"Ανθρωπος ανθρωπον γεννᾷ: Human is Generated by Human', in G.R. Dunstan (ed.), *The Human Embryo: Aristotle and the Arabic and European Traditions* (Exeter: University of Exeter Press, 1990), 20–31.
11. J. Sharp, *The Midwives Book: Or the Whole ART of Midwifry Discovered* (London: S. Miller, 1671), 92–3
12. *Ibid.*, 117–20.
13. Aristotle, *The Generation of Animals*, 772b13.
14. Thijssen, *op. cit.* (note 2).
15. *De Animalibus*, book XVIII, part 2, ch. 2. Albert used the term *sperma* for both the male and female contributions to conception and for the mixture of the two.
16. Thijssen, *op. cit.* (note 2), 237–46.
17. N. Remy (ed. M. Summers, transl. E.A. Ashwin), *Demonolatry* (Secaucus, NJ: University Books, 1974), 21, wrote of 'duplications and superfluities of parts of the body... it is agreed that they are due to an excessive abundance of semen'; see also P. Boaistuau, *Histoires Prodigieuses...* (Paris: V. Sentenas, 1560), fo. 142v.
18. E. Fenton, *Certaine Secrete Wonders of Nature...* (London: H. Bynneman, 1569), fo. 13v.
19. A. Paré (ed. and transl. J.L. Pallister), *On Monsters and Marvels* (Chicago and London, University of Chicago Press, 1982), 33.

20. L.M. Sinistrari (ed. and transl. M. Summers), *Demoniality* (London: The Fortune Press, 1927), 24.

21. J. Needham, *A History of Embryology* (Cambridge: Cambridge University Press, 1959),187.

22. Fenton, *op. cit.* (note 18), fo. 136v.

23. Appendix, 1534, 1546b.

24. See A.R. Hall and M.B. Hall (eds and transl.), *The Correspondence of Henry Oldenburg* (Madison: University of Wisconsin Press, 1965–77), II, 277. During most of the twentieth century the alternative 'fission' theory was prevalent, largely because of extrapolation from the results of experimental studies on lower vertebrates, but recent work has shown that human conjoined twins almost certainly do result from secondary union of initially separate embryonic discs: see R. Spencer, 'Theoretical and Analytical Embryology of Conjoined Twins: Part I: Embryogenesis', *Clinical Anatomy*, xiii (2000), 36–53.

25. Remy, *op. cit.* (note 17), 11.

26. *Ibid.*, 67.

27. Paré, *op. cit.* (note 19), 47.

28. J.W. Ballantyne, 'Antenatal Pathology and Heredity in the Hippocratic Writings', *Teratologia*, ii (1895), 275–87. Arguably Hippocrates also accepted maternal impressions, though Ballantyne disputed this.

29. See J.D., *A Discription of a Monstrous Chylde...* (London: L. Askel for F. Godlyf, 1562); Appendix, 1562a.

30. Philobiblon Society (eds), *Ancient Ballads & Broadsides...* (London: Whittingham and Wilkins, 1867), 40–2; Appendix, 1562c.

31. As does R.F. Oaks, 'Things Fearful to Name: Sodomy and Buggery in Seventeenth-Century New England', *Journal of Social History*, xii (1978), 268–81; Thijssen, *op. cit.* (note 2), suggests that in seeking natural explanations for monsters Albert was of the same school of thought as Bacon.

32. J.E. Salisbury, *The Beast Within: Animals in the Middle Ages* (New York: Routledge, 1994), 146.

33. *Ibid.*, 145.

34. Paré, *op. cit.* (note 19), 67.

35. *Ibid.*, 67, from Cardan's *De Rerum Varietate* (Basel: S.H. Petri, 1581), book XIV, ch. 64.

36. W. Turner, *History of the Most Remarkable Providences* (1697), quoted by E. Fudge, 'Monstrous Acts: Bestiality in Early Modern England', *History Today*, l (2000), 20–5.

37. K. Park and L.J. Daston, 'Unnatural Conceptions: The Study of Monsters in Sixteenth and Seventeenth-Century England and France', *Past & Present*, xcii

(1981), 20–54.

38. 'Harelip' was current in the sixteenth century; see *A Midsummer Night's Dream*, V, i, 418.

39. This opinion was based on Aristotle, *Generation of Animals*, 769b10–25: 'The likeness of monstrosities to animals is merely resemblance. Their differing gestation periods prevent mixtures of one animal in another'.

40. F. Liceti, *De Monstrorum Caussis, Natura, & Differentiis* (Padua: P. Frambott, 1634), 191. An opinion again based on Aristotle, who stated that if both male and female formative faculties were weak the foetus could resemble an animal; see Blane, *op. cit.* (note 10).

41. Bayle, 'Dissertationes Physicae in Quibus Principia Proprietatum in Mixtis, Aeconomia in Plantis & Animalibus, Causa & Signa Propensionum in Homine &c. Demonstrantur', *Journal des Savans* (1677), 161–3.

42. This does not however apply in the example of an ape, as a human baby resembles a foetal ape.

43. V. Nutton, 'The Anatomy of the Soul in Early Renaissance Medicine', in G.R. Dunstan (ed.), *The Human Embryo: Aristotle and the Arabic and European Traditions* (Exeter, University of Exeter Press, 1990), 136–57.

44. G. Mauquest de La Motte (transl. T. Tomkyns), *A General Treatise of Midwifry...* (London: J. Waugh, 1746), 192.

45. *Ibid.*, 235–6.

46. There is very extensive literature on maternal impressions, an introduction to which is G.M. Gould and W.L. Pyle, *Anomalies and Curiosities of Medicine* (New York: Sydenham, 1937), 81–5.

47. Fenton, *op. cit.* (note 18), fo. 13r.

48. *Ibid.*, fo. 15r–v.

49. Remy, *op. cit.* (note 17), 25.

50. Paré, *op. cit.* (note 19), 41–2.

51. Fenton, *op. cit.* (note 18), ff. 13v–14[16]r.

52. J.A. Hünerwolff, 'De Fœmellis Duabus Monstrosis', *Miscellanea Curiosa*, series 2, ix (1690), 170–1.

53. *Praegnantem enim operari per multam apprehensionem, atque foetum nonnunquam transformare omnio, imo ab humana natura in belluinam [sic] transfigurare...*: A. Löw, 'Foetus, quà Caput, Monstrosus', *Miscellanea Curiosa*, series 2, ix (1690), 200–2.

54. Remy, *op. cit.* (note 17), 25.

55. An example is the exchange of views between the London surgeon and (later) physician Daniel Turner (1667–1741) and the Paris-born but London-based physician and author of *The Power of the Mother's Imagination Described* James Blondel (d. 1734). For a discussion of their correspondence see P.K. Wilson, *Surgeon 'Turned' Physician: The Career and Writings of*

Daniel Turner (1667–1741) (PhD, University College London, 1992). In 1712, the Italian physician Francesco Nigrisoli (1648–1727) published another comparatively early expression of doubt about the possibility of maternal impressions: F.M. Nigrisoli, *Considerazioni Intorno alla Generazione de' Viventi* (Ferrara: B. Barbieri, 1712).

56. 'Extrait d'une Lettre de Monsieur le Prieur de Lugeris en Champagne, Sur un Enfantemant Arrivé au Mois de Mai Dernier', *Journal des Savans* (1690), 53–4.

57. O. Niccoli, '"Menstruum Quasi Monstruum": Monstrous Births and Menstrual Taboo in the Sixteenth Century', in E. Muir and G. Ruggiero (eds), *Sex and Gender in Historical Perspective* (Baltimore: Johns Hopkins University Press, 1990), 1–25.

58. *Op. cit.* (note 32).

59. See Bauhin's classification, Chapter 3, 79.

60. See Salisbury, *op. cit.* (note 32), 79, for early modern beliefs on the sexuality of animals. For the supposed sinfulness of dorsal intercourse see R.M. Warnicke, *The Rise and Fall of Ann Boleyn* (Cambridge: Cambridge University Press, 1989), 195.

61. One of the earliest references to the 'crime' (rather than the 'sin') of bestiality is from fourteenth-century Majorca: see Salisbury, *op. cit.* (note 32), 100. It was not regarded as a serious crime in England until the sixteenth century, when it became punishable by death and it also became a capital crime in Sweden at about the same time: see Fudge, *op. cit.* (note 36).

62. Animal trials were largely ignored by historians until the publication of E.P. Evans's seminal *The Criminal Prosecution and Capital Punishment of Animals* (London: Heinemann, 1906).

63. P. Beirne, 'The Law is an Ass: Reading E.P. Evans' *The Medieval Prosecution and Capital Punishment of Animals*', (www.colchsfc.ac.uk/english/barnes10.htm, viewed 19 April, 2002).

64. The relevant documents and background have been carefully analysed in D. Cressy, *Travesties and Transgressions in Tudor and Stuart England: Tales of Discord and Dissension* (Oxford: Oxford University Press, 2000), 9–28.

65. Much literature has been published on the 'rabbit breeder', an excellent introduction to which is J. Bondeson's 'Mary Toft the Rabbit Breeder', in his *A Cabinet of Medical Curiosities* (London: I.B. Tauris, 1997), 122–43.

66. Such as the authors of the German theses mentioned in Chapter 3, 87.

67. M. Summers deals with the meaning of these terms at length in the introduction to his translation of Sinistrari's *Demoniality*, where he states that in Classical Greece: 'daemones formed the connecting link between gods and men'.

68. Sinistrari was a highly cultured and learned Franciscan theologian but capable of some odd opinions. See the introduction to Summers's translation of his *Demoniality*.

69. Remy, *op. cit.* (note 17), 20–1.

70. Which he knew from C. Massaeus, *Chronicorum Multiplicis Historiae Utriusque Testamenti...* (Antwerp: J. Crinitus, 1540).

71. Remy, *op. cit.* (note 17), 21.

72. Probably a hydatidiform mole.

73. *Ibid,* 21.

74. *Ibid.,* 22.

75. *Ibid.,* 11.

76. *Ibid.*

77. Remy was no theologian, and indeed his work contained the statement that monsters were not to receive Christian baptism but were to be killed immediately – an opinion, as the historian and priest Montague Summers noted, 'clean contrary to the teaching of the Church'.

78. J. Bulwer, *Anthropometamorphosis...* (London: W. Hunt, 1653), 514, apparently accepted the possibility of monsters being produced by inter-species unions and ridiculed the notion that devils could conceive human offspring in similar terms: 'If the faculty of generation had been allowed to Devils, the world had long since been full of Devils'.

79. Appendix, 1547b.

80. Bulwer, *op. cit.* (note 78).

81. Paré, *op. cit.* (note 19), 3–4.

82. Fenton, *op. cit.* (note 18), fo. 12v. This belief probably originated from traditions of menstrual taboo: 'Because a child conceived during the menstrual flow takes its nourishment and growth – being in its mother's womb – from blood that is contaminated, dirty, and corrupt, which having established its infection in the course of time, manifests itself and causes its malignancy to appear': Paré, *op. cit.* (note 19), 5. Levin Lemne (1505–68) also warned against copulation 'when her courses run, not observing natures rules; for he strives against the flux, and fails against the stream. Our people by a proverb call it pissing against the moon': quoted in R. Hole, 'Incest, Consanguinity and a Monstrous Birth in Rural England, January 1600', *Social History,* xxv (2000), 183–99.

83. J. Maubray, *The Female Physician...* (London: J. Holland, 1724), 373.

84. Philalethes, or A Lover of Truth and Learning, *The Sooterkin Dissected ...* (London: A. Moore, 1726).

85. Maubray's description of the sooterkin may have been an intentional, and indeed successful, attempt to obtain publicity for *The Female Physician* by including some remarkable material (he also mentioned Countess Margaret

of Henneberg's 365 children and he later attended the birth chamber of the most celebrated of eighteenth-century England's producers of bizarre births, the 'rabbit-breeder' Mary Toft).

86. *Problems,* 878a18–24. Not, of course, the work of Aristotle. The earliest edition was printed in 1475 in Rome.

87. See Y.V. O'Neill, 'Michele Savonarola and the *Fera* or Blighted Twin Phenomenon', *Medical History,* xviii (1974), 222–39.

88. C. Peucer, *Commentarius de Præcipuis Divinationum Generibus...* (Wittenberg: J. Lufft, 1553), 326; see Appendix, 1531b.

89. S. Batman, *The Doome Warning All Men to the Judgement...* (London: R. Nubery, 1581), 412.

90. *Ibid.,* 363 (Batman's translation).

91. First printed in 1558; English translation as *Natural Magick...In Twenty Bookes* (London: T. Young and S. Speed, 1658), 28.

92. *Ibid.,* 28.

93. R. Josselin (ed. E. Hockliffe), *The Diary of the Rev. Ralph Josselin, 1616–1683* (London: Camden Society, 1908), 32.

94. E. Topsell, *The History of Four-footed Beasts and Serpents* (London: E. Cotes, 1658), 595–6.

95. J. Cleveland, *A Character of a Diurnal-Maker* (London: 1651).

96. H.E. Rollins (ed.), *The Pack of Autolycus...* (Cambridge: Harvard University Press, 1927), 185.

97. Sharp, *op. cit.* (note 11), 111.

98. T.L., *The Wonder of Wonders, or, The Strange Birth in Hampshire* (London: J. Hose and E. Oliver, *c.*1675), reprinted in Rollins, *op. cit.* (note 96), 188–9.

99. L.W., *True Wonders, and Strange News from Rumsey in Hampshire...,* reprinted in Rollins, *Ibid.,* 191–4.

100. J. Gélis, *History of Childbirth...* (Polity Press: Oxford, 1991), 259. This suggestion is also made by O'Neill, *op. cit.* (note 87), although with some confusion over the meaning of the term *mola.*

101. La Motte, *op. cit.* (note 44), 24.

102. Remy, *op. cit.* (note 17), 21.

103. Needham, *op. cit.* (note 21), 83.

104. For a discussion of the relation of the sooterkin to the spontaneous generation controversy see A.W. Bates, 'The Sooterkin Dissected: The Theoretical Basis of Animal Births to Human Mothers in Early Modern Europe', *Vesalius,* ix (2003), 6–14.

105. J. Rueff, *The Expert Midwife...* (London: E.G. for S.E., 1637), 138.

6

From the Womb to the Tomb[1]

> Whoever is born anywhere as a human being, that is, as a rational mortal creature, however strange he may appear to our senses in bodily form or colour or motion or utterance, or in any faculty, part or quality of his nature whatsoever; let no true believer have any doubt that such an individual is descended from the one man who was first created.[2]

So far, we have considered monstrous births from the point of view of those who wrote about them, giving emphasis, as they did, to their appearance and meaning, particularly their theological significance. The extensive literature on monstrous births is also a reflection of their social importance; it tells us something of the social context of their lives and of responses to them. Monstrous births were not for the most part illustrated as passive objects of contemplation; like Vesalius's anatomical plates they look back at the reader and they inhabit the same neoclassical landscape that he does. Even if they were stillborn, illustrations showed them older than their years, as they would have appeared had they lived (Figure 6.1, overleaf). We know that they attracted large crowds, including the well-educated, who were perhaps wealthy enough to acquire the body of a monster for themselves, and who left a record of what they saw and why they considered it significant. However, there were many others whose motives for going to see a monster were not recorded, and whose reactions were probably complex and sometimes ambivalent.

Delivery

Almost all early modern sources disregard the actual birth of monstrous babies; their arrival in the world was presented without mention of the now obvious fact that many must have had difficult deliveries. A monster would usually have been unsuspected until the time of birth, and if the pregnancy were close to full-term then double monsters and others bulkier than normal would have been at risk of obstructed labour. Several accounts describe fresh (that is, non-macerated) double monsters that died, presumably asphyxiated or traumatised ('…the sage women had used to much force and violence', wrote Fenton of one dead child)[3] during prolonged deliveries. Thomas Bedford, writing in 1635, lamented the lack of a 'skilfull hand' that might

Figure 6.1
'[A] girl was born whose whole body was well formed except the head, which
had a most horrible appearance: a secret eye was present in the back of the
head; the other eye was in the head above the future crown. This slightly larger,
human eye had neither lids nor lashes.' A painter who had seen the child alive
and after death made an engraving which was owned by Cardinal Barberini.
Liceti, De Monstrorum *(1634).*

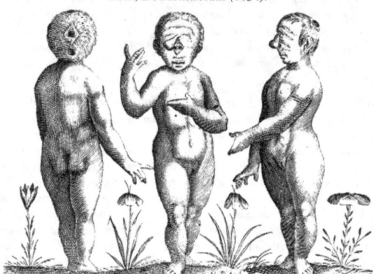

have enabled one pair 'living and lively some few houres before they were
borne... to see the light, if not to enjoy it',[4] and Garden wrote of a double
monster born in Aberdeen in 1686: 'It is thought they might have been
brought forth alive, but that they stayed so long in the Birth; for that both
heads presenting together, the Midwife thought they had been Twins, and
thrust one of them always back.'[5] Although some such as Francois Rousset
(in 1582) proposed the use of Caesarean section to save both mother and
child, risk of maternal deaths prevented its general use in Europe before the
eighteenth century, apart from a few, possibly anecdotal, successes.[6]

Those assisting at the delivery would have been the first to see a
monstrous birth and for most of the early modern period this would have
meant that midwives or the mothers' neighbours and friends were the usual
witnesses, although by the latter part of the seventeenth century the male
surgeon-accoucheur had appeared on the scene. Midwives were usually
women of mature years who had borne children themselves and had
undergone some form of training or licensing. In England, the Bishop of the

diocese in which they worked licensed them with the assistance of a panel of established midwives, although by the middle of the seventeenth century a secular licensing process was available in London via Surgeons' Hall. In *The Breviary of Helthe,*[7] Henry VIII's physician Andrew Borde characterized the ideal midwife as 'wyse and discrete', and licensing appears to have been concerned as much with the social requirements of the job as with an applicant's obstetric skills. An English midwives' oath of 1567 was chiefly concerned with preventing various superstitions ('sorcery or incantation') and Roman Catholic practices, and with enjoining midwives to obtain from unmarried mothers the name of the child's father.[8]

If no midwife were available, female neighbours showed a 'willing forwardnes'[9] to help, and the mid-sixteenth-century room of confinement could be a busy place:[10] an illustration on the title page of Rueff's *De Conceptu* shows, in addition to the pregnant woman, seven adults (three of whom are enjoying a large meal), two small children and a dog.[11] But a woodcut showing labour in progress, with a midwife modestly working with her hands beneath the patient's skirts while two other women comfort the mother and astrologers cast a natal horoscope,[12] shows that, despite the number of people present, there may have been no eye-witnesses to the birth itself, an important point when considering the possibilities of deception and concealment in relation to monstrous births. Illustrations such as these were of course symbolic; the celebratory meal took place, if at all, after the delivery and astrologers would probably not have worked in the birthing chamber itself. It has been claimed that most births in early modern times were all-female events, perhaps intentionally so because they were one of the few situations in which important proceedings took place in the absence of male witnesses,[13] but as most of the accounts of the birthing chamber and illustrations of it were made by men, their exclusion from the birthing process and its nature as a female 'ritual' have been questioned.[14] Almost all writers on monstrous births were men, and while those with a medical background may have been familiar with childbirth it was a mystery to some; in one mid-sixteenth-century ballad what looks to a modern observer to be a morphologically normal, though macerated, baby[15] was presented as a monster, and both the writer and a man who had seen it described its umbilical cord as though it were an unusual structure.[16]

Midwives were perhaps more likely to have been involved with monstrous births if labour was difficult, as apart from being experienced there were special techniques that they could use. Embryotomy (cutting off the limbs or puncturing the head to remove the brains in order to facilitate passage of the infant) was specifically forbidden by the English oath of 1567, but the necessity for this prohibition suggests that some (unlicensed?)

midwives were familiar with the method and were at least tempted to try it. The restriction seems to have been relaxed in the seventeenth century, when they were permitted to open the head if the baby had died.[17] By this time the use of instruments was an accepted part of the practice of the majority of men-midwives, most of whom were based in large towns. Percival Willughby of Derby (1596–1685) recorded 'two or three' examples where a living child was deliberately killed by embryotomy, each time with the sanction of a minister of religion, during his forty-nine years of obstetric practice between 1630 and 1678 and the French man-midwife Guillaume Mauquest de la Motte[18] stated in an account of his practice at the end of the seventeenth century that female midwives performed embryotomy in obstructed labours, but did not use the crotchet (a blunt hook with which to apply traction), though it seems that the latter was by choice rather than because they were forbidden from doing so. La Motte described several cases of embryotomy performed by surgeons[19] and emphasised that it was not usually permitted while a child lived: 'there was no hope left but in the instruments, and these we are forbid to use without a certain knowledge of the child's death.'[20] The only account of the use of these techniques in the delivery of a monstrous birth is of a double monster born in England in 1555 (Figure 6.2), 'so huge above order, that it was impossible to draw him whole from the bellie of his mother',[21] which had to be dismembered to effect delivery: 'the thighs which were apart were broken and pulled from the Mother when she was in travaille.'[22] As the child's entrails and liver were hanging out it must have been obvious that it was already dead before the procedure began.

In the context of huge infant mortality rates – never less than one in ten and in a bad year seven in ten *live-born* infants never reached one year of age[23] – stillbirths were, as a very broad generalization, not something over which much concern was shown. At the time of the English Civil War midwives were instructed in disposing of them:[24]

> If any childe be dead-born, you yourselfe shall see it buried in such secret place as neither hogg nor dogg, nor any other beast may come unto it, and in such sort done, as it may not be found or perceived, as much as you may; And that you shall not suffer any such childe to be cast into the Jaques or any other inconvenient place.[25]

Most of the mothers' concerns probably related to future fertility; Gélis has suggested that stillbirths were often kept secret because of 'guilt' or 'fear of barrenness'.[26] A stillborn monster must have been doubly alarming because of the prospect of being accused of sexual or other misconduct as well as being thought incapable of having normal children – it has been suggested that Henry VIII's change of attitude towards Anne Boleyn was

Figure 6.2
A double monster born at Genoa (Appendix, 1555a),
delivered by embryotomy and, by convention, depicted as if living. Edward
Fenton, Certaine Secrete Wonders of Nature *(1569).*

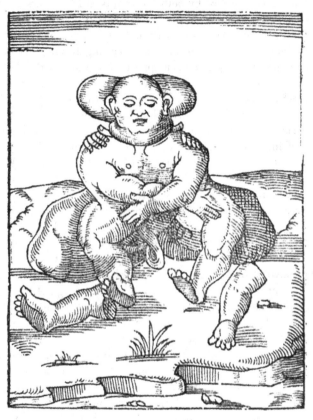

partly due to her having given birth to a monster[27] – and it is easy to imagine, though there is no evidence, that women concealed stillborn monstrous births if they could. The wife of a man in a cautionary story in the Puritan *The Theatre of God's Judgements* (1597), who was punished for hunting on the sabbath by the birth of a child with a dog's head, tries initially to conceal the birth.[28] Ben Jonson's play *The Magnetic Lady* (written in 1632) turns on a midwife's plot to conceal a birth[29] and its (male) audience was probably accustomed to, if uneasy about, humour concerning the possibilities of midwives keeping 'women-matters' to themselves.

Baptism

Popular sixteenth-century accounts of monstrous births by Protestant writers often related that the child had been baptised, and the baptism of monsters seems to have been expected by both Protestants and Catholics alike. The *Rituale Romanum* recommended that the ordinary baptised a monster, and when a child with two faces was born at Bononia in January 1514, the Cardinal Bishop himself performed the rite.[30] The highly public ceremony in the cathedral would have provided an opportunity to display the child as an edifying example of the Church's teaching that, as St Augustine had written, all people, whatever their appearance, were members of the race of Adam, and therefore potentially of the Church,[31] a message with renewed significance at a time when non-European races were potential converts. As well as signifying acceptance into the Christian community, the baptism of monsters was also used to make a point about the validity of infant baptism, a question that generated a huge body of literature in the sixteenth and early seventeenth centuries from Catholics, Lutherans and Zwinglians alike, who were united in their opposition to Anabaptists. In Catholic and the majority of Protestant churches, live-born children were baptised by a priest or minister as soon as they could conveniently be taken to church but a newborn child considered likely to die could, according to canon law, be baptised by anyone. Midwives were well placed to do this and it had always been expected of them; the English poet Robert Mannyng (*c.*1288–*c.*1338) had written that a midwife who neglected this duty might have 'loste a chylde both soule and lyfe', and after the Reformation English midwives received training in the administration of baptism.

A considerable amount of debate took place over the proper form to use when administering baptism to monstrous births. In general, this centred either on whether the child was to be considered human or whether double monsters were to be baptised twice or only once. Again, these concerns were directed at the Anabaptist heresy, because if double monsters had a single soul then repetition of baptism, a practice associated with Anabaptists, was to be avoided.[32] Another cause of difficulty not confined to monsters was uncertainty over whether a dying child retained some sign of life; this was (and still is) solved by giving conditional baptism in order to avoid attempting to administer the sacrament after death. In a letter to the *Journal des Savans* in 1690 a French priest referred to the conditional baptism, with the qualification 'if thou art alive',[33] of a child with a 'great deformity of the head', and raised an ethical question that remains today: can a child without a brain be said to be alive and could such a child possess a soul if the putative seat of that soul (the pineal gland) was lacking? A second form of conditional baptism with the qualification 'if thou art a Man' was probably intended for monstrous animals that resembled human foetuses;[34] there is no record of a human birth in the sixteenth or seventeenth century having received this form of baptism.

Exhibition

The Victorian physician, historian and man of letters Henry Morley wrote that, in Restoration England: 'the taste for monsters became a disease'.[35] Morley speculated that monstrous births were shown at fairs and were the year-round stock in trade of London showmen who for the rest of the year earned a living from exhibiting them in other parts of the city.[36] The type of show that Morley envisaged bears more than a passing resemblance to a Victorian 'freak show' and fostered an image of the exploited monster ogled by indifferent crowds. Public exhibition of monstrous births certainly occurred throughout the early modern period; it was recorded of conjoined twins born in Vienna in 1475:

> [B]ecause their parents were poor, they were carted around to several cities in Italy, in order to collect money from the people, who were burning to see this new spectacle of Nature.[37]

For the poor there was a strong financial incentive to exhibit monsters, so much so that the birth of a monster could be considered a blessing for the parents, but parents' motives cannot be generalised and some well-to-do parents also sought publicity: in sixteenth-century Germany Ulrich, Grave [Earl] of Muntfort, summoned his artist, Master Matheysen Miller of Lindau, to draw his monstrous child, and 'ordered it printed'.[38] The birth of a monster was a significant event; as they were often held to be a sign of divine intervention they had the impact of a miracle and hundreds or even thousands of people might have gone to see them while many more read of them or heard the news: 'This monster lived two days... and was seen alive by many hundreds of the neighbouring places, which flocked to see so strange a creature.'[39] Word of mouth alone was sufficient to attract a crowd in a short space of time: 'Not many hours passed, before the reports of this strange byrth was bruited abroad, and the eares of the inhabitants there-about dwelling, so filled with the newes thereof, that they came in multitudes to behold it'. One of the purposes of broadsides that described monstrous births was to act as advertisements ('[c]ome take a view good people all')[40] and provide directions: 'This childe beforsaid (the day of the date under written) was to be seene in Gleve Alley, in Suthwark, beeing alive and x week olde and iiij dayees, not unlikely to live long.'[41] There were even souvenirs: a majolica bowl produced in Italy in the early sixteenth century depicts a female double monster (Figure 6.3, overleaf).[42]

Figure 6.3
A tin-glazed earthenware bowl, Italian c.1515,
depicting female conjoined twins.

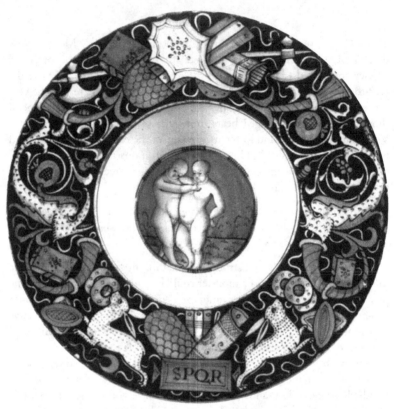

The evidence that monstrous births were exhibited at fairs is not strong. Bartholomew Fair, held in London since mediaeval times, has been emphasised as a location for the display of monstrous births,[43] and the expression 'a Bartlemew faire babie' became current for a fake.[44] The few surviving printed advertisements for monsters on display in London taverns and fairs suggest a degree of trickery, though perhaps with the connivance of the audience, who were seeing a show rather than a sign from God. These advertisements had no illustrations, partly perhaps to save money but also to excite the imagination of the reader, and were quite general so they could be used on a number of occasions; the date and place being inserted by hand. There is little doubt that anyone paying to inspect 'a monster... being Humane upwards, and Bruit downwards... so exactly stuffed'[45] would see nothing more than a clever example of the taxidermist's art. The following advertisement is perhaps more promising:

> A changeling child. To be seen next door to the Black Raven in West Smithfield, during the time of the fair. Aged 9 or more, a foot and a half high, legs and arms no bigger than a man's thumb, seems so grave and solid, as if it were 60. You can see the whole anatomy of its body by setting it against the sun. It never speaks, but cries like a cat. It has no teeth but is the most voracious and hungry creature in the world. Taken by a Venetian vessel from a Turkish galley.[46]

Quite apart from its romantic origins (it is more likely to have been taken from a poor local family), the physical description is unconvincing and the age probably much exaggerated to make the child look smaller for its age than it actually was.[47] Twins aged 21 years with two bodies but one head, described in another pair of advertisements, though not anatomically impossible, are unlikely to have survived to that age and, had they done so, one would expect them to have earned their livelihood by exhibiting widely, yet there seems to be no other record of the case.

Most monstrous births were 'exhibited' at their birthplace by their parents, where they could easily attract a crowd; 500 or more a day in the case of the double monster born at Isle Brewers in Somersetshire, so many that 'Mr A.P.', who reported the case to the Royal Society, had difficulty in getting close enough to see them,[48] and it was feared the children's lives would be shortened by constant examination. A thousand people saw a double monster born near Salisbury in 1664:

> This *Monster* lived two dayes and then dyed, and is Imbalmed, and to be brought to London to be seen. There hath been Lords, Ladys, and much Gentry to see it; The Father (being a poore man) had twenty pound given him the first day, by persons of Quality. I Josiah Smith, Practitioner of Phisick, saw them all three alive.[49]

Visitors often gave money to view such cases, either in payment or as an act of charity; the mother of a child born in Kent in 1615 was: 'relieved by much money, which out of Christian compassion many bestowed on her.'[50] In 1682, an eye-witness account of a double monster born in Ostend was considered interesting enough to publish for the London market:[51] a merchant and his friends paid to see the twins, whose parents had been offered a great sum of money for them to be 'carried about' for exhibition, and were permitted to make a thorough examination, with the parents' consent. The most demanding living was to be had by begging in the street: 'An observing Divine, a Traveller, and friend of mine... saw in *Cheapside*

London, but a few daies before, a child that was born without Armes, and had two little hands, which it could move, standing out of its shoulders, a poore woman had the child in her armes, begging with it.'[52] It was also possible to make a living by begging door-to-door: 'this mayde went from dore to dore searching for a living, to whom they gave more willingly for the noveltie of so strange a creature and so new a spectacle',[53] and sometimes such a person would be paid to move on by a community afraid of maternal impressions.[54]

A larger audience could be obtained by moving the child to a nearby city or town, and in 1583 a child with 'two heads and two backbones' was brought to Shrewsbury in its coffin.[55] Many children, like the case seen by Evelyn (see below), continued to be exhibited after death;[56] a double monster, almost certainly dead, was brought up to London in 1565, 'wheare it was seene by dyvers worshipfull men and women of the cytie. And also of the Countrey.'[57] Monstrous births seem to have been regarded as public events and there is evidence that, at least if they were stillborn, they could be brought out for viewing whether the parents liked it or not: 'this as it was still-borne was exposed unto publick view to the infinet amazement of the beholders, and to the great griefe of the Parents.'[58] The influential and well to do could acquire the bodies of monsters directly from the parents, or by exhumation. A cyclopic child born in 1624 at Firme, Italy, which 'fortunately' died almost at once, was exhumed on the orders of the prefect of Genoa, but the face had already decomposed.[59]

The secondary literature on monstrous births often gives the impression that exhibition was their usual fate, but, of course, the cases recorded are those that were publicised. Perhaps others were cared for in private if the parents lacked the desire, or the financial necessity, to exhibit them. It is also by no means certain that public exhibition was the degrading experience that we, from the position of a society where such things are no longer permitted, might imagine it to be. A broad range of people were interested in seeing monstrous children: monarchs, cardinals, priests, merchants and even nuns, one of whom recorded in her diary that 'a foreigner' had been paid to show them an embalmed male baby with 'two child's faces, and for the rest a single body, very beautiful to see'.[60] Montaigne's essay *On a Monstrous Child* preserves his impression on seeing a child exhibited:

> I saw two dayes since a child whom two men and a nurse (which named themselves to be his father, his uncle, and his aunt) carried about with intent to get some money with the sight of him, by reason of his strangenesse. In all the rest he was as other children are: he stood upon his feete, went and prattled in a manner as all others of his age. He would never take nourishment but by his nurses breast; and what in my presence was offred to

148

be put in his mouth he chewed a little and put it all out againe. His puling differed somewhat from others: he was just fourteene monthes olde. Under his paps he was fastned and joyned to another childe, but had no head, and who had the conduite of his backe stopped; the rest whole. One of his armes was shorter than the other, and was by accident broken at their birth. They were joyned face to face, and as if a little child would embrace another somewhat bigger. The joyning and space whereat they were closed together was but foure inches broad, or thereabouts; in such sort that if you thrust up the imperfect childe you might see under the others navill; and the seame was betweene the paps and his navill. The navill of the imperfect one could not be seene, but all the rest of his belly might. Thus, what of the imperfect one was not joyned, as armes, buttocks, thighes, and legges, did hang and shake upon the other, whose length reached to the middle-leg of the other perfect. His nurse told me he made water by both privities. The members of the little one were nourished, living, and in the same state as the others, except only they were lesse and thinner.[61]

The eyewitness accounts that survive are predominantly those left by the well-to-do; we know that Samuel Pepys, Robert Hooke and John Evelyn (all Fellows of the Royal Society) went to see monsters, and Eveyn left the following account:

September 13 I saw in Southwark at St. Margarites faire, a monstrous birth of Twinns, both femals & most perfectly shaped, save that they were joyn'd breast to breast, & incorporated at the navil, having their armes thrown about each other thus [drawing]. It was reported quick in May last, & produced neere Turne-style Holbourn: well exent[e]rated & preserved till now: We saw also a poore Woman, that had a living Child of one yeare old, who had its head, neck, with part of a Thigh growing out about Spina dorsi: The head had the place of Eyes & nose, but none perfected. The head monstrous, rather resembling a greate Wenn; and hanging on the buttocks, at side whereoff, & not in the due place, were (as I remembred) the excrements it avoided, we saw also Monkeys & Apes daunce, & do other feates of activity on the high-rope, to admiration: They were galantly clad alamode, went upright, saluted the Company, bowling, & pulling-off their hatts: They saluted one another with as good grace as if instructed by a Daucing Master.[62]

Monsters who lived to adulthood almost certainly had to earn a living by exhibiting themselves and therefore left documentary evidence. After a childhood spent travelling and earning money for a parent or guardian ('A Spaniard came to Florence, who had with him a boy of about thirteen, a kind of monstrosity, whom he went around showing everywhere, gaining much money'),[63] the few who reached adulthood could set up independently. One well-known example was Lazarus Colloredo and his parasitic twin brother John-Baptiste.[64] Their progress around Europe was marked by the appearance of ballads, but it is not clear whether these publications were organised by Lazarus himself, or whether they were opportunistic, the printers taking advantage of the Colloredos' visit to sell hastily produced accounts of them. *The Two Inseparable Brothers* (1637) describes Lazarus as an Italian gentleman, then about 17 years of age. He was born in Genoa in 1617 and examined by, amongst others, Caspar Bartholin the elder.[65] Paul Dubé, a country physician in Montargis, wrote that Lazarus was condemned to death but spared because his execution would have killed his innocent brother, and Lazarus himself was wont to tell this story, which sounds like a fiction designed to draw an audience.[66]

The 20-year-old Lazarus visited England, and on 4 November 1637 the Master of the Revels, Sir Henry Herbert, granted a licence 'to Lazarus, an Italian, to shew his brother Baptista, that grows out of his navell, and carryes him at his syde. In confirmation of his Majesty's warrant, granted unto him to make publique shewe.'[67] After a London audience with Charles I,[68] Lazarus exhibited himself in Norwich over Christmas 1639: 'This daie Larzeus Colleretto have leave to shewe a monster until the day after twelfe, he shewing to the Court a lycense signed with his Maties own hand.'[69] Thereafter he probably toured England en route to Scotland where we have an account, again discovered by Rollins, of his *modus operandi*:

> When he cam to the towne he had tuo servandis auaiting upone him, who with him self were weill clad. He had his portraiture with the monster drawin, and hung out at his lodging, to the view of the people. The one servand had ane trumpettour who soundit out at suche tyme as the people should cum and sie this monster, who flocked aboundantlie into his lodging. The uther servand receaved the moneyis fra ilk persone for his sight, sum less sum mair. And efter there was so muche collectit as culd be gottin, he with his servandis, shortlie left the toun, and went southuard agane.[70]

A picture emerges of a comfortable if peripatetic life for Lazarus, at the expense of his twin:

> And if you nip it by the arme,
> Or doe it any little harme,
>   (this hath been tride by many,)
>
> It like an infant (with voyce weake)
> Will cry out though it cannot speake,

150

As sensible of paine,
Which yet the other feeleth not...[71]

This simple experiment enabled the visitor to investigate the extent to which Lazarus and John-Baptiste were separate individuals, one of the traditional points of interest concerning double monsters:

> I will onely remember unto you a very handsome young man, late (if not now) in Towne [London], whose picture hath been publickely set out to the common view, and himselfe to be seene for money; who from one of his sides hath a twin brother growing, which was borne with him, and living still; though having sence [sensation] and feeling, yet destitute of reason and understanding: whence me thinks a disputable question might arise, whether they have distinct lives, so they are possessed of two soules; or have but one imparted betwixt them both.[72]

This type of twinning, now called thoracopagus parasiticus, is compatible with a normal life expectancy. Boaistuau had written of a similar case: a man, aged 40 in 1530, with a twin attached at the umbilicus. He carried the twin's body in his arms and 'great troupes' came to see him. He too travelled widely and was seen in Valence, Paris, and Montlehery[73] Another similar monster was reported by Rueff to have travelled 'all over the world'.[74]

Paying to see a monster enabled the visitor to satisfy his curiosity to the limit. Infants were picked up and palpated and some died from excessive handling. Adults were questioned – James Paris Du Plessis asked Lazarus Colloredo and the 'Yorkshire hermaphrodite' 'many questions' – and sometimes submitted to intimate examination: 'its viril Herge did Erect by Provocation' Du Plessis noted of the hermaphrodite.[75] In spite of these intrusive examinations, the evidence that we have suggests that congenitally malformed adults who were able to provide for themselves were regarded with interest and perhaps admiration. There is nothing to indicate that they were feared or ridiculed, as some historians have suggested,[76] and the tendency was for their accomplishments to be emphasised. The skill of Thomas Schweiker (1540–1602), a man born without arms, at writing with his feet was his stock in trade during life (he was depicted writing 'Blessed be God in all his works') and a sheet of parchment said to have his writing on it was on display at the mint at Worms more than a century after his death, when his calligraphy was still being praised as 'very Beautiful'.[77] This was a typical description of the capabilities of individuals with this type of deformity, who were said to use their feet 'marvellously well'.[78] Du Plessis noted that a child born without lower limbs 'jumps, dances and shows artfull tricks that any other person can do with thighs and legs. He speaks divers

151

different languages as High Dutch, Low Dutch, Sclavonian, French and English', while: 'A Man with a Head Growing out of his Belly... spoke and Rit Several Languages as Latin, French, Italian High Dutch and Pritty good English.'[79] As well as showing a favourable, even exaggerated, regard for their intellectual abilities, their linguistic talents suggest that they were widely travelled. The physical beauty of monstrous births was also given remarkable emphasis; conjoined twins 'were so well made in all the other Members, that the Painter, who was employed to draw them, affirm'd, that if they were done in Ivory, he would have paid any money for them'.[80] Despite the numbers of clergy, Protestant and Catholic, among the observers and collectors of monstrous births, the churches could not but disapprove of those who 'prostituted' malformed children for 'covetousnesse', or who bought or sold the body of a child for exhibition and so 'kept [it] from the grave'.[81] The situation was not helped by the fact that unbaptised children, including stillbirths, were officially denied Christian burial and should have been handed over to the midwife for disposal, though some clergy ignored the letter of the law and buried stillbirths, even monsters.[82]

The monetary value of monsters living and dead provided a motive for deception, and accounts of children intentionally maimed for exhibition date back to classical Rome: 'Finding a different savagery for each, this bone breaker cuts off the arms of one, slices the sinews of another: one he twists, another he castrates.'[83] The faking of illness for gain was a particular concern of Paré's and he claimed that the faking of monstrosities was still going on and proposed corporal punishment for offenders.[84] Fenton also claimed that fakes were being created:

> [V]acabunds... travelling through al provinces... as soone as their children
> be borne, and whilest their sinewes & bones be tender and flexible, with smal
> force, wil not stick to breke their arms, crush their legs, & puffe up their
> belly with some artificial pouder, defacing their noses with other parts of the
> face: & sometime pecking out their eyes, & all to make them appear
> monstrous.[85]

Another unsubstantiated seventeenth-century account mentions parents put to death for mutilating a live infant.[86] Despite the lurid tales that were circulated, there is only one example of a faked monstrous birth reported by an eyewitness, and this appears to have involved the mutilation of a stillborn infant. In Denmark in 1684 a soldier's wife gave birth to a child which died immediately: when it was subsequently exhibited there were fleshy excrescences on the legs, six toes on the right foot, a tail '1/4 of a Zealandish ell long', and excrescences on the forehead resembling 'laces', which one observer thought 'seemed to be very artificially done'. The fake was sufficient to draw a crowd to see the child: 'which the Painter, who 3 Days after it was dead, did draw the Scheme, testifieth to have been almost spoiled or rotten by the touching of so many Hundreds of People'.[87]

Dissection

At length it dy'd, and was convey'd,
    For Chyurgeons to Dissect,
And what Report thereof had said,
    They found it in Effect[88]

Many reported cases of monstrous births underwent postmortem examination; sometimes their bodies were described as having been 'opened', which may have referred to autopsy but could also have described part of the process of embalming. Contemporary accounts did not always distinguish *autopsy* and *anatomy* and these terms were sometimes interchangeable. From a modern perspective, the abnormal anatomy of birth defects *is* their pathology and one may wonder why it is necessary to distinguish anatomy from autopsy in a historical context. Most historians of anatomy do make a distinction, despite the lack of a clear distinction in the language used at the time, because the social implications of anatomy and the autopsy are thought to have differed. Public anatomies were punitive as well as educational and to be dissected was generally seen as undesirable. Autopsies were different in that they were usually carried out not in public but before an invited (and socially select) audience; they had some cachet from their association with the nobility, and in the seventeenth century other people's autopsies (such as Harvey's dissection of Old Parr) were fashionable spectacles.[89]

A brief chronology of anatomical and autopsy practice in Europe may help to set the scene. Medico-legal autopsies, to determine the cause of death, had been performed in the Middle Ages (one of the earliest recorded was in 1286 at Cremona). Mondino dei Lucci (*c.*1275–1327) is the first anatomist known to have taught from the human body and his *Anathomia*, based on lectures delivered around 1316, remained the standard text for over 200 years. The University of Montpellier began public anatomical dissection in 1366, Venice in 1368, Florence in 1388, Lérida in 1391 and Paris in 1478.[90] By the sixteenth century anatomy was a subject with which every educated man was expected to be familiar: 'the knowledge and true understanding of mans body... is also of great use to the Professors of Divinitie, Philosophy and all other good Literature and more particularly necessary for the faculties and Artes of Phisicke and Chirurgery'.[91] The longstanding notion that the church held back the development of anatomy has now been effectively challenged[92] and it appears that anatomical learning was hampered chiefly by lack of cadavers. As almost no one voluntarily gave a body for dissection, the only means of obtaining cadavers was to rely on compulsion: Montpellier was granted the right to the body of one executed criminal a year in 1375; the same privilege was granted to Lérida in 1391 by King John I;[93] James IV granted the Edinburgh Guild of Surgeons and Barbers the bodies of executed criminals for dissection in 1506; Henry VIII granted the Company of Barbers and Surgeons the right to the bodies of four hanged felons annually, and John Caius (1510–73), the founder of the Cambridge college who graduated in medicine from Padua in 1541, obtained a royal grant for the dissection of two felons' bodies annually in 1565.[94] One reason that Vesalius made such progress was that his supply of material was unusually good.[95] Few anatomists were this fortunate and at most schools dissections were infrequent; at Tübingen there was only one every three years and even in a major school such as Paris at the beginning of the seventeenth century, only four bodies a year were dissected.[96] The alternative to compulsion was theft, and as early as 1550 the people of Padua were demanding stricter laws against the stealing of bodies for dissection.[97]

The autopsy, usually performed by the physician or surgeon who had attended the patient during life, fared little better: the Swiss physician Felix Platter (1536–1614), who made an early attempt to classify disease according to symptoms, witnessed only eleven autopsies in the space of five years up to 1557. Anatomical knowledge is a prerequisite for the performance of an autopsy but despite the shortage of cadavers it would have been quite possible for students to acquire the skills needed; at Oxford, following the visitation of Edward VI in 1549, the statutes laid down that a student had to see two human dissections before obtaining his BM and perform two before being admitted to practice, which is more than is expected of UK medical students today.[98] Comparatively few medical practitioners were university educated, and the autopsy was a means for them to demonstrate publicly that they possessed the learning and skill to dissect the body. The status conferred on the physician by this knowledge is suggested by the portraits in which they were shown engaged in anatomical dissection.[99]

One of the earliest accounts of an autopsy on a monstrous birth dates from 1533, when 'two daughters attached to each other' were born on the island of Hispaniola (now Haiti and the Dominican Republic), then a Spanish colony. They were baptised Johanna and Melchiora and lived for only eight days. The priest who baptised them gave conditional baptism[100] to the second twin, an ingenious solution which nevertheless left doubts in the minds of the parents – had the twins one soul or two? To help resolve the problem they agreed to an autopsy, apparently the first in the New World.[101] The procedure was conducted in a formal manner, reminiscent of the anatomy schools of the European universities, two physicians supervising while delegating the manual task of cutting to a surgeon: 'Joan Camacho who held a Bachelor's Degree and was an excellent surgeon made an incision with a knife in the presence of two doctors of medicine: Hernando de Sepulveda and Rodrigo Navarro.' The girls' father was asked whether they had shown any differences in behaviour when alive, as '[t]his will prove, even without having them cut open, that they were two separate persons and two souls.' Different behaviour, even in infants, was thought to be at least as useful as anatomy in determining individuality. Anatomical solutions were hampered by differing opinions as to the seat of the soul; almost every major organ had been proposed, with the most favoured options being either the ventricles of the heart or the brain, but the liver was another possibility. The prosectors took care to describe a 'groove' separating the 'fused' livers (the only shared organ) into two parts, so that neither girl wanted any major organ. After the autopsy, the parents were told that Johanna and Melchiora were two when they 'passed from this life to celestial glory where, God willing, we shall see them.'[102]

Autopsies on monstrous births were performed in areas where adult autopsies were already accepted. In Spain and its colonies, France, and Italy they are recorded early in the sixteenth century, but in England, where the autopsy did not become fashionable until the seventeenth century, they were unusual before 1670.[103] The principal application of the autopsy to monstrous births in Europe was in the investigation of double monsters, to help solve the problem of one-in-two. The question of whether double monsters were one or two individuals was by no means as straightforward as it might appear; the classical solution, derived from Aristotle, was that when there was one heart there was one child: double monsters with two heads four arms and four legs ought, according to this rule, have been regarded as one person and book writers and contributors to journals tended to follow this classical precept. Fenton described a double monster with two heads, four arms and three legs as a 'childe',[104] and a 'biceps monstrum' described in *Miscellanea Curiosa* in 1672 was said to have a single soul.[105] Paré dissected double monsters to determine whether one or two hearts were present and, citing Aristotle as an authority that those with two hearts were two individuals, speculated that they were formed by crowding of seed within the uterus.[106] The view outside the academic world was that one head equalled one child and in practice, each head was baptised separately. In ballads, monstrous births with two heads were usually described as two children but if the heads were joined they were described in the singular as a 'child', whether or not two hearts were present.[107]

If the two elements of a double monster showed behavioural differences, as in the case from Hispaniola, this was usually seen as proof that they were two individuals; a point made by Jean Riolan with regard to the double monster born in Paris in 1605 and earlier monsters that had lived long enough to show different personalities.[108] Their different 'affections' were often noted by observers:

> That Double Child was Baptised with two Names, Peter and Paul, they had not Boath the same Affections nor Passions, the one wept Whilst the other Laffed, The one Slept Whilst the other Waked, the one was Hungary whilst the other Refused Victuals, the one Excremented whilst the other was hard Bound or Constipated &c, it Lived two Yeares and 20 Days, see Mr. M. Milsons Voyages in Germany and Italy Tome 2. Letter 31. Page 342. Dated from Florence the 23d of May 1688.[109]

Behavioural differences were generally given preference over anatomy in determining individuality, even if major organs such as the heart were shared, as it was in Riolan's case. A double monster born at Heidelberg was baptised John and Jerome and lived a day and a half. At autopsy, 'they found in the belly but one hart', but in spite of this there was no revision of the opinion formed of the children when living: they were two individuals.[110] The merchant who went with his friends to see the double child in Ostend wrote: 'That they are distinct in life, soul and brains appear plainly from the actions which they have.'[111] The autopsy also contributed to speculations on the cause of double monsters. In 1544 in Milan a 'well formed' and 'corpulent' double monster died during a prolonged labour; the surgeon Gabriel Cuneus made 'an anatomy' and found two uteri, two intestinal tracts except for a shared rectum, two livers and one heart, 'the which moveth us to think... that nature would have created two, saving that by some defecte she imperfected the whole.'[112]

The social significance of the autopsy is important for the evaluation of attitudes to monstrous births. If autopsies were regarded as degrading – literally 'a fate worse than death'[113]– then this would suggest that monstrous births were perhaps accorded a lower status than were morphologically normal infants, which rarely seem to have undergone postmortem examination. The autopsy was a continuation of the relationship of the physician with his patient and their family, and objections were respected; an autopsy on a 12-year-old child who died from tuberculosis, reported in the first volume of *Miscellanea Curiosa*, was abandoned when a female relative changed her mind and withheld consent. The author remarked that people:

'very rarely allow them [autopsies] unless special persuasion has been used,'[114] and in a commentary on the report, Sachs, the editor, observed that difficulty in procuring cadavers for autopsy:

...is a common evil in Germany, as is the complaint that some are too frequently overscrupulous with regard to the dead... Let it not be thought that opening the body defiles the honour of burial, since by skilful section... the members are shown which in good persons were organs of the Holy Spirit, and the mighty works of God are shown respect.[115]

In the same year, another contributor to *Miscellanea Curiosa* wrote of a monstrous birth: 'I desired to have the skeleton, but the laws of that land required me to have the goodwill of the parents of the child; nor did they permit a meticulous examination. I hope this brief account satisfies your curiosity...',[116] while seventeen years later another examined a monster, but 'time was short' and 'the girl's father witheld his consent; in fact neither pleading nor the offer of money could induce him to give it in order to obtain the little body for the anatomist's knife'.[117] The following year, the parents of a monster that had been examined by a physician 'were very concerned and snatched the body away to the grave immediately' in order to prevent an autopsy.[118]

Reactions to the post mortem examination of the body were dependent upon its context and on the exact nature of the procedure. Katherine Park has explored the paradoxical similarities between the humiliating public dissection of the bodies of criminals and dissection of the bodies of the saints. One difference is that anatomical dissection was seen as destructive, whereas the ultimate aim of dissection of the saintly body was its preservation (albeit piecemeal in reliquaries across Europe). It was the public and destructive nature of anatomy, argues Park, which constituted its punitive element.[119] If there was a dichotomy between destructive and preservatory treatment of the body (as there is at present: many people desire to be embalmed, some consent to an autopsy, very few accept anatomical dissection) the dissection of monstrous births belongs, I suggest, in the latter group. It was intended not to destroy the body but to display its structure in a way that could be preserved by description, illustration or embalming. The father of a double monster joined at the head 'took the child's two hearts and kept them as a souvenir.'[120]

Embalming monsters prolonged their life as objects for exhibition, and once embalmed the body of a monstrous birth became, like the saintly body, not only incorruptible, but also capable of being possessed and sold.[121] In 1670 the physician Jacomo Grandi attempted to purchase a double monster, but was unable to afford the price asked, so instead he was given the specimen to embalm and had to be content with eviscerating it through an abdominal incision as part of the embalming process:

> I could not dissect them as I would, because they were deliver'd to me to embalm, and the indigent Father of them, who look'd for gain, would not let me have them but for a great Sum of money. Wherefore, not to spoil them for the purpose design'd, having only open'd them upwards from the Navel, which was common to them both, I took out the Intestins, the Stomack, the Heart, the Lungs.[122]

Although this was not a complete autopsy, he was still able to obtain some of the information about their anatomy that an autopsy would have provided. They had a single heart: 'though greater and rounder than ordinary; so that Nature seemed to have united the Matter of two into one.' The embalmed specimen was then returned to the father, presumably for exhibition. Grandi successfully acquired the body of a second child with pelvic malformations, which he dissected 'in the presence of many Noblemen and Physitians at my house'. This social exclusivity – less of a public dissection than a private view – may have made agreeing to the autopsy more acceptable (and less reminiscent of public dissections of criminals) to the next-of-kin.

Infanticide

In ancient Greece and Rome, monstrous births were normally killed.[123] This can be seen partly as a eugenic approach (though many would never have reached reproductive age anyway) to prevent the birth of further monsters, but also as a response to the fear that monstrous births were indications of a breakdown in the cosmic order.[124] In Greece, deformed children were killed by exposure, whereas in Rome they were drowned in the Tiber (or burned first and their ashes scattered there), and the Sabines drowned children of doubtful sex: 'the halfe males were abominable, and were commanded forthwith to be carried by rafte into the sea',[125] drowning being perhaps intended to cleanse the taboo of a monstrous birth by symbolically carrying away pollution and preventing re-birth.[126] Early modern authors referred to these practices with disapproval:

> The auncient *Romains* following the ordinance of *Romulus*, used to cast suche monsters into *Tyber*, burning their bodies and blowing away the cinders: wherein the Emperor *Mauritius* (although he were a Christian) followed in this the lawes of the Auncients, who forthwith upon the sighte of any monstrous childe, caused it not only to be killed, but kissed the knife wherewith he committed the butchery.[127]

No early modern writer endorsed infanticide for monstrous births but given the secrecy in which it would necessarily have taken place it may be impossible to discover its true incidence. Infanticide was a capital crime for all involved and in a case from England in 1568 where a mother, midwife and parson had conspired in killing a child, all were condemned although only one had performed the murder.[128] Although there were many people present at confinements, there may have been no actual eyewitnesses to the birth (see above, 141). The concept of birth rituals and their female exclusivity[129] may have been overstated but there were undoubtedly times, such as the case of Agnes Bowker, where those present concealed the truth of what really went on. The indication from legal records is that infanticide was a relatively rare event. At Canterbury in the 1470s only four cases were heard over ten years, two of which were overlayings and probably accidental.[130] In Nuremberg, there were eighty-seven executions for infanticide in 250 years and in Geneva twenty-five in a hundred years,[131] while in Amsterdam, only twenty-four accusations of infanticide were brought before the magistrates between 1680 and 1811.[132] Scotland had the highest figure, and even there only thirty-four women were investigated for infanticide between 1661 and 1700, less than one a year.[133]

Niccoli described two documented examples of infanticides of monstrous births in the sixteenth century: one in Florence in 1506, which 'by order of the Signoria was not fed and died', and another in Venice in 1513, who was 'let die'.[134] These cases do not seem to have resulted in prosecutions and a legal (and perhaps a moral) distinction may have been drawn, at least in practice, between infanticide and 'letting die'. On the basis of these two examples, Niccoli claims that 'these were patterns of behaviour for which there is long-standing testimony and which continued into the eighteenth century and probably longer.' Nevertheless, the humane treatment of other monstrous births shows that such patterns of behaviour were not societal norms. Broadsides show that, even when the parents' personal sin was said to be an initiating factor in the deformity, the child was not seen as sharing their guilt, but as an innocent victim, born, like the man born blind in the gospel, to show the power of God, and there is no suggestion that they were treated any less well than their normal contemporaries. In *A Most Straunge, and True Discourse...*[135] a monstrous child was initially supposed to have been stillborn, but when it showed signs of life the midwives treated it 'as a childe ought to be used',[136] and a child born at Much Horkesley in 1562 was drop fed until mature enough to suckle; despite his deformities he was described as 'well favoured, and of good and chearful face', and the final piece of information in the ballad is that at the time of writing he was doing well.[137]

The treatment of monstrous births in the early modern period was not dictated by humanitarian considerations; monsters were valued as signs and curiosities, and they were also of potential financial value. Of course being valued as an emblem of the power of the creator is not the same as being valued as an individual, but neither is it the same as being marginalised, feared or ridiculed. It is impossible to know if infanticide was performed covertly, but we can say that there was more concern over parents faking monstrous births (an equally serious crime) than concealing them. It is salutary to remember that in most European counties, the types of malformations described in this book (usually now diagnosed antenatally) are regarded as grounds for termination of pregnancy, and conjoined twins may be separated, against the wishes of their parents, even if the death of one twin is a certain result. The reasons for society's change of attitude are potentially very complex, but the growth during the seventeenth century of the concept of the monster as a mistake may have been a factor in relegating the monstrous to a peripheral and less-valued role.

Afterlife

For some monstrous births, death was not the end of their exposure to the public gaze. Embalming could prolong the time for which they could be shown to the public, usually by their parents, until, perhaps, they disintegrated through repeated handling. In the mediaeval period, embalming had been largely confined to the clergy (their embalmed and uncorrupted bodies, when exhumed, gave off the odour of sanctity) but by the sixteenth century the practice had spread to high-status lay people, to enable their burial inside churches, formerly a clerical preserve. By the end of the seventeenth century an interest in Egyptian antiquity provided a further boost for embalming; it was an expensive process (a surprising number of physicians, surgeons and assistants was required properly to embalm one body in the classical fashion), and one way in which medical practitioners could continue to be paid for their services even after their patient's death. Consequently, physicians and surgeons were protective of their right to embalm and tried to prevent those without medical training, such as wax-chandlers (who supplied the necessary wax) and, by the end of the seventeenth century, undertakers, from doing the embalming themselves. By the late-seventeenth century bodies were being preserved for some time before burial, for example if family members away from home wished to return for a final viewing, and embalming was beginning to be used for preserving medically interesting material: anatomical specimens and monstrous births could take their place in the then fashionable cabinets of curiosities, where they were advertisements for the skill of the embalmer.

Most seventeenth-century cabinets of curiosities displayed a preserved foetus or two; Ole Worm had one,[138] and Paul Hermann several (so far as I am aware, there is no surviving example of an *abnormal* foetus from before the eighteenth century).[139] A foetal specimen in the *Kunstkammer* of Frederick III of Denmark was alleged to be one of Countess Margaret's 365 children (the other 364 seem to have disappeared).[140] These collections were the personal property of noblemen or scholars but they were anything but private, and Aldrovandi boasted that 'an infinite number of gentlemen' had visited his cabinet of curiosities.[141] Before the eighteenth century most objects preserved in cabinets were dried or skeletalised[142] (Paré's collection was preserved in this way). Humidity was the enemy of preservation and moist humours were:

> ...excrementations and also alimentations, by which the least defect of Heat is easily turned into putrefaction... whence it is that foul Bodies, Trees cut down at Full Moon, being full of their sap, and Fruits gather'd before their maturity, very easily corrupt.... Wherefore they who would embalm bodies well, must make use of several means.... Humidity must be absum'd by Hot Drugs, amongst which, Wormwood and Scordium hold the first place [along with] Balsames Cold, Dry and penetrating, which may preserve the figure, colour, and consistence in the dead body.[143]

In 1677, Robert Boyle published the results of experiments on the preservation of dog and chick embryos in spirits.[144] These 'wet' specimens were still something of a novelty in 1681: 'I also saw in the cabinet of curiosities [of Vescher in Amsterdam] all sorts of embryos, one of which I saw inside the womb, because of its transparency on account of the property of the water in which it was preserved.'[145]

Paul Hermann's collection is of particular interest because the values given to the specimens when it was sold have been recorded.[146] Although the figures written next to many of the specimens in the index catalogue[147] are not the prices of individual lots but rather notes made as a means of reckoning up the total price, they do give us some insight into the high monetary value (in 1711) of preserved human material such as:

The skeleton of a foetus	£1 2s
The skeleton of a five month foetus	£7 10s
Two small human foetuses	£1 8s
An infant of Egyptian appearance, preserved in balsam, male	£3 18s

One motive for collecting was to increase one's intellectual and social prestige, a point well made by Findlen: '[t]hrough the possession of objects, one physically acquired knowledge, and through their display, one symbolically acquired the honor and reputation that all men of learning cultivated.'[148] Another reason to collect (and to classify) was to impose organization, and collecting 'was one way of maintaining some degree of control over the natural world and taking its measure'.[149] Collecting and classifying were related activities; early collections were not displayed haphazardly but were ordered, often according to aesthetic criteria.[150] The contents of the cabinet of Ole Worm, for example, were arranged in groups; minerals in one part, plants in another, and so on. Phrases such as 'A World of Wonders in one closet shut'[151] suggest a desire to organize nature on a human scale. Catherine the Great criticised one of the curators of the museum set up by her grandfather-in-law, Peter the Great, for attempting just that: 'I often quarrelled with him about his wish to enclose Nature in a cabinet – even a huge palace could not hold her.'[152]

Foetal material differed in one key respect from most of the curiosities, animal and mineral, that found their way into collections: it was potentially unique, and it was ephemeral. Whereas animals, plants and minerals have a continuous existence in the world, and are brought into collections only for convenience, monstrous births are unpredictable events and will be lost to decay or ill usage if not preserved and protected from damage. Anyone who wants to study human malformations in the flesh and in significant numbers can only do so in a museum. The creators of museums can be seen – like the authors of learned journals – as adding to the store of knowledge, taking their cue from merchants who accumulated and preserved goods in anticipation of future demand.[153] The collection and preservation of specimens made them available for examination by future generations of students and those collections that have survived are still of use today, an example being the recent re-cataloguing and re-examination by Dutch pathologists of eighteenth- and nineteenth-century specimens in the Museum Vrolik.[154]

Of course, the seventeenth century cabinet was not created as a resource for future teratologists; although its contents became a source for classification it was not intended as such. As Findlen writes: 'While we perceive the museum of natural history to be alternately a research laboratory or a place of public education, they understood it to be a repository of the collective imagination of their society.'[155] A museum was 'the place where the Muses dwell',[156] or a place, as Jean-Baptiste Lamark (1744–1829) later dismissively wrote, 'for amusement'.[157] Although museums were highly ordered places, their contents were not classified in the same way that monsters were in books. Like the public anatomy hall at Leiden they were: 'so set in order that every thing may easily be found in their places', yet exhibits were eclectically juxtaposed. In the entrance hall the visitor passed, in sequence: 'A Crocodile', 'A Norway house', 'The skin of an Animal from Brasil', 'The Snout of an unknown Fish' and 'Some Indian Darts'.[158] The museum translated natural philosophy from a 'bookish' to a 'tactile, theatrical' culture;[159] to use a word beloved of modern educators, it made knowledge 'accessible'.

The collector who most obviously combined 'anatomical' and 'aesthetic' interpretations of human material was Frederik Ruysch (or Ruijsch, 1638–1731), *praelector* of anatomy and surgery of the Guild of Surgeons in Amsterdam and one of the most dedicated collectors of anatomical specimens in Holland. As chief of the midwives' guild, and their anatomical lecturer, Ruysch was well placed to have access to stillbirths, and he assembled an impressive collection both of malformed and normal foetal material.[160] By 1710, his museum contained more than 1,300 (mostly 'wet') anatomical specimens; the first catalogue was published in 1691, and the specimens were described in detail in a series of quartos published between 1701 and 1715. These list such exhibits as a phial containing a human foetus (item 4), a 'human foetus, in its natural colours, four months after conception' (item 7), and 'conserved in a phial of liquor, the arm of a human foetus representing the living specimen, in its hand a child's heart, the arteries of which have been carefully filled' (item 14). In 1717 Ruysch sold his entire collection to Peter the Great (it was not uncommon for natural philosophers to assemble a collection with the intention of selling it) and it was shipped to St Petersburg.[161] Peter continued to add to the collection (in the so-called 'monster decree', he ordered all monstrous births to be handed over),[162] his stated purpose being a desire to educate himself and others. In his characteristically idiosyncratic way; Peter, like many rulers whose temporal power was secure, wished to associate his rule with culture and learning, and he retained throughout his life a rather child-like curiosity towards the unusual. On a visit to Libau in 1697, after he had paid a call on the local apothecary, he wrote: 'Here I have seen a great marvel which at home they used to say was a lie: a man here has in his apothecary's shop in a jar of spirits a salamander which I took out and held in my own hands: this is word for word exactly as has been written.' Of his *kunstkammer*, he said simply: 'I want people to look and learn'.[163] The museum had introduced the possibility of direct observation as a new way of establishing credibility: seeing was believing; though sometimes, as with Peter's salamander, seeing and believing could be very different.

Ruysch had more complex motives for collecting. While it was in Holland, his museum associated him with learning, attracted distinguished visitors and demonstrated that his medical knowledge was science-based rather than empirical ('medicine', he wrote, 'is not the origin but rather the

Figure 6.4
One of Ruysch's dried anatomical tableaux showing foetal skeletons grieving (they have handkerchiefs of placental membranes) over disordered human remains. A memento mori to the layman, for the anatomist this scene celebrates the capacity of preserved human material to evade the degradations of time.

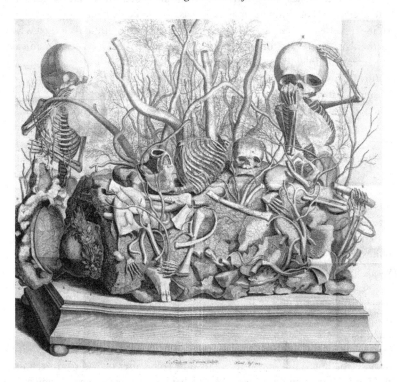

offshoot of experiment'),[164] and when sold it brought income and further publicity. Some of the human foetal material was presented in the form of anatomical tableaux in which skeletons were set in landscapes in which the rocks and vegetation were made from dried adult tissues such as arteries and meninges. These displayed Ruysch's technical skill in the preparation of detailed and durable specimens (not so durable as the wet specimens, since none has survived); several of the skeletons were posed as if playing musical instruments (again made up of body parts) and others held symbols of folly or of the brevity of life (Figure 6.4) as if to contrast the transience of foetal life with the durability and order of the anatomical museum in which the specimens 'represented permanence in the face of the forces of decay'.[165] The *vanitas* theme of these tableaux was common in art of the period, particularly Dutch still life painting, and although it is anachronistic to say that Ruysch's work crossed the boundary between anatomy and art, it is apparent that Ruysch and his audience saw anatomy as a medium for moral instruction as well as for medical learning. Ruysch's foetuses were not presented as passive objects of contemplation or as victims of the anatomist's knife; they looked back at the audience, standing, as had their predecessors in ballads and wonder books, in a landscape and telling the audience their moral message, for which Thomas Bedford's words seem as appropriate as they did for his sermon on a monstrous birth: 'They are shewed that they may... though, peradventure dead, yet speake'.[166]

Notes

1. *Ab Utero ad Tumulum*, the motto of one of Ruysch's dioramas.
2. Augustine, Bishop of Hippo, *The City of God*, book XVI, ch. 8.
3. E. Fenton, *Certaine Secrete Wonders of Nature...* (London: H. Bynneman, 1569), fo. 36v.
4. T. B[edford], *A True and Certain Relation of a Strange Birth...* (London: A. Griffin, 1635), 7.
5. G. Garden, 'Two Monstrous Births in Scotland', *Philosophical Transactions*, xv (1686), 1156; Appendix, 1686b.
6. In one of the better documented cases from France in 1667 both mother and child lived, see La Motte (transl. Thomas Tomkyns), *A General Treatise of Midwifry...* (London: James Waugh, 1746), 435.
7. A. Borde, *The Breviary of Helthe...* (London: W. Middleton, 1547).
8. For the text of the oath see J. Towler and J. Bramall, *Midwives in History and Society* (London: Croom Helm, 1986), 56–7.
9. Anon., *Strange Newes out of Kent...* (London: T.C. for W. Barley, 1609), sig. B.
10. A. Paré (ed. and transl. J.L. Pallister), *On Monsters and Marvels* (Chicago and London: University of Chicago Press, 1982), 11, describes a 'crowd' at the place of confinement.
11. Reproduced in Towler and Bramall, *op. cit.* (note 8), 54.
12. Reproduced in O. Hagelin, *The Byrth of Mankynde...* (Stockholm: Svenska Läkaresällskapet, 1990), 23.
13. A. Wilson, 'The Ceremony of Childbirth and its Interpretation', in V. Fildes (ed.), *Women as Mothers in Pre-Industrial England: Essays in Memory of Dorothy McLaren* (London: Routledge, 1990), 68–107; *Idem, The Making of Man-Midwifery: Childbirth in England 1660–1770* (London: UCL Press, 1995); J. Sanders, 'Midwifery and the New Science in the Seventeenth Century: Language, Print and Theatre', in E. Fudge, R. Gilbert and S. Wiseman (eds), *At the Borders of the Human: Beasts, Bodies and Natural*

Philosophy in the Early Modern Period (Basingstoke: Macmillan, 1999), 74–90.

14. C. James, *Ritual and Ceremony? The Social Context of Early Modern Childbirth* (BSc, University College London, 2003), copy in Wellcome Library, London, WL 2003/JAM.

15. Appendix, 1562a.

16. See J.D., *A Discription of a Monstrous Chylde...* (London: L. Askel for F. Godlyf, 1562).

17. D. Wilson, *Signs and Portents: Monstrous Births from the Middle Ages to the Enlightenment* (London: Routledge, 1993), 19–22.

18. La Motte was born and worked at Valognes, France.

19. La Motte, *op. cit.* (note 6), 249–50.

20. *Ibid.*, 321.

21. P. Boaistuau, *Histoires Prodigieuses...* (Paris: Jean de Bordeaux, 1571), fo. 124v.

22. S. Batman, *The Doome Warning All Men to the Judgement...* (London: R. Nubery, 1581), 373 [374].

23. Unbaptised infants such as stillbirths are excluded from these figures; see C.M. Cipolla, *Before the Industrial Revolution: European Society and Economy 1000–1700* (London: Routledge, 1993), 285.

24. Two well-known passages from the *Malleus Maleficarum,* in which midwives were alleged to have misused their position to murder children, mark the beginning of the myth of the witch-midwife: H. Kramer and J. Sprenger (ed. and transl. M. Summers), *Malleus Maleficarum* (London: J. Rodker, 1928), 140–1, 269. Midwives continued to feature in cheap literature as the perpetrators of child-murder, for example, Anon. *The Cruel Midwife...* (London: R. Wier, 1693). Recent studies have found no connection between witchcraft and midwifery in early modern witch trials: D. Harley, 'Historians as Demonologists: The Myth of the Midwife-Witch', *Social History of Medicine,* iii (1990), 1–26.

25. From an oath taken in England in 1649, reproduced in Towler and Bramall, *op. cit.* (note 8), 59.

26. J. Gélis, *History of Childbirth: Fertility, Pregnancy and Birth in Early Modern Europe* (Polity Press: Oxford, 1991), 217.

27. See R.M. Warnicke, *The Rise and Fall of Ann Boleyn* (Cambridge: Cambridge University Press, 1989), 202–3, 246. The evidence that Ann gave birth to a monster is not compelling, resting as it does largely on the assertion of a hostile early biographer, Nicholas Sander, that she delivered a 'shapeless mass', but the claim points to a link between sexual immorality and monstrous births.

28. T. Bridoul, *The School of the Eucharist* (London: R. Taylor, 1687), 17.

29. See Sanders, *op. cit.* (note 13), 82–6.

30. Appendix, 1514c.

31. Men with serious physical deformities were debarred from the priesthood, not due to survival of Judaic laws on physical perfection of the priesthood, as is sometimes supposed, but for the practical reason that they would have been unable to celebrate mass.

32. Anabaptists did not intentionally repeat baptism but their denial of the validity of infant baptism caused them to do so. The Anabaptist fanatics who preached the kingdom of heaven on Earth in Saxony, Westphalia and The Netherlands had been savagely and effectively suppressed by 1535, but opposition to infant baptism lived on in many Protestant groups.

33. Le Prieur de Lugeris, 'Extrait d'une Lettre de Monsieur le Prieur de Lugeris en Champagne, Sur un Enfantemant Arrivé au Mois de Mai Dernier', *Journal des Savans* (1690), 53–4.

34. The rubric from the *Rituale Romanum* stated: *In monstris vero baptizandis, si casus eveniat, magna cautio adhibenda est: de quo si opus fuerit Ordinarius loci, vel alii periti consulantur, nisi mortis periculum immineat. Monstrum, quod humanam speciam non prae se ferat, baptizari non debet: de quo, si dubium fuerit, baptizetur sub hac conditione: 'Si tu es homo, ego te baptizo...,* [With regard to monsters, they should certainly be baptized: if this misfortune comes about, great caution is to be employed; and so it should be done by the Ordinary of the diocese, or another experienced person should be consulted, unless there is immanent danger of death. But if the monster itself is not considered to be human, it ought not to be baptized, or, if there is doubt, baptised under this condition: 'If thou art a Man, I baptise thee...']; see N. Remy, *Demonolatry* (Secaucus: University Books, 1974), 26.

35. H. Morley, *Memoirs of Bartholomew Fair* (London: Chapman and Hall, 1892), 246.

36. See also P. Semonin, 'Monsters in the Marketplace: The Exhibition of Human Oddities in Early Modern England', in R.G. Thomson (ed.), *Freakery: Cultural Spectacles of the Extraordinary Body* (New York: New York University Press, 1996), 69–81. In 1665 some 750,000 people lived in the London area: see R.D. Altick, *The Shows of London* (Cambridge, MA: Belknap Press, 1978), 34.

37. Paré, *op. cit.* (note 10), 9.

38. H. Burgkmair the Elder, *Disz Künd ist Geboren Worden zu Tettnang* (Munich, 1516), reproduced in L. Daston and K. Park, *Wonders and the Order of Nature, 1150–1750* (New York: Zone Books, 1998), 186.

39. Anon., *The True Picture of a Female Monster Born Near Salisbury* (1644), reprinted in H.E. Rollins (ed.), *The Pack of Autolycus...* (Cambridge: Harvard University Press, 1927), 140.

40. Anon., *Natures Wonder?...*, reprinted in Rollins, *Ibid.*, 141; Appendix, 1664b.

41. Anon., *A True Description of a Childe with Ruffes...*, reprinted in Philobiblon Society (eds), *Ancient Ballads & Broadsides...* (London: Whittingham and Wilkins, 1867), 360; Appendix, 1566b.

42. Currently in the Wallace collection, London, catalogue number C13. They are described in the catalogue as 'two small naked girls embracing': see A.V.B. Norman, *Wallace Collection Catalogue of Ceramics 1: Pottery, Maiolica, Faience, Stoneware* (London: Trustees of the Wallace Collection, 1976), 57–8. I am very grateful to the curator, Mrs Suzanne Higgott, for her helpful discussion of this object.

43. Semonin, *op. cit.* (note 36), 75–80; K. Park and L. Daston, 'Unnatural Conceptions: The Study of Monsters in Sixteenth and Seventeenth-Century England and France', *Past & Present*, xcii (1981), 20–54: 34. See also Morley, *op. cit.* (note 35), 317–32.

44. Anon., *A Wonder Woorth the Reading...* (London: 1617), sig. A3r.

45. From a collection of broadsides in the British Library, N.TAB. 2026/25.

46. *Ibid.*

47. Later a common practice with dwarfs such as the 'Sicilian fairy', see J. Bondeson, *A Cabinet of Medical Curiosities* (London: I.B. Tauris, 1997), 186–215.

48. Appendix, 1680b.

49. Rollins, *op. cit.* (note 39), 140–5, 241: 'It was alive 24 hours, and cried and did as all hopefull children do; but, being showed too much to people, was killed.' This was the first monstrous birth to be reported in a learned journal: Anon., 'Extrait d'une Lettre Escrite d'Oxfort, le 12 Novembre 1664', *Journal des Savans*, i (1665), 11–12; Appendix, 1664b.

50. D. Cressy, *Travesties and Transgressions in Tudor and Stuart England: Tales of discord and dissension* (Oxford: Oxford University Press, 2000), 46.

51. Appendix, 1682.

52. J. Bulwer, *Anthropometamorphosis...* (London: W. Hunt, 1653), 302; Appendix, 1654.

53. C.J.S. Thompson, *The Mystery and Lore of Monsters* (London: Williams and Norgate Ltd., 1930), 42.

54. See Lycosthenes' case in Bavaria; Appendix, 1538b.

55. Cressy, *op. cit.* (note 50), 46.

56. F. Bouchard, 'Infante Monstroso Lugduni in Viam Publicam Die V Martii A. MDCLXXI Exposito', *Miscellanea Curiosa*, series 1, iii (1672), 14–16.

57. H.L. Collmann (ed.), *Ballads & Broadsides Chiefly of the Elizabethan Period...* (Oxford: Oxford University Press, 1912), 113; Appendix, 1565a.

58. Anon., *The Most Strange and Wovnderfvll Apperation of Blood in a Poole at*

Garraton... (London: I.H., 1645).

59. Appendix, 1624.
60. Quoted in L. Daston and K. Park, *Wonders and the Order of Nature, 1150–1750* (New York: Zone Books, 1998), 191, their translation; Appendix, 1550a.
61. M. de Montaigne (transl. J. Florio), *The Essays* (London: M. Bradwood, 1613).
62. J. Evelyn (ed. G. de la Bédoyère), *The Diary of John Evelyn* (Woodbridge: Boydell, 1995), 114–15.
63. Lucca Landucci, quoted by Daston and Park, *op. cit.* (note 61), 190; their translation.
64. Appendix, 1617a.
65. Who described him in his *Historiarum Anatomicarum Rariorum* (Amsterdam: J. Henrici, 1654). Wilson, *op. cit.* (note 17), 88, identified Dubé's account of 1650 as a reference to the Colloredo twins.
66. A similar plot was used in the film *Chained for Life* (dir. H. Fraser, 1951), which featured the conjoined twin sisters Daisy and Violet Hilton.
67. Rollins, *op. cit.* (note 39), 8.
68. J. Bondeson, *The Two-Headed Boy, and Other Medical Marvels* (Ithaca: Cornell University Press, 2000).
69. From the Norwich Mayors' Court Books, 21 December 1639, quoted in J.T. Murray, *English Dramatic Companies, 1558–1642* (New York: Russell and Russell, 1963), II, 359.
70. Rollins, *op. cit.* (note 39), 9; see also Wilson, *op. cit.* (note 17), 180; Bondeson, *op. cit.* (note 68).
71. Parker, *Two Inseperable Brothers*, reprinted in Rollins, *op. cit.* (note 39), 13.
72. Anon., *A Certaine Relation of the Hog-faced Gentlewoman* (London: J.O., 1640), sig. A4.
73. Appendix, 1530b.
74. Appendix, 1529a.
75. Du Plessis, *A Short History of Human Prodigious & Monstrous Births...* (1730), BL MS Sloane 5246, 33–4, 61.
76. For example, Semonin, *op. cit.* (note 36), 78–80: 'They [monsters] were characters of comic horror intimately connected to an ancient tradition of folk humour... The monsters in the marketplace of early modern England embodied elements of an ancient comic tradition.' See also J. Teelucksingh's review of J. Bondeson's *The Two-headed Boy, and Other Medical Marvels* in *Social History of Medicine*, xv (2002), 166–7.
77. Appendix, *c.*1580.
78. Appendix, 1528.

79. Du Plessis, *op. cit.* (note 75), 31–2, 58. His manuscripts do not suggest that he had an expert knowledge of these languages.

80. J. Grandi, 'An Extract of an Italian Letter...', *Philosophical Transactions*, v (1670), 1188–9; Appendix, *c.*1670a.

81. See Bedford, *op. cit.* (note 4), 13.

82. See Anon., *op. cit.* (note 9), sig. Biii.

83. Seneca (transl. M. Winterbottom), *Controversiae* (Cambridge: Loeb Classical Library, 1974), 423.

84. Paré, *op. cit.* (note 10), 74–84.

85. Fenton, *op. cit.* (note 3), fo. 14[16]r.

86. Bulwer, *op. cit.* (note 52). The technique described would be likely to have led to rapid death of the child from infection.

87. C. Krahe, 'The Description of a Monstrous Child, Born Friday the 29th of February 1684 at a Village Called Heisagger, Distant About 4 English Miles from Hattersleben, a Town in South-Jutland, under the King of Denmark's Dominion', *Philosophical Transactions*, xiv (1684), 599–600; Appendix, 1684a.

88. Anon., *op. cit.* (note 40).

89. Harvey also dissected his own father and sister; see W. Harvey, *Lectures on the Whole of Anatomy* (Berkeley: University of California Press, 1961), 13.

90. R.K. Spiro, 'A Backward Glance at the Study of Postmortem Anatomy', *International Surgery*, lvi (1971), 27–40.

91. H.M. Sinclair and A.H.T. Robb-Smith, *A Short History of Anatomical Teaching in Oxford* (Oxford: Oxford University Press, 1950), 10.

92. Though perhaps not entirely dispelled. Examples of the encouragement of anatomy by the Catholic Church are many: see, for example, A. Carlino, *Books of the Body: Anatomical Ritual and Renaissance Learning* (Chicago: University of Chicago Press, 1999), 223, and G.M. Weisz, 'The Papal Contribution to the Development of Modern Medicine', *The Australian and New Zealand Journal of Surgery*, lxvii (1997), 472–5.

93. The criminal was to be drowned so the body was uninjured; see T. Puschmann (ed. and transl. E.H. Hare), *A History of Medical Education From the Most Remote to the Most Recent Times* (London: H.K. Lewis, 1891), 247.

94. R. Richardson, *Death, Dissection and the Destitute* (London: Routledge and Kegan Paul, 1987), 32.

95. Cadavers came from hospitals as well as scaffolds, and obliging judges chose the date and mode of executions to suit his requirements. When he wished to dissect a virgin, Pope Cosimo I (1519–74) made available the body of a nun: Puschmann, *op. cit.* (note 93), 327–8.

96. R. French, 'The Anatomical Tradition', in R. Porter and W.F. Bynum (eds), *Companion Encyclopedia of the History of Medicine* (London: Routledge,

1993), 81–101.

97. Puschmann, *op. cit.* (note 93), 327.

98. Sinclair and Robb-Smith, *op. cit.* (note 91), 10.

99. A well-known example is Jan van Neck's *The Anatomy Lesson of Dr Frederik Ruysch.*

100. Usual practice if it was not known whether a person had been previously baptised.

101. F.A. Jimenez, 'The First Autopsy in the New World', *Bulletin of the New York Academy of Medicine,* liv (1978), 618–19.

102. Quoted from A. Peña Chavarría and P.G. Shipley, 'The Siamese Twins of Española (The First Known Post-Mortem Examination in the New World)', *Annals of Medical History,* vi (1924), 297–302, their translation. The desire to establish whether the twins had a single soul may reflect a response to the statements of the doctrine of the immortality of the soul, which the fifth Lateran Council had pronounced a dogma of the Church in 1512.

103. Appendix, 1670a. An exception is Appendix, 1552a.

104. *Op. cit.* (note 3), fo. 141r

105. *Una animum tamen erat:* J. Scultetus, 'De Duobus Monstris', *Miscellanea Curiosa,* series 1, iii (1672), 346–51.

106. Paré, *op. cit.* (note 10), 14: Appendix, 1546b.

107. I. Blickstein, 'The Conjoined Twins of Löwen', *Twin Research,* iii (2000), pp. 185–8.

108. J. Riolan, *De Monstro Nato Lutetiae Anno Domini 1605* (Paris: Olivarum Varennaeum, 1605).

109. Du Plessis, *op. cit.* (note 75), 38–9.

110. Batman, *op. cit.* (note 22), 338; Appendix, 1544a.

111. From an anonymous pamphlet, c.1682, BL N.TAB.2026/23, 3; Appendix, 1682.

112. C. Schott, *Physica Curiosa...* (Würtzburg: J. Hertz for J.A. Endter and Wolff, 1662), I, 659.

113. Richardson, *op. cit.* (note 94), 32.

114. G. Segerus, 'De Phthisici Pueri Anatome', *Miscellania Curiosa,* series 1, i (1670), 53–6, quoted in S. Jarcho, 'Problems of the Autopsy in 1670 A.D.', *Bulletin of the New York Academy of Medicine,* xlvii (1971), 792–6, his translation.

115. *Ibid.*

116. *Bina cernebantur corda:* C Rayger, 'De Anatomia Monstri Bicipitis', *Miscellanea Curiosa,* series 1, i (1670), 21–3.

117. *[S]ed temporis brevitas & voluntas monstrosae puellae Patris obstabant, hic enim nec precibus nec nummis a philiatris oblatis se permoveri patiebatur, ut corpusculum defunctae cultro Anatomico subjici permitteret...*: J.M. Hoffmann,

'De Foetu Monstroso', *Miscellanea Curiosa*, series 2, vi (1687), 333–6.

118. *Parentes desiderio nostro pertinacissime sese opponebant, & cadaver ad sepulturam absque mora abripiebant:* J.M. Hoffmann, 'Foetu Monstroso ex Imaginatione Matris', *Miscellanea Curiosa*, series 2, viii (1689), 483–5.

119. K. Park, 'The Criminal and the Saintly Body: Autopsy and Dissection in Renaissance Italy', *Renaissance Quarterly*, xlvii (1994), 1–33.

120. *Ibid.*; Appendix, 1547a.

121. Relics are, of course, never actually sold, and any money paid is considered to cover only the cost of the reliquary.

122. Grandi, *op. cit.* (note 80).

123. The Roman Laws of the Twelve Tables stated: 'A father shall immediately put to death a son recently born, who is a monster, or has a form different from that of the human race': quoted in J.B. Friedman, *The Monstrous Races in Mediaeval Art and Thought* (Cambridge, MA: Harvard University Press, 1981), 179.

124. *Ibid.*, 179.

125. This occurred around 188 BC; see Batman, *op. cit.* (note 22), 76.

126. Gélis, *op. cit.* (note 26), 262.

127. Fenton, *op. cit.* (note 3), 124r.

128. P.C. Hoffer and N.E.H. Hull, *Murdering Mothers: Infanticide in England and New England 1558–1803* (New York: New York University Press, 1981), 7.

129. L. Gowing, 'Secret Births and Infanticide in Seventeenth-Century England', *Past & Present*, clvi (1997), 87–115.

130. Hoffer and Hull, *op. cit.* (note 128), 3–5.

131. *Ibid.*, 5–6.

132. S. Faber, 'Kindermoord in het Bijzonder in de Achttiende Eeuw te Amsterdam', *Bijdragen en Mededelingen Betreffende de Geshciedenis der Nederlanden*, lxxiii (1978), 224–40.

133. D.A. Symonds, *Weep Not for Me: Women, Ballads, and Infanticide in Early Modern Scotland* (University Park: Pennsylvania State University Press, 1997), 236–7.

134. O. Niccoli (transl. L.G. Cochrane), *Prophecy and People in Renaissance Italy* (Princeton: Princeton University Press, 1990), 33.

135. R.J., *A Most Strange and True Discourse...* (London, 1600).

136. Appendix, 1599b.

137. Appendix, 1562c.

138. O. Worm, (1655) *Museum Wormianum Seu Historia Rerum Rariorum...* (Amsterdam: L. and D. Elzevir, 1655), 343.

139. Though there are some fine 'wet' specimens of normal foetal material from Ruysch's collection, beautifully illustrated in R.W. Purcell and S.J. Gould. *Finders, Keepers: Eight Collectors* (London: Pimlico, 1993), 24–31.

140. See J. Bondeson and A. Molenkamp, 'The Countess Margaret of Henneberg and Her 365 Children', *Journal of the Royal Society of Medicine*, lxxxix (1996), 711–16.

141. P. Findlen, *Possessing Nature: Museums, Collecting, and Scientific Culture in Early Modern Italy* (Berkeley: University of California Press, 1994), 17. In 1595 Aldrovandi's museum contained 11,000 animals, fruits and minerals and 7,000 plants; see G. Olmi, 'Science-Honour-Metaphor: Italian Cabinets of the Sixteenth and Seventeenth Centuries', in O. Impey and A. Macgregor (eds), *The Origins of Museums...* (Oxford: Clarendon Press, 1985), 5–16.

142. See H.J. Cook, 'Time's Bodies: Crafting the Preparation and Preservation of Naturalia', in P. Findlen and P. Smith (eds), *Merchants and Marvels* (London: Routledge, 2001), 223–47.

143. T. Renaudot (ed. and transl. G. Havers) *A General Collection of Discourses of the Virtuosi of France...* (London: T. Dring and J. Starkey, 1664), 185.

144. *Philosophical Transactions*, xii (1677), 199.

145. *J'ay veu encore dans le Cabinet de ce mesme curieux toutes sortes d'Embrions, & un entre autres qui se voit dans la matrice à cause de la transparence qu'elle a par le moyen de l'eau dans laquelle ce curieux la conserve: Hansen*, [Untitled letter from Oxford] *Journal des Savans* (1681), 46–7: 47.

146. P. Hermann, *Catologus Musei Indici...* (Leiden: J. du Virie, 1711). Hermann (1646–95) was born in Halle, the son of Johann Hermann, a well-known organist. He was to make one of the earliest scientific collections of plant specimens from Ceylon, where he was medical officer to the Dutch East India Company between 1672 and 1677. After his return to Europe, Hermann took up the Chair of Botany at the University of Leiden in 1679 and spent the rest of his life there. In 1711 his entire collection was sold to a Mr James Petiver and transported to London.

147. BL 1004.c.4.

148. Findlen, *op. cit.* (note 141), 3.

149. *Ibid.*, 4.

150. Olmi, *op. cit.* (note 141).

151. Quoted in Findlen, *op. cit.* (note 141), 17.

152. Purcell and Gould, *op. cit.* (note 139).

153. Cook, *op. cit.* (note 142).

154. See the series of papers by R.-J. Oostra *et al.*, *American Journal of Medical Genetics*, lxxvii (1998), 100–15, 116–34; lxxx (1998), 46–59, 60–73, 74–89.

155. Findlen, *op. cit.* (note 141), 9.

156. Quoted in Findlen, *op. cit.* (note 141), 48.

157. *Ibid.*, 398.

158. F. Schuyl, *A Catalogue of All the Chiefest Rarities in the Publick Anatomie-Hall, of the University of Leyden* (Leyden: D. vander Boxe, 1723), 3.

159. Findlen, *op. cit.* (note 141), 9.

160. F. Ruysch, *Catalogus Musaei Ruyschiani...* (Amsterdam: J. Waesberg, 1731). His *Observationem Anatomico-Chirurgicorum Centuria* (Amsterdam: H. and T. Boom, 1691) included monstrous births.

161. Some cabinets of curiosities were made with a view to being sold; see P. Findlen, 'Inventing Nature: Commerce, Art and Science in the Early Modern Cabinet of Curiosities', in P. Findlen and P. Smith (eds), *Merchants and Marvels* (London: Routledge, 2001), 223–47. It is estimated that 47% of Ruysch's collection remains in St Petersburg, mostly in the Imperial Academy of Science: B. Baljet and R.-J. Oostra, 'Historical Aspects of the Study of Malformations in The Netherlands', *American Journal of Medical Genetics*, lxxvii (1998), 91–9; some has been redisplayed in the Museum Vrolik, currently located in the Academic Medical Centre at the University of Amsterdam.

162. H.E. Muller-Dietz, 'Anatomische Praparate in der Petersburg "Kunstkammer"', *Zentralblatt fur Allgemeine Pathologie und Pathologische Anatomie*, cxxxv (1989), 757–67. A similar legal requirement to collect together human malformations existed in Prussia in the eighteenth and nineteenth centuries: P. Krietsch, 'Zur Geschichte des Pathologischen Museums der Charite Berlin, 2, Mitteilung: Die Sammlung von Missbildungspraparaten ("Monstra")', *Zentralblatt fur Allgemeine Pathologie und Pathologische Anatomie*, cxxxii (1986), 335–47.

163. O. Neverov, '"His Majesty's Cabinet" and Peter I's *Kunstkammer*', in O. Impey and A. Macgregor (eds), *The Origins of Museums: The Cabinet of Curiosities in Sixteenth- and Seventeenth-Century Europe* (Oxford: Clarendon Press, 1985), 54–61.

164. *Medicinam non originem tantum, verum etiam incrementum ab Experientia sumpsisse...*

165. Cook, *op. cit.* (note 142), 241.

166. Bedford, *op. cit.* (note 4), 12.

7

Retrospective Diagnosis

At the turn of the nineteenth century, two American physicians, George Gould (1848–1922) and Walter Pyle (1871–1921), produced a book called *Anomalies and Curiosities of Medicine*. This work, intended as a summary of interesting cases gleaned from the written historical record, is reminiscent of the *Centuria*, assemblages of cases presented by the hundred in book form, that had been popular two centuries earlier. Unusually for a time in which most medical writers emphasised progress, Gould and Pyle presented historical material as though it were evidentially equivalent to the case reports of their contemporaries. Their approach is open to criticism for neglecting to evaluate the comparative worth of historical sources or to see them in context, but it was not uncritical. They relied instead on the internal evidence of the accounts themselves and favoured those that were plausible from a nineteenth-century medical point of view. One of their claims was that early modern accounts of monstrous births were not just a literary genre, but that they were intended as descriptions, and records, of real events, which could be 'classified among some of our known forms of monsters'.[1]

It may be helpful to consider three arguments against the reading of these accounts as records of actual cases: that they were fakes, intended to mislead; that they were 'poetical' accounts without a factual basis; or that, although inspired by actual cases, no attempt was made at anatomical description. We have seen that there were accusations that monstrous births were themselves faked, and the prospect of selling ballads to an audience eager for new monsters might have prompted literary deception. However, there is nothing to suggest that spurious descriptions of monstrous births were ever produced, and while the possibility can never be entirely excluded, circumstantial evidence points towards the writers' intention of accuracy: witnesses were named, exact locations given, the reader was encouraged to see for himself, different accounts of the same case appeared, artists were commissioned to make likenesses, and the monsters were sometimes dissected and often seen by many people. The distinction between actual cases and 'poetical' ones is only slightly more problematic; 'poetical' accounts did not have lists of witnesses, dates and places, they were not dissected, and they were often anatomically implausible. Furthermore, poetical accounts

175

were, I suggest, often indicated as such by the inclusion of improbable detail: we do not believe that a 77-year-old can bear a child and any more than did the reader of 1581 (see Chapter 1, 33). The third objection is the most problematic; if accounts of monstrous births were records of real events, they were not necessarily descriptions in the modern sense. Many were reported as signs and emblems rather than things, and, like the Ravenna monster, their anatomy was less important than their meaning.

In order to use the internal evidence present in accounts of monstrous births to substantiate a claim that they were based on observation, I have used the technique of retrospective diagnosis. That a modern observer with experience of human birth defects can recognise in the great majority of early modern accounts malformations with which he is familiar supports a claim that these descriptions were attempts, and successful ones, to describe the anatomy of actual cases – they are just too close to modern types of birth defects to have been invented. The criterion of 'plausibility' as an indicator of veracity creates its own problems. When Malgaigne wrote of an account recorded by Paré and others of a man with a second head in his abdomen – '[a]ll these stories are probably imaginary, because no such monstrosity has ever been authenticated'[2] – he appears to have been unaware that a similar case had been described by Du Plessis.[3] After a recent report by Biswas and others, Paré's original appears less unlikely.[4]

Retrospective diagnosis is questionable both on pragmatic grounds (the various diagnoses that have been offered for the Ravenna monster cannot all be correct) and because it imposes a conceptual framework which (based as it is on cytogenetics, X-rays and other techniques) is simply not appropriate for material collected in the early modern period. At its most sophisticated, there is a danger that it can become a kind interpretative game, and with sufficient ingenuity it is possible to suggest retrospective diagnoses for almost all illnesses, even those of fictional characters.[5] Many of the criticisms of retrospective diagnosis, and many of its most ambitious uses, have been in the field of infectious disease, where arguably a plague is a historical event that cannot be equated with a modern diagnosis, but all disease and the way it is perceived changes over time, and some historians would deny that retrospective diagnosis is ever a legitimate approach. So-called constructionist theory sees disease as primarily a social phenomenon, understandable only within a specific socio-cultural setting. The extreme position would be to deny the duality of object and representation in knowledge of monstrous births: in other words, representation is everything and we can say nothing of the supposed reality underlying it.[6] A counter-argument for the validity of retrospective diagnosis is that birth defects are essentially anatomical variations, less prone to subjectivity than accounts of disease: the perception that a child has four legs or two hearts is less subjective than labelling it as having diphtheria or depression. This is not to say that anatomical terms are static, although it is noticeable that their use has tended to escape constructionist criticism even though understanding of anatomy has changed at least as much as understanding of disease.

The present-day study of birth defects is still largely based on their morphology; cases can be reviewed at second hand because pictures and a description are sufficient to make a diagnosis and indeed some birth defects are so rare that classification depends on comparing new cases with published accounts. Early modern observers described monstrous births and classified them without assigning them a name or diagnosis, but most modern 'diagnoses' are descriptive and so can be applied quite appropriately to older material – it does not significantly change our understanding of a two-headed child to call it dicephalus. Some malformations are now recognised as syndromic – two or more occur together in predictable associations – and it is possible to identify similar associations in older descriptions. Retrospective diagnosis also demonstrates the differences between monsters and modern birth defects and is a reminder that our study of monstrous births from the sixteenth and seventeenth centuries is determined by what contemporary writers chose to record. Some types that one might expect to find are not represented; for example Down's syndrome, the commonest present-day malformation syndrome, affecting some one in 600 births, does not appear to have been described earlier than the nineteenth century[7] and, along with many other conditions which led to relatively mild morphological changes, probably fitted into the broad range of 'normality' in the early modern period. Preauricular appendages (supernumerary ear lobes), a common minor malformation, were not described until Saviard reported two cases, one his own niece, in 1702 (interestingly, he reported that some people did not want them removed, on the grounds that they had been born with them).[8]

The appendix lists human monstrous births born between 1500 and 1700 that were reported in contemporary European publications. This list is unavoidably incomplete, and excludes undated examples (partly on the grounds that they were not necessarily born during the period under consideration). The English literature is well represented, as is that of France, largely owing to the important recent work of Wilson[9] in this area. Holländer reviewed the German literature in the 1920s but it was rather neglected until Irene Ewinkel's *De Monstris*.[10] Italy has received less attention, though Niccoli recently researched the early fifteenth century.[11] Cases from outside these areas are represented largely owing to their having been reported as news items in one of the aforementioned countries soon after they occurred. Every student of human teratology is indebted to the work of Gould and Pyle in the preparation of the index to the library of the Surgeon General (and, as a by-product, *Anomalies and Curiosities of Medicine*). I have omitted cases that could not be assigned (at least approximately) to a date and have excluded non-human monstrous births, even if contemporary writers regarded them as human, as these require knowledge of veterinary pathology for their interpretation.

The retrospective diagnoses given are, like all diagnoses, an opinion, one that might be revised or discarded if more information became available. They are intended to enable readers unfamiliar with perinatal autopsy appearances to compare monstrous births with modern accounts of birth defects,[12] and to direct the attention of those interested in the more recent history of birth defects to the older literature. I have reproduced contemporary descriptions, which speak for themselves, where space permits. Once reported in print, all cases of birth defects become part of the historical record: readers may decide for themselves how far the status of the authors, the content or the distance in time of the report from the present affect their value as evidence. I have tried to favour common entities over rare ones, except when the description of the case brought to mind a modern equivalent with similar features: a subjective process of pattern recognition.

Conjoined twins

Double monsters were the commonest reported monstrous births:[13] they were described anatomically in terms of the number and arrangement of heads, limbs and, if dissected, viscera, and these descriptions, along with iconographic evidence, can be used to assign them to groups in the modern classification of conjoined twins proposed by Spencer.[14] This classification is based on the concept of 'conjoined' twins having become fused *in utero* and the categories are named in terms of the site of 'union' of the twins. Of the seven groups, only thoracopagus (joined at the chest) and omphalopagus (joined at the abdomen) are not always separable on the basis of external appearances, because they are differentiated by whether the thoracic viscera are shared, and these have therefore been combined into a single 'thoraco/omphalopagus' group.

Of the thoraco/omphalopagus group, fifteen were identifiable as thoracopagus, either from specific description of union 'from the neck to the navel'[15] or from the presence of a shared heart.[16] Although the earliest reports are of same sex twins – an illustration from 1511 clearly shows both twins as female[17]– accounts from the mid-sixteenth century recorded conjoined twins of opposite sexes,[18] or one male and one of 'indistinct sex'. Conjoined twins of opposite sexes have not been reported in modern times, and are all but

Figure 7.1
The separation of conjoined twins. Miscellanea Curiosa, *1689.*

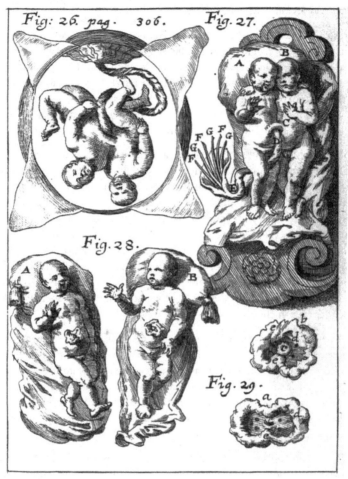

impossible biologically because they are 'identical' twins, formed from a single fertilised egg.[19]

Only two cases were unequivocally omphalopagus type: one pair of male twins underwent an autopsy and was found to share no organ except the liver.[20] The second, an extreme type known as xiphopagus and joined by 'skin' only, were surgically separated, the only example of this procedure in the early modern period: a tight ligature was passed around the joining band, which was then cut (Figure 7.1): the first surgical separation of conjoined twins.[21]

Parapagus twins (joined side-to-side) constitute the largest group.[22] Six of these cases were of diprosopus type (one head with two faces),[23] only one of which had an autopsy, which showed:

[An] exceptionally big head [that] seemed to be made up of two other heads put together; it had four eyes, two hooked noses, two mouths, two tongues and two ears. The interior was also double: it contained two brain-pans, separated by a cartilaginous partition, and two little brains, quite complete. The interior of the chest also contained two lungs and three hearts; the other viscera were single. This little monster lived for an hour, and would perhaps have lived longer if the midwife had not dropped it.[24]

We might also note in this group a female child said to have two eyes, two noses and three mouths[25] (there are no well-documented cases of more than one supernumerary mouth). Some parapagus twins showed malformations of one or both heads,[26] which are common in this type of twinning. Autopsies of parapagus twins revealed something of the tremendous diversity of anatomical variations possible in this group.[27] Parapagus twins, especially the tetrabrachius dipus type, tend to have the longest life expectancies. Brief though the description is of adult parapagus twins who came to Basel, probably to exhibit themselves, in 1538, it gives the impression that they were self-sufficient members of society and not dependent upon charity:

There was one borne, and grew to the perfect stature of man having two heades and foure shoulders, so that one heade was before, the other behinde, of a wonderful likenesse one to another: they were both bearded and looked one upon another, their appetite to meate was alike, their hunger alike, their voyce very like, they had one desire to the same wife, the whiche he had, and had the same waye of voyding excrements, and he was thirtie yeares old when he came to Basil.[28]

The cephalopagus group includes fourteen examples of what is now known as cephalothoracopagus janiceps,[29] a complex form of twinning where the heads and thoraces are fused, often resulting in a large head with two faces; the analogy with Janus was first made in a case from 1555. The autopsy of another revealed separate livers, two spleens and a single heart – an uncommon arrangement.[30] Two had apparent abdominal wall defects.[31] The barber-surgeon René Ciret gave the skeletons of one pair to Paré.[32]

The rarest types of conjoined twins are craniopagus (joined at the head), of which three examples were identified,[33] and pygopagus (joined at the sacrum), of which there were two examples, the later of which underwent an autopsy.[34] A case of 1613 may have been rachipagus (back to back) twins, however the description is insufficient to be certain and pygopagus twins may have been illustrated as rachipagus type.[35]

Ischiopagus twins (joined at the ischium, typically with one head at each end of the long axis), of which there were eight examples,[36] can show various arrangements of the lower limbs, one pair of which may be fused (tripus):

> In England, not far from Oxford, we are informed that a certain birth
> occurred with two heads, four arms and hands, one belly and a single set of
> female genitals. From one side two feet came out sideways, and from the
> other side, a single, or more correctly a double foot, having ten digits. At the
> second hour of the fifteenth day first one then the other died. They had
> rarely cried. One had a cheerful demeanour, while the other was sleepy and
> sad. The twenty transverse digits were the same length and breadth
> precisely.[37]

The proportion of the total cases of each major anatomical type of twinning is similar in the early modern literature to the data of Spencer;[38] the latter, derived from a very extensive survey of some 1,200 conjoined twins in modern times, showed 5% craniopagus, 37% thoraco/omphalopagus, 11% cephalopagus, 28% parapagus, 11% ischiopagus and 5% pygopagus. Excluding cases of uncertain conjunction, between 1500 and 1700 there were three cases of craniopagus twins (3%), twenty-nine cases of thoraco/omphalopagus (32%), fifteen cephalopagus (16%) thirty-four parapagus (37%), eight ischiopagus (9%) and three pygopagus (3%).

Five cases of double monsters could not be assigned to a specific type of union: in two it was not possible to determine their anatomy from the illustration and text;[39] others were given very brief descriptions such as 'joined laterally'.[40] There is a tantalising account of conjoined triplets: 'an infant having three heads, three chests, six arms, and the same number of feet was born... this monster had three souls in its breast, as the three hearts suggested.'[41] Human tricephalus is extremely rare – parasitic twins (see below) account for most reported cases[42]– and although the interpretation cannot be rejected solely on the grounds of rarity, it must at least be regarded as uncertain. Another unusual account describes an apparent rachipagus parasite attached to one of a pair of thoraco/omphalopagus twins:

> Their bellies were growne and Joyned together, from their breastes to their
> Navells.... And of the backe partes, from the shoulders of the supposed
> manchild, was a lumpe almoste as bigg as the head, was softe, and verily
> thought by the Middwife to be the Coddes and members, beinge turned on
> the backe partes, wronge placed, and out of eyther side of the sayd Lumpe
> was a small legg and a foote, and the feet were turned backwardes, but noe
> thighes to be seen, and had no fundament nor passage for water, but had a

prettie face, and head, shoulders, body, breaste, Armes, handes and feete, but the daughter was a large Child, and had all the Proportion of a Child.[43]

The changing terminology of these cases, from double monsters to conjoined twins, does not necessarily reflect how they were conceptualised. In the sixteenth century, double monsters were understood in terms of excess of seed, so for example cephalothoracopagus twins were 'so huge above order' that it was suggested they were formed from a quantity of 'matter' sufficient to form two children, which might have happened had their substance not been mingled, 'so that which shoulde have served for two made but one creature'.[44] A century later, fusion of two foetuses was supposed. 'Mr A.P.' wrote that that conjoined twins arose at 'the time of the first Formation of the Foetus' if the 'navel-strings' became joined. He thought that the 'bigness' of the afterbirth in a case of thoraco/omphalopagus twins supported this hypothesis, and tried to see if 'there might be distinct, though joined umbilical Vessels', however 'There was such a Crowd of People there, that I could not give myself that Satisfaction I desired.'[45] Although the 'fusion' hypothesis is now again in favour, for most of the twentieth century a 'fission' hypothesis (partial division of the egg) was favoured despite the twins being referred to as 'conjoined'.

Parasitic twins

This term is used to describe conjoined twins where there is a marked discrepancy in size and one is poorly or partially formed. The smaller twin is known as the parasite because it is dependent upon the circulation of its larger twin (the autosite). Parasites are usually located at one of the sites of union of conjoined twins; Spencer therefore classifies them in the same way and I have followed her scheme.[46] Observers in the early modern period were preoccupied with the parasite's response to stimulation and the possibility of a shared nervous system between parasite and autosite. According to Spencer the heart and neural tube (brain and spinal cord) are the structures least likely to be present in parasites, but she notes that sensory and/or motor nerve supply is well documented in some parasites, which can therefore respond to stimuli, although they do not seem to possess consciousness. Perhaps surprisingly given the longstanding interest in the subject, there have been no detailed anatomical studies of the nervous systems of parasitic twins.

Thoracopagus parasites are the commonest form in the early modern literature, the parasite usually being complete except for the head.[47] They are capable of prolonged survival. Some degree of limb deformity – contractures due to spastic paraparesis – is common and this is presumably what was described as: 'hands like feet that had been shaped into hands'.[48] All of the cases were male and they seem to have made a living by exhibiting themselves. Some were widely travelled: one man was seen in Valence, Paris and Montlehery, and according to Boaistuau he later appeared 'whole' and was asked what had become of the monster.[49] A case seen by Du Plessis resembled the Colloredo brothers in its mode of union:

> This man was á Tall and well Shaped man, att his Navel came out of his Body a head and neck Down to the Breast, the face Perfectly well Shaped with Eyes nose mouth chin forehead and Ears, all well Shaped and a Live but Could not Speak Eat nor Drink nor open its Eyes though he had two Eyes and Showed no Sign of Life it had a good Colour and two Long locks of Hair on its head, of a Black Colour, and a Downy Beard it had Teeth wee Could not see if it had a Toung for it did not Speak... He was Born about the year 1678, near Ratisbonn in Germany and was seen by me James Paris in London in the Year 1698, in the Mounth of December.[50]

An extreme form of omphalopagus parasitic twinning in which a parasitic head is present on the ventral abdomen is represented by three cases.[51] This type of parasitism is rare and there have been few cases in the modern literature.[52]

Craniopagus parasites are represented by a single example. Bondeson and Allen[53] first drew attention to this Hungarian case of 1620 in their discussion of a later case of craniopagus parasiticus, although the description is not sufficient to make a definitive diagnosis. A Bavarian case of 1538, a woman with two heads who lived into adulthood, was probably a cephalopagus parasite rather than a dicephalic.[54] '[A] well-formed child with an extra head like the head of a cat'[55] may also belong in this group. A broadside of 1645 also describes possible parasitic twinning – one child arising from the 'upper part' of another – but the exact mode of union is unclear.[56]

Fetus amorphus

The scope for malformation is considerably increased if a foetus can parasitise a normally functioning co-twin via anastomosis of their chorionic circulations (the parasite is termed *chorangiopagus parasiticus* or *fetus amorphus*). Essentially, these are identical twins in which one foetus fails to develop a functional heart, relying on the circulation of its co-twin via the placenta and without being joined to it. No two examples of fetus amorphus are identical, and a complex morphological classification has been developed.[57] Fetus amorphus is shown in an anonymous pamphlet of 1551 and a ballad of 1564,[58] and there were two other cases.[59] Fetus amorphus is a possible explanation for some sooterkin reports (the sooterkin always accompanied a normal pregnancy).

Craniofacial malformations

By the late-seventeenth century, 'cleft' lip and maxilla (palate) was being described in modern terms.[60] Prior to this, it can be inferred from a variety of descriptions; children said to have the head of a cat,[61] or the mouth of a dog, leopard or sheep,[62] may be interpreted as having cleft lip. Some descriptions suggest more severe facial clefting.[63] A child with 'awrie mouth' and 'a cloven or double tongue' may represent an association between cleft lip and palate and bifid tongue.[64] Double tongue alone (a relatively common malformation, showing great variability) was also described.[65] Despite its present frequency (of the order of one in a thousand live births), descriptions suggestive of cleft palate or facial cleft are relatively few. Nor is the lack of reports attributable to the comparatively minor nature of the defect from a modern perspective: contemporary accounts indicate that these disfiguring abnormalities had fatal consequences due to feeding difficulties[66] and were seen as serious malformations ('God be thanked, death supervened').[67] Perhaps there has been an increase in their incidence.

Cyclopia (a single, mid-line eye) is readily identifiable.[68] It is now considered to be part of a spectrum of failures of facial development due to an abnormality of the brain in which there is a single cerebral hemisphere – holoprosencephaly – of which cyclopia is the most extreme outcome. Descriptions compatible with less severe holoprosencephalic facies include 'an infant very clearly of the female sex... entirely lacking ears, eyes and nose, having only a mouth in the face'[69] and a similar child born eleven years later in which '[t]he eyes and nose were utterly absent'.[70] The complex of malformations in a third child which had the navel 'where the nose should stand', eyes 'where should stand the mouth: betweene the which was a certaine opening: hys eares stode on either side the chinne, and his mouthe at the ende of the same' suggests cyclopia with additional malformations, possibly otocephaly.[71] Cyclopia with encephalocoele (a sac containing fluid or cerebral substance that herniates through a defect in the skull) is also reported.[72] Encephalocoeles (described as fleshy masses) can also occur alone[73] and as part of malformation complexes (see below).

Monstrous births were commonly described as having the head of a frog, or another animal such as a dog, cat, cow or ape;[74] or as being without a head.[75] These probably correspond to the relatively common malformation of anencephaly. The head and eyes are present in these infants, but the calvarium and brain are absent and consequently the eyes appear large and protruding ('the eyes of an ox'), though they are of normal size. The first autopsy of an anencephalic, which included a detailed anatomical description and engravings of the head and skull, was published in 1671.[76] The longest-lived of these anencephalics survived only four or five days.[77]

A traditional type of monster called a blemmye was depicted with a proboscis, eyes in the chest, and ears on the shoulders.[78] They were mentioned by many early modern writers and described by Liceti as follows:

> Ambroise Pare acknowledges that in the town of Franca in Vasconia there was a girl without a head, having ears behind her shoulder-blades, a nose between them on her spine resembling a little proboscis, eyes in her shoulders, looking backwards, a strange, high, tongue where the throat ought to have been, a portrait of which monster by Fontano Agenesi, physician, who himself will dogmatically claim to have seen it.[79]

Schenck described a blemmye from an illustration:

> [A]round the neck region was a subcutaneous swelling. At the rear of the body was a single rudimentary stalk like a nipple, coming out from the spiral line [it is unclear what structure is meant here], and depending from the middle of the rostral end was something not unlike a copy of an elephant's curved proboscis... the head was entirely absent.[80]

Blemmyae do not suggest any modern malformation complex, although they may just possibly have been derived from cases of anencephaly combined with cyclopia[81] or iniencephaly,[82] however both are rare and iniencephalics appear to have been described differently elsewhere.[83] Blemmyae have a long iconographic history (among the monsters in distant lands in mediaeval world maps) but were apparently without emblematic significance, and their origin is obscure.

Multiple congenital malformations

So-called complex or multiple congenital malformations offer the most scope for retrospective diagnosis. In the twentieth century, many 'new' congenital malformation syndromes were described when predictable associations of congenital malformations were discovered. Once the link between the elements of the syndrome has been made, it is often possible to see the pattern in earlier cases. While the search for similar historical cases is a valid and indeed a necessary approach when a novel syndrome is proposed, overconfident retrospective diagnosis without considering alternatives, particularly if the syndrome is rare, is a pitfall. The monster of Ravenna[84] has already been discussed at length and the reader is referred to the sources in Chapter 1 for a discussion of some suggested diagnoses. A male child born at Much Horkesley near Colchester with parts of its limbs missing, an absent penis and 'absent' (short?) tongue has been interpreted by Anderson[85] as the earliest description of Hanhart complex.[86] This is one possibility, but intra-uterine amputations due to amniotic bands should also have been considered, particularly as there is no evidence of micrognathia or of other affected family members (limb reduction defects of this type may be inherited according to an autosomal recessive pattern): the original report mentions that this was the first child conceived between these parents, though both had other normal children.[87] A child with multiple malformations including cleft lip and a spinal defect (*spina bifida*) was diagnosed as showing arthrogryposis multiplex congenita or Larsen syndrome,[88] but the description of 'stumps on the hands' suggests syndactyly and this, coupled with the apparent microcephaly shown in the illustration (Figure 2.4, 53), is compatible with trisomy 13, though again it is not possible to reach a definitive diagnosis.[89]

Roberts' syndrome is a good example of how re-examination of the older literature can reveal earlier accounts of 'new' syndromes. The eponymous description of the syndrome of facial malformations and limb defects was made in 1919,[90] but more recently further cases have been identified from the literature before that date. Mayer's case of 1829 was classified as Roberts' syndrome by Van Den Berg and Francke, who in an extensive review of the literature identified five other examples of the Roberts' syndrome before Roberts.[91] Geoffroy Saint Hilaire's description of 'seal limb' syndrome in 1838 ('hands or feet of unusual size and commonly even completely normal, which, supported by excessively short limbs usually emerge directly from the shoulders or hips') also seems to anticipate Roberts.[92] A foetus described by Virchow in 1898 has recently been interpreted as Roberts's syndrome after re-examination of the museum specimen[93] and another Roberts foetus has been identified amongst the specimens in the teratological collection of the Museum Vrolik in Amsterdam.[94] A retrospective diagnosis of Roberts's syndrome has also been proposed in a case reported in Germany in 1737.[95]

A detailed description of the autopsy of a male infant discovered on public exhibition at Leipzig by François Bouchard in 1672 appears to describe the same syndrome. Bouchard, professor of medicine at the University of Besançon in France, sent an account of his findings to *Miscellanea Curiosa*.[96] The account is given in full as it shows the technique of description of a monstrous birth at its most developed, allowing the reader to virtually witness the autopsy:

A monstrous child exposed in a public street at Leiden on 5 March 1671

A monster is anything that appears outside the normal course and order of nature, such as a child with two heads, or which has three or more arms or other superfluous members, mutilated or maimed.

A prodigy is that which goes totally against nature, such as if a woman gives birth to a beast, whether four-footed, aquatic, flying, reptilian, or of some other kind. These can be seen in *Historia de Monstris* of Ulyssis Aldrovandi and in Ambroise Pare's book 25, *de Monstris.*

Among the causes of monsters authors place the Glory of God, in which group are those born blind, and His anger; because men and women do not live according to the laws of God and of nature laid down for them. This often happens in these times, just as the prophet Esdras says.

The remaining causes of monsters are many, from defects of material to the force of the imagination on the formative faculty.

The present monster has an unusually large head, the hair of the head being as long as that of a child of ten or twelve months. Unnaturally, the brain floated in serum without water, this was owing to hydrocephalus or water-tumour. The two superolateral parts of the cranium were unnaturally prominent, because of contact with the floating brain.

The quantity of water in the head had also separated the cranial bones from one another.

His ears were both ugly and defective in their composition, shape, and site, like a single mass (as the figures show), without any cartilage, but with two small foramina, and very much compressed, as is the face.

The upper lip is fissured on both sides, and its bone made of two parts, like that of a rabbit; skin and flesh surround the middle part. This same upper lip has one incisor tooth on the left side, still covered by a small piece of skin.

His nipples were somewhat low-set, but otherwise normal.

His hands resemble those of an ape, without thumbs, and only two of the fingers of the right hand have their nails. The third has neither bones nor joints, but there was a proximal phalanx at its base.

The left hand also lacks a thumb, and has only two digits with nails; the third is mutilated, and the first and last bones are lacking.

His hands are linked to the humerus or arm-bone by simple ligaments, both lacking the bones that make up the first part or forearm.

He has a good back as far down as the coccyx.

The anterior part of his lower belly is reasonably natural; from the umbilicus to the penis is a space the breadth of three fingers, and the same from there to the extremity.

From the posterior parts around the coccyx has grown out an extra piece of flesh which appears very pliant, and from there to its end it resembles more nearly the tail of a duck or a goose: it bears neither femora or tibiae.

His feet arise directly from the os coccyx, are attached there by simple ligaments, and resemble the feet of a duck.

The ductus from the mouth to the chest is fair and open, as is the other canal that leads from the mouth to the stomach. The way from the stomach to the extremity is completely open, and is healthy and free everywhere.

The ureters or canals that carry urine from the kidneys to the bladder are both patent and free, as is the canal from the bladder to the tip of the penis.

The whole abdomen was swimming in blood from a ruptured umbilical vein, which probably happened during the mother's difficult labour and delivery, which happened against nature, in that the feet came out first, and, on account of the violence in dragging him out (because the head was so large egress was not possible) the vein ruptured.

Otherwise the remaining parts were nobly formed and healthy, and if he had been able to come forth into the light uninjured he would have been undoubtedly capable of begetting offspring as well-formed as he was, to the small extremities and other defective parts, since I see the maimed and crippled all conceive freely because of their complete parts.

The monster here could never have carried itself upright, nor have sat down, and furthermore his hands were too little for him to have learned a trade, as these observations make clear.'[97]

The detailed engraving of the case appears to show micrognathia and cryptorchidism (Figure 7.2). The principal findings may therefore be summarised as hydrocephalus, bilateral cleft lip, malformed ears, tetraphocomelia with absence of the forearm bones and all long bones of the legs, and oligodactyly with absent thumbs. Minor findings include low-set nipples and possible hypertrichosis. These features allow a reasonably confident diagnosis of Roberts' syndrome, of which hydrocephalus is an uncommon but recognised association.[98]

The autopsy findings indicate that the child would have died shortly after delivery. It was therefore exhibited dead in the public street; Bouchard probably purchased the body from the parents in order to perform the autopsy. His report emphasizes the patency of the oesophagus, trachea and gastrointestinal tract, suggesting awareness of the association between atresia and other abnormalities of these structures and skeletal defects. The test for hydrocephalus described by Bouchard has not, to my knowledge, been

Figure 7.2
An engraving of a child with tetraphocomelia. Note, in addition to the
features described by Bouchard, cryptorchidism and micrognathia.
Miscellanea Curiosa, *1672).*

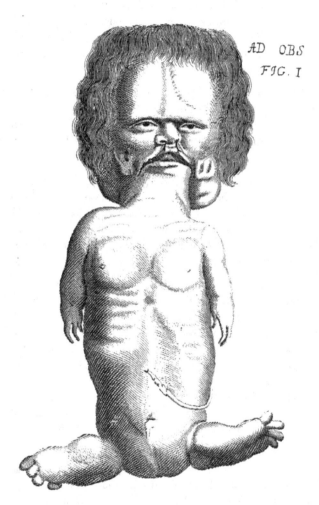

described earlier than 1673, though Bouchard does not treat it as innovative. It depends upon the observation that the specific gravity of the hydrocephalic brain is less than that of the normal, owing to its greater water content.[99] The brain therefore floated in 'serum'.[100]

It is interesting to compare a similar account from the sixteenth-century literature, a child born to Annis Figge at Chichester in Sussex:

> In Februarie the firste day, at Chichester in the Countie of Sussex was borne in the suburbes a monstrous chylde of liltle shape of body, trussed together, the head verye great, bigger than the body, the body in compasse 9 inches, the arme an inche long, and two inches about the face, of indifferet favour, on the cheeke and chin the likenesse of a blacke beard, the legs wanted thighs, the toes crooked.[101]

Although there are features suggestive of Roberts' syndrome, particularly absent long bones in the leg, it is not possible to render a firm diagnosis.

Four accounts of monstrous births described features suggestive of Meckel–Gruber syndrome. The first is a child born in Piedmont, which:

> ...the face being well-proportioned in all its parts... was found to be monstrous on the rest of the head, in that five horns approximating to those of a ram came out of it, the horns being arranged one against the other on the top of the forehead and at the rear a long piece of flesh hanging along the back, like a maiden's hood. It had around its neck a flap of double-layered flesh like a shirt collar all of one piece, the extremities of the fingers resembling the talons of some bird of prey, its knees like hams.[102]

Another was born the following year: 'with a single head, from the occiput of which a large piece of flesh hung down: in the mouth were two tongues...'.[103] The descriptions suggest occipital encephalocoele with malformations of the hands and lower limbs in the first case and lobulated tongue in the second. In neither however are the details sufficient to make a definitive diagnosis. An even more tentative attribution is a macerated child born at Old Sandwich in Kent,[104] though the description does suggest encephalocoele, polydactyly and limb deformity. Perhaps the best candidate for this syndrome may have had a posterior encephalocoele, a large abdominal wall defect with the liver, stomach and intestines exteriorised, right-sided cleft lip, and mutilated digits"[105]

> Another horrible accident in pregnancy happened at Arnstadt... a girl gave birth to a stillborn child. Except for the calvarium and forehead, the membranes of the brain formed a high, red crest, with a fleshy sac hanging down from the occiput, prominent eyes, a rounded left ear and harelip. The palate and also the nose were disfigured on the right side.... From a round hole in the breast the heart hung out exposed and divided into two parts, a shapeless liver and a huge stomach lay underneath, the intestines were displaced above the fissure in the left hypogastrium, the fingers were partly mutilated, and bent back towards the nails. This monster was quickly taken

away and buried; I myself had the opportunity to look carefully all over it, the internal parts as well as the external.[106]

Urogenital malformations

Monstrous births described as of uncertain sex, or with features of both sexes probably showed sexual indifference due to immaturity and not true hermaphroditism in its modern sense. It is possible that other malformations were also interpreted as representing the presence of external genitalia of both kinds. The following can be interpreted as exstrophic bladder in a male infant: 'an hermaphrodite or androgene was born, above the umbilicus well-favoured, but around the umbilicus was a mass of reddish flesh, beneath which was the female member, and beneath that, in an appropriate place, the male.'[107] Absence of the bladder was recorded at autopsy in a case with imperforate anus.[108]

Notes

1. G.M. Gould and W.L. Pyle, *Anomalies and Curiosities of Medicine* (New York: Sydenham, 1937), 1–4, 163.
2. Appendix, 1516a; see A. Paré (ed. and transl. J.L. Pallister), *On Monsters and Marvels* (Chicago: University of Chicago Press, 1982), 187.
3. Appendix, 1686a.
4. S.K. Biswas *et al.*, 'An Unusual Case of Heteropagous Twinning', *Journal of Pediatric Surgery*, xxvii (1992), 96–7, described a 'spherical' umbilical swelling with 'facial features'.
5. One example must suffice: A.N. Williams, 'Cerebrovascular Disease in Dumas' *The Count of Monte Cristo*', *Journal of the Royal Society of Medicine*, xcvi (2003), 412–14.
6. J. Arrizabalaga, 'Problematizing Retrospective Diagnosis in the History of Disease', *Asclepio*, liv (2002), 51–70.
7. Except in art: A.S. Levitas and C.S. Reid, 'An Angel with Down Syndrome in a Sixteenth-Century Flemish Nativity Painting', *American Journal of Medical Genetics*, cxvi A (2003), 399–405; also J.M. Berg, and M. Korossy, 'Down Syndrome Before Down: A Retrospect', *American Journal of Medical Genetics*, cii (2001), 205–21.
8. J.W. Ballantyne, 'Preauricular Appendages', *Teratologia*, ii (1895), 18–36.
9. D. Wilson, *Signs and Portents: Monstrous Births from the Middle Ages to The Enlightenment* (London: Routledge, 1993).
10. I. Ewinkel, *De Monstris...* (Tübingen: Niemeyer, 1995).
11. O. Niccoli (transl. L.G. Cochrane), *Prophecy and People in Renaissance Italy* (Princeton: Princeton University Press, 1990).
12. Those interested in so doing are directed to the standard textbooks on birth

defects: E. Gilbert-Barness, *Potter's Pathology of the Fetus and Infant* (St Louis: Mosby, 1997); J.S. Wigglesworth and D.B. Singer (eds), *Textbook of Fetal and Perinatal Pathology* (Massachusetts: Blackwell Science, 1998); K.L. Jones (ed.), *Smith's Recognizable Patterns of Human Malformation* (Philadelphia: W.B. Saunders, 1997).

13. There are seventeen reports between 1665 and 1700. The population of the British Isles, France, Scandinavia, Italy and Germany together was in the order of sixty million – see R. Mols, 'Population in Europe 1500–1700', in C. Cipolla (ed.), *The Fontana Economic History of Europe: The Sixteenth and Seventeenth Centuries* (London, 1974), 38 – suggesting anything from 600,000 to 2,000,000 births a year. If the incidence of conjoined twins were the same as in recent years, that is, between 1 in 50,000 and 1 in 100,000 births, it is apparent even from these approximations that the great majority went unreported.

14. R. Spencer, 'Conjoined Twins: Theoretical Embryological Basis', *Teratology*, vl (1992), 591–602.

15. Appendix, 1543a, 1550b, 1552a, 1555b, 1566a, 1635, 1680b.

16. Appendix, 1544b, 1546b, 1572b, 1605, 1628, c.1670a, 1670a, 1685.

17. The artist advanced their age and depicted them as children rather than newborn infants: Appendix, 1511a.

18. Appendix, 1547a, 1552a, 1555a, 1566a, 1570b.

19. Appendix, 1614. For possible reasons see I. Blickstein, 'The Conjoined Twins of Löwen', *Twin Research*, iii (2000), 185–8, and A.W. Bates, 'Conjoined Twins in the Sixteenth Century', *Twin Research*, v (2002), 521–8.

20. Appendix, 1692b.

21. The only successful example; separation of twins joined at the forehead had been attempted in Worms in 1495 after the death one of them, but the hurt she receyved in the separation from her dead sister was the onely cause she died immediately': see E. Fenton, *Certaine Secrete Wonders of Nature...* (London: H. Bynneman, 1569), fo. 15v. On the successful surgery, see Appendix, c.1689; R.G. Harper *et al.*, 'Xiphopagus Conjoined Twins: A 300-Year Review of the Obstetric, Morphopathologic, Neonatal, and Surgical Parameters', *American Journal of Obstetrics and Gynecology*, cxxxvii (1980), 617–29.

22. Appendix, 1512b, 1514b, 1517b, 1531a, 1536a, 1538a, 1543b, 1544a, 1552c, 1553c, 1565d, 1567, 1579c, 1581, 1597a, 1598, 1599a, 1620a, 1631, 1658a, 1664a, 1668a, 1669a, 1677a, c.1681, c.1685, 1687, 1691a.

23. Appendix, 1514c, 1540a, 1550a, 1579a, c.1657, 1684b.

24. J.B. Salgues, *Des Erreurs et des Préjugés Répandus dans la Société* (Paris: F. Buisson, 1810–13), III, 118–19; see also J. Gélis, *History of Childbirth:*

Fertility, Pregnancy and Birth in Early Modern Europe (Oxford: Polity Press, 1991), 268.

25. Appendix, 1617d.
26. Appendix, 1579c, 1599a, *c.*1685.
27. Appendix, 1544a, 1597a, 1664a.
28. S. Batman, *The Doome Warning All Men to the Judgement...* (London: R. Nubery, 1581), 330; Appendix, 1538a.
29. Appendix, 1529b, 1536c, 1540b, 1555a, 1560, 1565a, 1569a, 1576a, 1578a, 1579g, 1606b, 1661, 1674b, 1680a.
30. Appendix, 1540b; see T.H. Grundfest and S. Weisenfeld, 'A Case of Cephalothoracopagus', *New York State Medical Journal,* l (1950), 576–9; A.W. Bates and S.M. Dodd, 'Anomalies in Cephalothoracopagus Synotus Twins and Their Implications for Morphogenesis in Conjoined Twins', *Pediatric and Developmental Pathology,* ii (1999), 464–72.
31. Appendix, 1555a, 1578a.
32. Paré, *op. cit.* (note 2), 15; Appendix, 1569a.
33. Appendix, 1563, 1620b, 1682.
34. Appendix, 1545b, 1675b.
35. Rachipagus twinning had been thought not to occur, but was recently rediscovered: R. Spencer, 'Rachipagus Conjoined Twins: They Really Do Occur!', *Teratology,* lii (1995), 346–56.
36. Appendix, 1570a, b, 1572a, 1575a, 1585a, 1610, 1617c, 1664b.
37. *[I]n Anglia non procul ab Oxonia informis quidam partus natus est, capitis duobus, brachijs quatuor, manib. totidem, ventre vno, membro muliebri, sede vna. Ex vna parte pedes transuersi duo erant, ex altero vnus tantum, rite exporrectus, forma duorum pedum, digitos habens decem. Horum alter diebus quindecim, alter vero vno superuixit. Lachrymarunt hoc tempore raro. Alter ex his laetus ad modum, alter vero somniculosus & tristis extitit. Viginti digitos transuersos erat longitudo & latitudo ipsorum:* J. Rueff, *De Conceptu et Genratione Hominis...* (Zürich: C. Froschauer, 1554), 382.
38. R. Spencer, 'Theoretical and Analytical Embryology of Conjoined Twins: Part I: Embryogenesis', *Clinical Anatomy,* xiii (2000), 36–53: 42.
39. Appendix, 1511b, 1576b.
40. Appendix, 1534; other unclassifiable twins are 1553b and 1593a.
41. *[I]nfans tria habens capita, tria pectora, sex brachia, totidemque; pedes, natus est, qui ex triplicis capitis ore & lac fugebat & vagiebat. Tres habuisse animas id monstrum ex triplici pectore, ex quo triplex cor infertur...:* L.G. Gerlin, *Disputatio Philosophica de Monstris* (Wittenberg: C. Tham, 1624), 8; Appendix, 1536b.
42. Spencer, *op. cit.* (note 38), 47–9.

43. D. Woodward, 'Some Difficult Confinements in Seventeenth-Century Yorkshire', *Medical History*, xviii (1974), 349–53.

44. Appendix, 1555a.

45. Appendix, 1680b.

46. Spencer, *op. cit.* (note 38), 47–9; *Idem*, 'Parasitic Conjoined Twins: External, Internal (Fetuses in Fetu and Teratomas), and Detached (Acardiacs)', *Clinical Anatomy*, xiv (2001), 428–44.

47. Appendix, 1513, 1514a, 1529a, 1530b, 1566c, 1571a, 1617a, 1678.

48. Appendix, 1529a.

49. P. Boaistuau, *Histoires Prodigieuses...* (Paris: V. Sentenas, 1560), fo. 83r.

50. Du Plessis, *A Short History of Human Prodigious & Monstrous Births...* (1730), 31–2.

51. Appendix, 1516b, 1677b, 1686a.

52. A baby boy with a cystic umbilical swelling with facial features may be a *forme fruste* of this condition: S.K. Biswas *et al.*, 'An Unusual Case of Heteropagus Twinning', *Journal of Pediatric Surgery*, xxvii (1992), 96–7.

53. J. Bondeson and E. Allen, 'Craniopagus Parasiticus: Everard Home's Two-Headed Boy of Bengal and Some Other Cases', *Surgical Neurology*, xxxi (1989), 426–34; Appendix, 1620b.

54. Appendix, 1538b.

55. Appendix, *c.*1681.

56. Appendix, 1645.

57. T. Sato *et al.*, 'Acardiac Anomalies: Review of 88 Cases in Japan', *Asia-Oceana Journal of Obstetrics and Gynaecology*, x (1984), 45–52; see J.P. Simonds and G.A. Gowen, 'Fetus Amorphus (Report of a Case)', *Surgery Gynecology Obstetrics*, xli (1925), 171–9, for a simpler classification, and Wigglesworth and Singer, *op. cit.* (note 12), 223, for a comparison of the two.

58. Appendix, 1551c, 1564.

59. Appendix, *c.*1690d, 1690b.

60. Appendix, 1668c.

61. Appendix, 1638.

62. Appendix, 1556d, 1568b, 1608c.

63. Appendix, 1557a.

64. J.A. Britto, R.H. Ragoowansi and B.C. Sommerlad, 'Double Tongue, Intraoral Anomalies, and Cleft Palate – Case Reports and a Discussion of Developmental Pathology', *The Cleft Palate–Craniofacial Journal*, xxxvii (2000), 410–15; Appendix, 1553a.

65. Appendix, 1659; see Wigglesworth and Singer, *op. cit.* (note 12), 763

66. Appendix, 1671.

67. Appendix, 1668c.

68. Appendix, 1551b, 1568a, 1624, 1670b.

69. Appendix, 1503.

70. Appendix, 1514d.

71. Appendix, 1568a.

72. Appendix, 1670b.

73. Appendix, 1530a, 1578c, 1686c, 1690a.

74. Appendix, 1517a, 1544c, 1556b, 1578d, 1646, 1665, *c.*1690c, *c.*1697a, b, 1698, 1700.

75. Appendix, 1525, 1557b, 1566d, 1579d, 1617b, 1642, 1666a, *c.*1667b, *c.*1673, *c.*1677, 1694.

76. Appendix, 1646.

77. Appendix, *c.*1697b.

78. Appendix, 1565c.

79. F. Liceti, *De Monstris...* (Amsterdam: A. Frisii, 1665), 131; Appendix, 1562b.

80. *[A]uersa corporis parte singulis scapulis rudimenta quaedam papillarum, ex spirali linea ductarum, apparent, ex quarum demissiore regione media rostellum incuruum elephantis proboscidi haud absimile exprimitur...capite in uniuersum careat:* J.G. Schenck, *Observationum Medicarum Rariorum...* (Leyden: J.-A. Huguetan, 1644), 7.

81. See R.C. Gupta, V.K. Gupta and S. Gupta, 'Human Cyclopia with Associated Microstoma and Anencephaly (A Case Report)', *Indian Journal of Ophthalmology*, xxix (1981), 121–3.

82. See J.B. Friedman, *The Monstrous Races in Medieval Art and Thought* (Cambridge, MA: Harvard University Press, 1981).

83. Appendix, 1640b, *c.*1679a.

84. Appendix, 1512a.

85. T. Anderson, 'Artistic and Documentary Evidence for Tetradysmelia from Sixteenth-Century England', *American Journal of Medical Genetics*, lii (1994), 475–7; Appendix, 1562c.

86. MIM 103300. The MIM number refers to the Mendelian Inheritance in Man coding: see V.A. McKusick, *Mendelian Inheritance in Man: Catalogs of Human Genes and Genetic Disorders* (Baltimore: Johns Hopkins University Press, 1998).

87. Anon., *The True Reporte of the Forme and Shape of a Monstrous Childe ...* (London: T. Marshe, 1562), reprinted in Philobiblon Society (ed.), *Ancient Ballads & Broadsides...* (London: Whittingham & Wilkins, 1867), 38–42.

88. T. Anderson, 'Earliest Evidence for Arthrogryposis Multiplex Congenita or Larsen syndrome?', *American Journal of Medical Genetics*, lxxi (1997), 127–9; Appendix, 1568b.

89. A.W. Bates, 'Birth Defects Described in Elizabethan ballads', *Journal of the Royal Society of Medicine*, xciii (2000), 202–7.

90. J.B. Roberts, 'A Child with Double Cleft Lip and Palate, Protrusion of the Intermaxillary Portion of the Upper Jaw and Imperfect Development of the Bones of the Four Extremities', *Annals of Surgery*, lxx (1919), 252–3.

91. D.J. Van Den Berg and U. Francke, 'Roberts Syndrome: A Review of 100 Cases and a New Rating System for Severity', *American Journal of Medical Genetics*, xlvii (1993), 1104–23.

92. H.O. Grundy *et al.*, 'Roberts Syndrome: Antenatal Ultrasound – A Case Report', *Journal of Perinatal Medicine*, xvi (1988), 71–5.

93. M. Urban *et al.*, 'Tetraphocomelia and Bilateral Cleft Lip in a Historical Case of Roberts Syndrome [Virchow, 1898]', *American Journal of Medical Genetics*, lxxii (1997), 307–14.

94. R.-J. Oostra *et al.*, 'Congenital Anomalies in the Teratological Collection of Museum Vrolik in Amsterdam, The Netherlands, I: Syndromes with Multiple Congenital Abnormalities', *American Journal of Medical Genetics*, lxxvii (1998), 100–15.

95. A.W. Bates, 'A Case of Roberts Syndrome Described in 1737', *Journal of Medical Genetics*, xxxviii (2001), 565–7.

96. F. Bouchard, 'Infante Monstroso Lugduni in Viam Publicam Die V. Martii A. MDCLXXI Exposito', *Miscellanea Curiosa*, series 1, iii (1672), 14–6.

97. The original text is given in A.W. Bates, 'Autopsy on a Case of Roberts Syndrome Reported in 1672: The Earliest Description?', *American Journal of Medical Genetics*, cxvii A (2003), 92–6.

98. See, for example: M.V. Freeman *et al.*, 'The Roberts Syndrome', *Clinical Genetics*, v (1974), 1–16; C.E.U. Ekong and B. Rozdilsky, 'Hydranencephaly in Association with Roberts Syndrome', *Canadian Journal of Neurological Science*, v (1978), 253–5; R.A. Pfeiffer and H. Zwerner, 'The Roberts Syndrome: Report of a Case Without Anomaly of the Centromeric Region', *Monatsschrift Kinderheilkunde*, cxxx (1982), 296–8 and Grundy *et al.*, *op. cit.* (note 92). The dramatic limb shortening and craniofacial abnormalities place this case at the severe end of the Roberts spectrum: Van Den Berg and Francke, *op. cit.* (note 91). The differential diagnosis includes Cornelia de Lange syndrome, which in a minority of cases shows phocomelia. The facial features – downturned angles of the mouth, depressed nasal bridge, micrognathia and possibly synophrys – resemble those of this syndrome, as does the apparent hypertrichosis and low posterior hair line, however hydrocephalus is not a feature of de Lange syndrome, and though occasional cases with lower limb defects have been recorded, limb defects of the severity of Bouchard's case are not seen; see L. Jackson *et al.*, 'De Lange Syndrome: A Clinical Review of 310 Individuals', *American Journal of Medical Genetics*,

xlvii (1993), 940–6 and R.A. Pfeiffer and J. Correll, 'Hemimelia in Brachmann–de Lange Syndrome (BDLS): A Patient with Severe Deficiency of the Upper and Lower Limbs', *American Journal of Medical Genetics*, xlvii (1993), 1014–7.

99. H.W. Bothe *et al.*, 'Relationship Between Specific Gravity, Water Content, and Serum Protein Extravasation in Various Types of Vasogenic Brain Edema', *Acta Neuropathologica* (Berlin), lxiv (1984), 37–42.

100. Hydrocephalic dog brain has a specific gravity of around 1.035, compared with a normal value of 1.043: see H. Hiratsuka *et al.*, 'Evaluation of Periventricular Hypodensity in Experimental Hydrocephalus by Metrizamide CT Ventriculography', *Journal of Neurosurgury*, lvi (1982), 235–40 and R.A. Fishman and M. Greer, 'Experimental Obstructive Hydrocephalus', *Archives of Neurology*, viii (1963), 156–61.

101. Batman, *op. cit.* (note 28), 415; Appendix, 1580c.

102. Paré, *op. cit.* (note 2), 10–11; Appendix, 1578b.

103. Liceti, *op. cit.* (note 79), 91; Appendix, 1579f.

104. Appendix, *c.*1609.

105. This underwent an autopsy; see J.A. Hünerwolff, 'De Foemellis Duabus Monstrosis', *Miscellanea Curiosa*, series 2, ix (1690), 170–1.

106. *Alius horribilis casus in praegnante contigit Arnstadii… pendulos intentis oculis contemplans, puellam peperit mortuam, absq; calvaria & fronte, membranis cerebri cristae instar erectis rubentibus, cum sacco de occipite pendente carnoso, oculis prominentibus, aure sinistra orbiculari, labio leporino, palatum etiam & narem dextram deturpante, collo rumente, foramine pectoris parro & rotundo, corde ex eo pendente foras nudo & bifida, hepate informe & ventriculo vasto subjacentibus, intestinis super scissuram in hypogastrio dextro non perviam aberrantibus, digitis partim mutilatis, partim recurris unguiculis adnatis. Humatio autem monstri festinata eripuit mihi pariter occasionem accurare perlustrandi internam partium cum externis connexionem: Ibid.*; Appendix, *c.*1690b.

107. *Tiguri Hermaphroditus vel androgynos natus est, supra vmbilicum egregie formatus, sed circa vmbilicum rubeam carnis massam habens, sub qua membrum muliebre, & infra hoc, loco convenienti, virile quoque.* Rueff, *op. cit.* (note 37), I, 382; Appendix, 1519.

108. Appendix, 1606a.

Conclusion

[W]ee carry with us the wonders we seeke without us: There is all *Africa* and her prodigies in us[1]

The history of monstrous births cannot be reduced to a single narrative; the uses to which they were put – theological exemplars, opportunities for the display of anatomical skill, sources of income and others – and the people who described them – theologians, physicians, men of letters – are too varied for that: popular prints such as those on the Ravenna monster were very different from descriptions of monsters in the journals of learned societies, and wonder books from more systematic accounts such as those of Liceti and Schott. One feature common to almost the entire early modern literature was the truth claims made by those who described monsters. Readers expected 'the true account', and writers of all classes sought ways to convey through text and images that the singular occurrences they had witnessed or heard of could be taken as true. For sixteenth-century readers the meaning of an emblem was not self-evidently placed there by its deviser, it was part of the natural property or signature of the things of which it was formed; monsters were to be interpreted 'rightly' because their meaning was inherent in them and when found enabled them to 'declare the truthe'.[2] The search for hidden 'truths' is perhaps the single theme underpinning the early modern (and later) interest in monsters.

Providence and plenitude

Can we in retrospect identify any property common to the monsters themselves? Montaigne, supporting his argument by quoting Cicero ('What one often sees one does not wonder at…')[3] argued that monsters and other wonders were remarkable because of their rarity, a claim also made by Liceti. This however does not explain why they attracted more interest than other natural rarities, or rare diseases. One modern interpretation is that monsters were exceptional because of their ambiguous or intermediate status. While this line of reasoning has contributed much to the analysis of some of the common types of monstrous births such as double monsters and hermaphrodites, it is, I suggest, insufficient fully to characterize the monstrous. Many of the monstrous births described in the early modern period, such as infants with no head, holes in the belly or back, fleshy swellings and other defects, cannot plausibly be seen as intermediates.[4] There is also an apparent inconsistency between monsters as outsiders, 'between' categories, and the many early modern classifications of monsters.

An alternative is that the monstrous was chaotic or formless,[5] but although some examples of monstrous births, such as *fetus amorphus*, are now seen as lacking in order, it is difficult to argue from early modern accounts that, for example, double monsters were thought to show less complexity or organisation than normal infants. Bizarreness and unnaturalness could be combined with internal order and symmetry, as in this double monster described by the Florentine historian Benedetto Varchi (1502–65):

> They were two females joyned and stuck together, one toward the other in such a way that half the chest of one along with that of the other made up a single chest, & thus they formed two chests, one joining up with the other; their backs were not shared, but each had its own: it had its head turned directly towards one of the two chests, & on the other side, in the place of the face it had two ears that were joined one to the other, & they touched....
> They found two hearts, two livers, & two lungs, & finally everything was doubled, just as for two bodies, but the windpipes, which began at the [level of the] heart, joyned up near the entrance to the throat and became one.[6]

The one feature common to all monstrous births, which separates them from deformities due to trauma or disease, is that they were congenital. They were as they were made, whether according to the will of God or a 'secondary plan' of nature. Monstrous births were part of the divine plan and as such they showed (*monstrat*, from which the word *monster* was derived) the unseen hand of God, the potter who had power over the clay,[7] and who formed the human body as He chose.

For Protestants, such unnatural happenings, outwith the normal course or laws of nature, were evidence of direct intervention by the Creator in the natural world. Because they appeared when and where they were needed, monsters were signs *par excellence* of divine providence, and so were invested with great significance, because if they were not evidence of God's continued involvement with his creation, then nothing was. This use of monstrous births was the basis of broadsides from Melanchthon and Luther onwards, reaching a peak in the mid-sixteenth century and continuing in a rather tired form in the output of Protestant faculties of theology in the seventeenth. To the seventeenth-century English cleric Thomas Bedford, monstrous births were 'the subject matter on which [God] stampeth the marks of his providence, either in hindering or in altering the ordinary course of nature'.[8] This is not to say that they were seen as being God-given in a way that 'normal' births or other events were not, but because their deformity drew attention to them they were the most obvious evidence of God's ongoing creative activity in the world 'in hindering, so also in altering and changing the course of Nature, doth God call man to an observation of his Providence'.[9] Nor were they miracles; Protestants agreed with Montaigne that although monsters seemed unnatural to men, they were not so to God. As a prefatory verse to Batman's translation of Lycosthenes put it:

> Al things are natural to God on hye,
> But here below in every mortal thing,
> Gainst natures lore some wonder forth doth spryng...[10]

While scholarly writers showed a greater interest in 'lower' causes (God, in most cases, being the higher cause), partly because of their utility in classification, we must not suppose that popular writers were ignorant of them; causes of monstrous births such as excess of formative material, heredity or maternal impressions were recognised by writers (and by readers) of ballads as well as by scholars, but they were not emphasised. Except for encyclopaedists like Aldrovandi, who aimed to lay the whole of their subject before the reader, most writers exercised some form of 'discursive self-restraint'[11] and considered only what seemed to be the salient features of monstrous births. Consequently, interpretations of monsters as signs or emblems and interest in their causes were often separated ('why' monsters were formed and what they signified was largely distinct from 'how' they were formed),[12] but they were not mutually exclusive: a monstrous birth could for example be seen both as the 'natural' (cause-and-effect) consequence of bestiality and as a divine warning against the sin.[13] A natural explanation for wonders did not preclude their interpretation as signs from God: 'I am not ignorant that such meteors proceed from natural causes', wrote the antiquary Ralph Thoresby in 1682, 'yet [they] are frequently also the presages of imminent calamities.' Providence revealed itself through natural events, because 'nature is God's minister'.[14]

To sixteenth-century writers of broadsides and wonder books, monstrous births were public displays, calls to 'the forgetful world' that in its over-familiarity sometimes took providence for granted; they were signs of God seeking the sinner, wisdom crying in the streets. Each one showed God's handiwork so clearly that it was, in a small way, an emblem of the Incarnation. Like the man born blind in St John's gospel (and like the Incarnation), monstrous births happened so that men might see and believe; God Himself was the truth under the veil of a monstrous birth, and to see one was to witness the power of God: 'These straunge and monstrous thinges, almighty GOD sendeth amongst us, that we should not be forgetful of his almighty power'.[15] The works of God could not be vain, and as each monster had its own time, place and form, so too it had its own meaning. Monsters were evidence of underlying order and purpose in the world and far from being used by 'disorderly people', they were a means to regulate behaviour: claims that they were signs from God in response to human sinfulness reinforced the links between natural and human laws. The association of monsters with wars, price rises and transgressive behaviour should not obscure the fact that for protestant writers (who had an interest in preserving moral order) they were tools for the inculcation of obedience by showing that disorder in human affairs provoked the anger of God.

Perhaps the greatest change that took place in the early modern world view was a shift away from reading the works of nature as signs. The importance of signs was not simply religious (and still less superstitious); they were an essential part of the process of understanding the world. For mediaeval thinkers, '[t]o understand and explain anything consisted... in showing that it was not what it appeared to be, but that it was a symbol or sign of a more profound reality, that it proclaimed something else',[16] and the approach taken in sixteenth-century popular literature and wonder books, where meaning was more important than causation, was in continuity with mediaeval modes of thought: '[M]onstrous births might mean many things, but they could not be allowed to mean nothing.'[17]

One explanation of the decline in the importance of signs sees an increasing division between popular and learned culture; while lay people continued to see things as signs or warnings, learned authors looked for their causes, and so, it has been suggested, there was a change in the interpretation of monstrous births from a relationship of sign and signified to one of cause and effect.[18] According to Foucault, a conceptual 'discontinuity' occurred roughly halfway through the seventeenth century that changed the description of monsters along with the rest of nature:[19] the gap that opened up 'between things and words' meant that signs came to be seen not as part of things themselves, but as modes of representation. When words ceased to be part of the world (as they had been when Paracelsus treated the names of things as part of their signatures) and became tools or labels by means of which to describe the world, natural history became not a reading of signs but a meticulous examination of nature. Thus, Aldrovandi presented the symbolic meanings of animals as part of their description, whereas later naturalists such as Buffon did not. This new form of ordering, according to Foucault, created a new modern science of order and classification in which, for example, the cabinet of curiosities ceased to be a 'show' and became an organized 'table'.[20]

We have seen that sixteenth-century ballads and wonder books interpreted monsters as religious signs and emblems. Their readers were interested in them not merely as singular occurrences but also for their meaning: monsters had to be made sense of, and it was up to the authors to establish the connection between the sign and the thing signified.[21] If the scrutiny of monstrous births underwent a transformation from a reading of signs to a process of observation and description, this raises the question of why, when they were no longer important as signs, people continued to describe them in such numbers. Francis Bacon famously mentioned monsters among the things that should be recorded as part of the advancement of knowledge,[22] but it is doubtful whether natural philosophers actually proceeded to accumulate observations along these principles. Science has always tended to progress by the formulation of hypotheses and the gathering of data to substantiate or refute them, rather than by an open-minded Baconian accumulation of observations to no preconceived purpose. I suggest that seventeenth-century natural philosophers had a purpose in describing monstrous births and that their unstated hypothesis was that monsters, far from being the exceptional events of popular literature, fitted into a continuum as part of an orderly creation.

The concept of monsters as examples of plenitude was first explicitly stated towards the end of the sixteenth century. In his essay *On a Monstrous Child*[23] Montaigne interpreted the monster not as a warning from God but as evidence of the hidden complexity and orderliness of creation: 'Those which we call monsters are not so with God, who in the immensitie of his work seeth the infinite of formes therein contained.... From out his all-seeing wisdome proceedeth nothing but good, common, regular, and orderly; but we neither see the sorting, nor conceive the relation.'[24] It is possible to see this view of monsters as part of a creation that was 'good, common, regular and orderly' in the works of Catholic writers such as Liceti and Schott, whose books of monsters, with their orderly classifications, were microcosms of the great book of nature, a response perhaps to the apocalyptic associations of the monstrous promoted by some Protestants.[25] Classifications of monstrous births were not disinterested description but a response to theological preconceptions. Much seventeenth-century, and later, classification was 'anthropocentric', that it to say its aim was utility; for example, Aldrovandi's classification of birds in his *Ornithologia* gave prominence to the attributes that men found useful, so there were categories for birds that sing well and birds used in hunting, but the same cannot be said of classifications of monsters such as those of Liceti and Schott, where the utility of the monsters was not a consideration. One common feature with Aldrovandi – and with emblems – was that these classifications were not regarded as artificial constructs but were attempts to work out the pattern that underlay an apparent chaos of observations. Classification was a process of discovery, part of a quest for order, and monstrous births could not have been more apt subject matter: what could have been more evocative of the orderliness of creation than for it to contain a place for even these most rare and exceptional of happenings? The diversity of creation that was manifest in monstrous bodies glorified God because the more diverse the creation, the more admirable the creator.[26]

Whether they were signs of providence or of plenitude, monsters spoke of the existence of God, and they were a powerful argument against atheism. The natural philosopher that wished to defend a pantheistic world view had to account for monstrous births. In 1616, Julius Caesar (Lucilio) Vanini's controversial *De Admirandis Naturae Reginae, Deaeque Mortalium Arcanis* [On the Secrets of Nature, Queen and Goddess of Mortal Beings] was published in Paris. Vanini (*c.*1584–1619) was a one-time Carmelite friar who, after taking holy orders in 1603, received a doctorate in canon and civil law at the University of Naples three years later. He devoted his time to scholarship and began to explore radical ideas, developing a naturalistic philosophy in which nature and its immanent laws were the same as divine providence and the world was governed by a necessary natural order. He denied the existence of miracles and claimed that all apparently extraordinary phenomena could be shown to have natural causes.[27] This included monstrous births, which he attributed to one of six causes: vehement imagination during sexual intercourse, inordinate lust, parents who are too much alike, a defect or excess of semen, malformation of the feminine receptacle and the influence of the stars.[28] By classifying monsters as 'natural' occurrences, Vanini discounted them as evidence of divine intervention in the world, in keeping with his argument that nature was a mechanism that, once set in motion, ran itself without the need for further intervention. This highly controversial position was unacceptable to his ecclesiastical superiors and he lapsed into Protestantism: finding the reformed church equally unsympathetic he returned to Catholicism as a secular priest but continued to teach his heretical views and, largely on the basis of his books, was condemned for atheism at Toulouse in 1619. Vanini's *De Admirandis* and Liceti's *De Monstrorum* were published in the same year and both men were influenced by the works of Aristotle, for whom they professed a great admiration (Vanini called him 'the God of Philosophers').[29] Liceti was as interested in natural causes of monsters as was Vanini and by reasserting the classical and mediaeval idea of the monster as a mistake (*peccata naturae*) he too was effectively denying their use as evidence of a divine plan, a problem that he prudently evaded by philosophically setting aside from his discussion the role of God as 'sole, efficient Cause'[30] and confining his attention to 'lower' levels of causation (see Chapter 3, 81). While *De Admirandis* was, like its author, burned, *De Monstrorum* duly received an *imprimatur*.

The creator in his creatures

The anatomical description of monsters was no less theologically based than their interpretation as signs. The role of anatomy as a vehicle for theological study has been persuasively argued by Camporesi, who saw it as: 'an essential discipline for knowing man as the Son of God, and the divine image in humanity... used by Catholic intellectuals and the Church to underscore the most extraordinary miracle ever performed by divine power: the creation of man.'[31] The complexities that anatomists discovered were an important tool of the counter-reformation, which 'used anatomy as a kind of subtle instrument for the rediscovery of God';[32] part of 'an edifying and devout mission' to explore the works of God, whose 'bold bizarreness of invention' the human body was.[33] Calvinists also discovered signs of divine plenitude in nature, as testified in the Dutch anatomist Jan Swammerdam's (1637–80) dedication of his study of the anatomy of the louse: 'I present to you herewith the Almighty Finger of God in the anatomy of a louse; in which you will find wonder piled upon wonder and God's Wisdom clearly exposed in one minute particle'. The atheist, it was felt, would be converted by the miracle of creation that anatomy could reveal (astronomy flourished for the same reason) and it literally had the blessing of the Church: 'When each is in his appointed position', wrote Tomaso Garzoni (*c.*1549–89) in his *Piazza Universale* (1587),[34] 'let the anatomical operation commence in the name of the Lord.'

Protestant theology had required that emblems, if used at all, should be clear and unambiguous: there was no room for subtle symbolism or 'allegorical fancies' of the sort popular with Catholics and other 'abusers of the Scriptures'. In Protestant societies, 'curiosity' and the search for 'illicit' knowledge were more often seen as vices than virtues. Certain subjects – notably divination, magic and witchcraft – were always suspect,[35] and to be a legitimate area of interest monsters had to have a 'true' meaning. The truth could be 'hidden' but it was an agreeable surprise rather than a mystery 'which nature had kept unknowne from us (as it should seeme of set purpose)'.[36] The search for unambiguous meanings in monsters seems in retrospect to have encountered a central problem in Protestant theology: the book of nature, like the scriptures, could be interpreted in more than one way. The 'sacred mysteries' of the Catholic church made its clergy and laity much more comfortable with the idea of hidden knowledge than were

Protestants who criticised even the use of church Latin as magical 'hocus pocus', and counter-reformation scholars strove to establish a 'licit' tradition of ancient knowledge supposedly handed down since the time of Adam,[37] a counterpart of the body of unscriptural tradition that was essential to the Catholic church's teaching.

The search for hidden truths took Catholic natural philosophers into areas that some regarded as off limits. The young Neapolitan nobleman Giovanni Battista della Porta (1535–1615) formed a learned society called the *Accademia Secretorum Naturae*, which met in his home to perform experiments of the kind he described in *Natural Magick* (1558). Although he made a firm distinction between the magic of sorcerers and magic as studied by himself and his associates, which was 'nothing else but the survey of the whole course of nature... [that] openeth unto us the properties and qualities of hidden things',[38] (this was very much the approach taken by the Jesuit Caspar Schott over a century later: 'licit' magic was the search for hidden knowledge), he was nevertheless denounced to Pope Paul V in the 1570s for involvement in witchcraft and summoned to Rome to explain himself. He returned after being cautioned and told to disband his academy, but continued his work, later becoming vice president of the Academy of Lynxes (whose emblem came from the title page of the 1589 *Magiae Naturalis*). *Natural Magick* proved popular and was translated into French, Dutch, Spanish and Arabic within a few years of its first appearance (the quotations here are from an anonymous English translation of 1658). It included instructions for the generation of monsters: 'let us see the wayes of engendering such monsters, which the Ancients have set down, that the ingenious Reader may learn by the consideration of these wayes, to invent of himself other wayes how to generate wonderful monsters'.[39] Although it is arguable whether, at least with respect to monstrous births, Porta expected readers to attempt actual experiments rather than philosophical speculation (he did not include accounts of his own or his contemporaries' experiments, and the descriptions of how to make monsters were taken from classical sources; his comment on the story of Laban's sheep that 'such experiments might be practiced' does not suggest that he had tried them himself), he indicated to the reader that it was not necessary passively to await the action of providence: man could create monsters whose very existence glorified God.

Whether through the anatomist's exploration of the secrets of the body's microcosm, the traveller's discovery of what from a European perspective had been previously hidden worlds (a sixteenth-century map of Africa unfolded to reveal a land of monsters[40]), or the natural philosopher's experiments, there was a fascination in the early modern period with bringing secret things to light, of which the study of monsters was part, because in monsters: 'Nature... cannot avoid sometimes betraying its secret'.[41] Anatomy was a work of discovery, creative rather than destructive, and Christ could be compared to the anatomist: 'O sinner, here is Christ, he has become your anatomist'.[42] As both priest and victim, Christ's image was also found in the anatomised body: a crucifixion scene from Berengario de Carpi's (1521) commentary on the *Anathomia* of Mondino depicted a flayed and crucified anatomy, an *écorché* Christ, with every muscle displayed for our inspection.[43] The work of the anatomist, the exposure of each organ, muscle and vessel, the laying bare of secrets, the probing of that which lay concealed not only revealed the wonders of creation but was also a metaphor for the action of the creator, laying bare the heart of the sinner, on his creation.

The anatomical description of monstrous births flowered with the advent of scholarly journals. The level of detail achieved in the richest late-seventeenth-century source of natural philosophical observations of monstrous births, *Miscellanea Curiosa*, is comparable to that in much more recent publications.[44] In Chapter 4, some comparisons were made between reports of monstrous births in broadsides and in scholarly journals. A significant difference was the greater descriptive detail that journals supplied. The reasons for this were many: more print space, anatomically skilled observers, more detailed means of illustration, and less urgency to get into print. Detailed description also advertised the writers' university-acquired anatomical expertise. Autopsy reports spread over several pages with meticulous engravings offered unprecedented access to information for physicians who were unable to see a case for themselves, and formed an archive to which later scholars could refer. No single observer can expect to encounter all the different types of human birth defects, and the modern student of dysmorphology must rely on the study of case reports and museum specimens, a good example of the scientific value of accumulating units of knowledge, an activity beloved of seventeenth-century collectors and derided as 'stamp collecting' later on.[45] However, this use of material had not been anticipated in the seventeenth century; observers did not intend their accounts of monstrous births as a resource for future dysmorphologists and they must have had other reasons for collecting and describing them. Unlike eighteenth-century taxonomists, whose morphological classification systems encouraged detailed description, it is doubtful that seventeenth-century observers were prompted to record monstrous births in more detail in order to classify them: no contributor to a journal referred to a system of classification. Description of monsters was a means of creating order where for ballad writers there had been only 'a caios of confusion, a mixture of things without any discription.'[46] *Miscellanea Curiosa* is replete with references to monsters and other natural phenomena as the works of the creator and the process of collecting and ordering knowledge can be seen as part of the quest for God in the order of the natural world. Monsters were no longer presented as signs or emblems in isolation; it was, as in the books of natural philosophers, the cumulative effect of such natural variety in which the reader was to see the hand of the creator.

To look into a volume of *Miscellanea Curiosa* with its variety of human, animal, vegetable and mineral rarities is in some way to reproduce the experiences of visitors to contemporary cabinets of curiosities. Despite the important work that has been done on these cabinets in recent years, the actual experience that visitors had remains elusive; museums were, as their name suggested, supposed to be the home of the muses, but were their contents intended to convey specific meanings? The contents of cabinets of curiosities may have been meant to inspire a general sense of wonder, perhaps as much at the monetary and intellectual scope of the collector as in the works of the Creator but they could also be seen as a representation of the diversity of the natural world ('a world of wonders') that was capable of being ordered and of conveying a message. The emblem, old-fashioned on the printed page, had found a new form. The few examples of anatomical specimens from before the eighteenth century that survive in museums are the work of Ruysch, and these, along with illustrative evidence for some of his preparations that have now been lost, show him to have been an emblem-maker *par excellence* in the tradition of the moralizing pamphleteers of the sixteenth century. In his tableaux, foetuses bemoaned their lot, pondering symbols of the brevity of life such as bubbles and mayflies, and making music, that most transient of pleasures, on instruments formed of dried body parts, while lamenting: 'ah, fate! ah bitter fate!' To modern observers, such preparations might appear 'bizarre',[47] but Ruysch had a message. As a source of material, access to the bodies of infants recovered from the sea was invaluable to him, but to a medical man devoted to the improvement of midwifery this evidence of concealed births, abortions and infanticide must have been an unpleasant spectacle that suggested the need for a moral lesson. Ruysch's anatomical preparations allowed him to confront people with foetuses presented not as corpses but, just as ballads and wonder books had, as living people able to speak for themselves. The detailed anatomical descriptions of his tableaux run to 116 pages,[48] but like printed emblems each had an appended motto, such as 'homo bulla' or 'mundus lachrymarum vallis'. The tableaux, like his more conventional 'wet' preparations, were intended to instruct the viewer morally as well as anatomically (so-called *anatomie moralisée*)[49] and so to raise the status of the stillborn infant. In one preparation, the skull of a prostitute is kicked by the leg of an infant and in another a foetal skeleton pointing to a uterus bore the words: 'this noble tomb could not hide him'.[50]

The 'hidden' truth of monstrous births was made known by perhaps the commonest single phrase that occurs in accounts of them, from sixteenth-century broadsides to the earliest scholarly journals at the end of the seventeenth century: 'blessed be God in His works'. However, no phenomenon subjected to the attentions of so many observers over hundreds of years could retain its attributes of singularity and wonder. In the sixteenth century monstrous births were important historical events – Stow recorded them alongside wars, coronations and executions in the annals of Britain – but by the end of the seventeenth century, accounts of them were commonplace in medical literature, and they were the stock-in-trade of showmen. The reader who finds that the catalogue of monstrous births becomes tedious with constant repetition of types (see Appendix) may perhaps share something of the loss of wonder experienced by readers of Liceti or Schott, or of the journals of learned societies. Monsters classified, recorded and preserved in collections seem to lose their strangeness, that apparent originality on the part of their creator that first supplied the reason to study them. Collections of monsters could no longer pile wonder upon wonder: only so many malformations were possible. The reintroduction in the seventeenth century of the classical concept of monsters as slips of nature was inimical to their use as signs of divine intervention or of divine plenitude and eventually robbed them of their meaning. The special place of monstrous births as signs of God or as part of a creation 'good, common, regular and orderly' was overturned by the possibility that nature could make a mistake. Lazarus Colloredo, a man with a parasitic twin whose birth had been brought to the attention of Liceti (who correctly supposed that he would live a long time) and who led the life of a gentleman by the expedient of exhibiting himself throughout Europe,[51] was described in 1815 as 'this horrid error of nature',[52] a view that differs little from the popular view of birth defects today, but in 1637 he had been presented with a different message in the tradition of Montaigne: 'Admire the Creator in His Creatures'.[53]

Notes

1. T. Browne, *Religio Medici* (London: A. Crooke, 1642), part 1, section 15.
2. J. Barkar, *The True Description of a Monsterous Chylde...* (London: W. Gryffith, 1564).
3. *On Divination*, book II, ch. 27.
4. See A. Paré (ed. and transl. J.L. Pallister), *On Monsters and Marvels* (Chicago: University of Chicago Press, 1982), 41–2; Anon. *The Forme and Shape of a Monstrous Child...* (London: J. Awdeley, 1568); J.G. Schenck, *Observationum Medicarum Rariorum...* (Leyden: J.-A. Huguetan, 1644), 12; C.F. Paullin, 'Observationes Medico-Physicae, Selectae & Curiosae, Variis Antiquitatibus Historico-Germanicis Bonâ Fide Interdum Conspersae', *Miscellanea Curiosa*, series 2, vi (1687), appendix, 53–4, and Anon., *Briefz Discours d'un Merveilleux Monstre Né a Eusrigo...* (Chambéry: F. Poumard, 1578).
5. G. Lascault, *Le Monstre dans l'Art Occidental, Un Problème Esthétique* (Paris: Klincksieck, 1973).
6. B. Varchi (1548) cited in Z. Hanafi, *The Monster in the Machine...* (Durham: Duke University Press, 2000), 18, 21.
7. Romans 9: 21, a popular text in accounts on monstrous births, see Chapter 2, 54.
8. T. B[edford], *A True and Certain Relation of a Strange Birth...* (London: A. Griffin, 1635),10.
9. *Ibid.*, 12.
10. S. Batman, *The Doome Warning All Men to the Judgement...* (London: R. Nubery, 1581), fo. v r.
11. J. Moscoso, 'Monsters as Evidence: The Uses of the Abnormal Body During the Early Eighteenth Century', *Journal of the History of Biology*, xxxi (1998), 355–82.
12. The Romans, whose interest in monstrous births was as prodigies, showed a similar lack of concern over how they arose: J.P. Davies, *The Articulation of Roman Religion in the Latin Historians Livy, Tacitus and Ammianus Marcellinus* (PhD, University College London, 1999), 125.
13. L. Daston, 'Marvellous Facts and Miraculous Evidence in Early Modern Europe', in P.G. Platt (ed.), *Wonders, Marvels, and Monsters in Early Modern Culture* (Newark: University of Delaware Press, 1999), 76–104.
14. From the dedicatory epistle to Lycosthenes' *Chronicon*, quoted in L. Daston and K. Park, *Wonders and the Order of Nature, 1150–1750* (New York: Zone Books, 1998), 183.
15. H.B., *The True Discription of a Childe with Ruffes...*(London: J. Allde, 1566).
16. E. Gilson, quoted by A.C. Crombie, *Augustine to Galileo* (London: Heinemann Educational, 1979), 37.

17. D. Cressy, *Travesties and Transgressions in Tudor and Stuart England: Tales of Discord and Dissension* (Oxford: Oxford University Press, 2000), 36.

18. O. Niccoli (transl. L.G. Cochrane), *Prophecy and People in Renaissance Italy* (Princeton: Princeton University Press, 1990), 190; R. Hole, 'Incest, Consanguinity and a Monstrous Birth in Rural England, January 1600', *Social History*, xxv (2000), 183–99.

19. M. Foucault, *The Order of Things* (London and New York: Routledge, 1989), 129–30.

20. *Ibid.*, 129–31.

21. As it had been in the time of Livy; see Davies, *op. cit.* (note 12), 211.

22. Bacon, *Novum Organon*, book II, aphorism 8.

23. *D'un Enfant Monstrueux*, first published in 1580. The discussion quoted was added in the 1595 edition.

24. M. de Montaigne (transl J. Florio), *The Essays* (London: M. Bradwood, 1613).

25. D. Wilson, *Signs and Portents: Monstrous Births from the Middle Ages to The Enlightenment* (London: Routledge, 1993), 107, argues that Bacon's own assumption that separate phenomena could be fitted into a larger picture reveals his acceptance, perhaps unconsciously, of the doctrine of plenitude.

26. Originally a Platonic concept, '[t]he "best soul" could begrudge existence to nothing that could conceivably possess it'; see A.O. Lovejoy, *The Great Chain of Being: A Study of the History of an Idea* (Cambridge: Harvard University Press, 1936), 50.

27. Vanini had 'studied much' the writings of the physician Jerome Cardan, also a student of monstrous births, whose horoscope of Christ Vanini referred to as 'impious': J.C. Vanini (ed. P. Bayle), *The Life of L… Vanini…With an Abstract of his Writings…* (London: W. Meadows, 1730), 10, 45. Cardan was fortunate to escape with no more severe punishment than imprisonment from which patronage gained him early release.

28. J.C. Vanini, *De Admirandis Naturae Reginae…* (Paris: A. Perrier, 1616), quoted in L. Thorndike, *A History of Magic and Experimental Science* (New York: Columbia University Press, 1941), VI, 571, her translation.

29. Vanini, *op. cit.* (note 27), 10.

30. F. Liceti, *De Monstrorum…* (Padua: P. Frambott, 1634), 51–2.

31. P. Camporesi, *The Anatomy of the Senses* (Cambridge: Polity Press, 1994), 101.

32. *Ibid.*, 93.

33. G. Ciampoli, *Del Corpo Humano* (1676), quoted in Camporesi, *op. cit.* (note 31), 94.

34. *Ibid.*, 132.

35. P. Harrison, 'Curiosity, Forbidden Knowledge, and the Reformation of

Natural Philosophy in Early Modern England', *Isis*, xcii (2001), 265–90: 265, 275.

36. E. Fenton, *Certaine Secrete Wonders of Nature...* (London: H. Bynneman, 1569), sig. A2v.

37. See Chapter 3, 83.

38. J.B. Porta, *Natural Magick* (New York: Basic Books, 1957), 2. There are chapters on 'interspecies conception' and 'sundry copulations, whereby a man gender with sundry kinds of Beasts' in order to 'produce new and strange Monsters'. Z. Hanafi, *The Monster in the Machine...* (Durham: Duke University Press, 2000), 41–5, argues that *Natural Magick* was intended as a practical manual for experimentation. The artificial production of monsters (experimentally rather than the creation of 'fakes') is not convincingly documented until three centuries later, in the work of Dareste, who was among the first to develop techniques for the culture and manipulation of embryos: C. Dareste, 'Recherches Sur les Conditions Organiques Hes hétérotaxies', *Comptes Rendus des Séances de la Societe de Biologie et de ses Filiales*, series 3, i (1859), 8–11; *idem, Recherches sur la Production Artificielle des Monstruosités ou essais de tératogénie expérimentale* (Paris: C. Reinwald, 1877).

39. Hanafi, *op. cit.* (note 38), 41–5

40. P. Parker, *Shakespeare from the Margins: Language, Culture, Context* (Chicago: University of Chicago Press, 1996), 240–1.

41. B. de Fontenelle, *Histoire du Renouvellement de l'Académie Royale des Sciences...* (Amsterdam: P. de Coup, 1709), 11.

42. *Ibid.*, 117.

43. R. French, *Dissection and Vivisection in the European Renaissance* (Aldershot: Ashgate, 1999), 3.

44. For example the detailed osteological illustrations in M. Hofmann, 'Anatome Partus Cerebro Carentis', *Miscellanea Curiosa*, series 1, ii (1671), 60–4.

45. This derogatory term may have originated with the physicist Lord Rutherford, who described taxonomists as 'stamp collectors'. Luis Alvarez used the term to describe palaeontologists; see R.W. Purcell and S.J. Gould's *Finders, Keepers: Eight Collectors* (London: Pimlico, 1993), 46.

46. Anon., *Strange Newes out of Kent...* (London: T.C. for W. Barley, 1609).

47. M. Kidd and I.M. Modlin, 'Frederik Ruysch: Master Anatomist and Depictor of the Surreality of Death', *Journal of Medical Biography*, vii (1999), 69–77.

48. F. Ruysch, *Observationum Anatomico-Chirurgicarum Centuria...* (Amsterdam: H. and T. Boom, 1691).

49. T.H.L. Scheurleer, 'Early Dutch Cabinets of Curiosities', in O. Impey and A. Macgregor (eds), *The Origins of Museums: The Cabinet of Curiosities in*

Sixteenth- and Seventeenth-Century Europe (Oxford: Clarendon Press, 1985), 115–20.

50. *Nec poterat Tumulo nobiliore tegi*: Ruysch, *op. cit.* (note 48).

51. See C. Wallrich, *Disputatio Physica de Monstris quam Deo Juvante* (Wittenberg: J. Borckardt, 1655); J. Bondeson, *The Two-Headed Boy, and Other Medical Marvels* (Ithaca: Cornell University Press, 2000), viii–xix; Liceti, *op. cit.* (note 30), 114, 274; T. Bartholin, *Historiarum Anatomicarum Rariorum* (Amsterdam: J. Henrici, 1654), 117.

52. H.E. Rollins (ed.), *The Pack of Autolycus...* (Cambridge: Harvard University Press, 1927), 7.

53. M. Parker, *The Two Inseparable Brothers* (London: T. Lambert, 1637).

213

Appendix:
Human Monstrous Births, 1500–1700

1503

In Hessen [Germany] an infant very clearly of the female sex was born, entirely lacking ears, eyes and nose, having only a mouth in the face.[1]

Possibly holoprosencephaly.

1511a

Born near the town of Neuweiler (Germany), 11 May, two boys: 'sewn together like lovers'.[2]

Thoraco/omphalopagus conjoined twins joined from the xiphisternum downwards. The illustration shows female external genitalia and hairstyles, but the text refers to them as a boy. The illustration may have been re-used. The viscera were described as joined, but this could have been deduced from external appearances and does not necessarily indicate that an autopsy was performed.

1511b

Germany: a female double monster having two faces side by side, three arms and four legs.[3]

Probably cephalopagus tribrachius tetrapus conjoined twins. The location of the third arm, originating from the left side of the thorax, suggests that the woodcut – in which the twins are depicted alive and in a landscape – was derived from the text.

1512a

At Ravenna a monster was born which had a horn on the head, two wings, no arms, one foot like a bird of prey, an eye in the knee, ambiguous sex, in the middle of its chest epsilon and a cross portrayed. (Rueff)

[A] monster was seen to be born having a horn on its head, two wings, and a single foot similar to that of a bird of prey, at the knee joint an eye, and participating in the natures of both male and female. (Paré)

Earlier illustrations depict the monster as male but later ones show an hermaphrodite. Two lower limbs later become one (Figure 1.1).[4] A possible diagnosis was suggested by M.T. Walton *et al.*: 'It appears to be an example of the sirenomelia sequence: severe caudal "regression," fusion of the lower limbs, hydrocephalus with bulging of the anterior fontanelle, upper limb deficiencies, and pterygium'.[5]

1512b

Germany: female twins, drawn by Dürer, also shown in an anonymous drawing.[6]

Parapagus tetrabrachius dipus conjoined twins.

1513

A 13-year-old boy, seen in Florence: 'he had another creature coming out of his body, who had his head inside the boy's body, with his legs and his genitals and part of his body hanging outside.'[7]

Thoracopagus parasite.

1514a

A male child born at Colmar, Alsace: 'from its chest arose a complete human body, of the same sex with all its members complete, hanging down to the knees, only the head fixed into the body…'.[8]

Thoracopagus parasite.

1514b

Sarzana (Italy), 11 March:

> A two-headed child was born…. There is a considerable quantity of long, black hair on the heads. Between the heads arises the hand of the third arm, but it by no means exceeds the ears in length, neither is the whole thing visible. The rest of the body was well-formed and without any blemish.[9]

Parapagus tribrachius dipus conjoined twins.

1514c

A girl born in Bologna, January, having two 'orifices' in the face and four eyes: 'Cardinal de Grassis then Bishop of Bononia made atonement to heaven, and called her Mary, and she lived for four days.'[10]

Diprosopus twins.

1514d

A female child born on 10 May 1514 at Bologna: 'The eyes and nose were utterly absent, relates Cornelius Gemma in his *Cosmocritice* [Anvers, 1575] his informant was a girl of low birth from Bologna near St. Peter's church, where it received the sacrament of baptism'.[11]

Possibly holoprosencephaly.

1516a

In Germany was seen a proper man, who had another head protruding from the umbilicus and which, in the fashion of this world, actually took food. Jacob Rueff related this. (Liceti)

...he lived to be an adult; and the head took nourishment just like the other. (Paré)[12]

Possibly omphalopagus parasite. A similar case is described by Du Plessis (see below, 1678). More recently Biswas, *et al.* described a 'spherical' umbilical swelling with 'facial features'.[13]

1516b

Born at Tettnang, Germany, 8 April, a baby girl with a supernumerary, well-formed lower limb. The child died after 9 days.[14]

Omphalopagus parasite.

1517a

...in the parish of Bois-le-Roy, in the Forest of Bière, on the road to Fontainebleau, a child was born having the face of a frog, who was seen and visited by Master Jean Bellanger, a surgeon in the company of the King's Artillery, in the presence of gentlemen from the court of Harmois: notably the Honorable gentleman Jacques Bribon. (Paré)[15]

Anencephaly.

1517b

Twins born at Landshut, Bavaria, with two heads, three arms and two legs. The shared arm was fused and pointed upwards. There was a single umbilicus. The external genitalia are not clearly shown.[16]

Parapagus tribrachius dipus conjoined twins.

1519

An hermaphrodite or androgyne was born at Zürich. Above the umbilicus was an extraordinary arrangement: there was a red fleshy mass around the umbilicus, beneath which was the female member, and beneath this, next to it, the male member. (Rueff)[17]

A male with exstrophic bladder.

1523a

A monster born at Lüneburg near Hamburg:

> [H]ad a human face, a long stretched out nose, the crown of the head was smooth and hairless like a monastic tonsure, with a circlet or crown as of a monk, and the neck of a crane. It had normal human arms, legs, feet and hands, a round, swollen belly; the arms were furnished with wings, and the legs were feathered....[18]

1523b

Germany: an anonymous broadside showing an infant with hydrocephalus (perhaps not congenital).[19]

1525

'Another at Wittenberg without a head.'[20]
Anencephalic.

1528

> Later a girl appeared elsewhere, who was entirely deprived of arms, the rest of the body very well formed. Her feet, by means of which she had thrived for many years, she used instead of hands, and marvellously well. (Liceti)[21]

Upper limb amelia.

1529a

> [In] the Mittelberg region of Germany a child was born, and in appearance and stature grew up as a man, the whole body having the proper form and shape of a man, except that it had from its breast another body hanging down, without head and arms, the forearms stretched out, hands like feet that had been shaped into hands.... (Rueff)

[A] little body with all its members hung down from the chest to the knees – only the head was in the other's body. This monster travelled all over the world. (Liceti)[22]

Thoracopagus parasite.

1529b

On 9 January at Esselingen, Germany: '...a child was seen with one head, four ears, four arms, and four legs and feet.' (Schott)[23]
Probably cephalothoracopagus conjoined twins.

1530a

A child born at Freiburg 'of horrific aspect... in the frontal and occipital areas were masses of hard flesh sticking out'.[24]
Possibly encephalocoele.

1530b

At Valencia, a man aged about forty years: '...out of whose bellie issued another man, all whole, reserving the head.' He carried the body in his arms and 'great troupes' came to see him. (Fenton)

[It] was said that he was the child of some fallen woman, who had prostituted herself to all and sundry. (Boaistuau)[25]

Thoracopagus parasite.

1531a

Born 26 August at Gossau, near Zürich, Switzerland: 'a monsterous Childe... with two heads, three armes, and so many feet.'[26]
Parapagus tribrachius tripus conjoined twins.

1531b

Augsburg, Germany: 'a woman gave birth first to a human head wrapped in membranes, second to a two-footed serpent, which had the head of a pike, the body and feet of a frog and the tail of a lizard, and thirdly a pig with all its parts complete.'[27]

1534

Born at (Bad) Sackingen, near Basel, twins 'joined laterally, who because of the mother's excessively protracted labour were pressed together at the beginning of life'.[28]

1535

'[In] the Brandenburg district, there was born a child whose body was wrapped with a mass of loose flesh, like a German military cloak…'.[29]

1536a

Born not far from Tegernsee, Germany 'a Chylde… with one bodye, two heades, three handes and three feete.'[30]

    Parapagus tribrachius tripus conjoined twins.

1536b

Born 30 August, Sicily: 'an infant having three heads, three chests, six arms, and the same number of feet was born… this monster had three souls in its breast, as the three hearts suggested'.[31]

    ?Conjoined triplets.

1536c

At Florence:

> [W]ere two females joyned and stuck together, one toward the other in such a way that half the chest of one along with that of the other made up a single chest, & thus they formed two chests, one joining up with the other; their backs were not shared, but each had its own: it had its head turned directly towards one of the two chests, & on the other side, in the place of the face it had two ears that were joined one to the other, & they touched….

> [They were dissected:] They found two hearts, two livers, & two lungs, & finally everything was doubled, just as for two bodies, but the windpipes, which began at the [level of the] heart, joyned up near the entrance to the throat and became one.[32]

Cephalothoracopagus janiceps asymmetros conjoined twins.

1537

In the village of 'Nepritz' near Wurzen on the Mulde 'an infant was born without feet'.[33]

1538a

'There was one borne, and grew to the perfect stature of man having two heades and foure shoulders, so that one heade was before, the other behinde, of a wonderful likenesse one to another'.[34]

    Parapagus tetrabrachius dipus conjoined twins.

1538b

I [Lycosthenes] saw also the like monster in Bavaria, the yere of Christ 1541 it was a woman of five and twentie yeares of age with two heades, one of which notwithstanding was very deformed: when she got her living by begging from doore to dore, she was commaunded (by reason of women with child) to departe out of the Countrey, in giving her money to paye hir charges. (Batman)

She lived to the age of twenty-five years 'which is not natural for monsters, who ordinarily live scarcely any length of time at all because they grow displeased and melancholy at seeing themselves so repugnant to everyone'. (Paré)[35]

Craniopagus parasiticus conjoined twins.

1540a

Hessen, Germany, 9 January: 'a childe was borne... with two heads turned towards the backe, whole faces standing one against the other, behelde eache other with a threatening countenaunce.'[36]

Diprosopus twins.

1540b

A boy born at Ferrara, Italy on 19 March, after a gestation of three months:

[A]s big and well-formed as if he were four months old, having both feminine and masculine sexual organs, and two heads, the one of a male and the other of a female. (Paré)

Secondarily, he had two faire heades well proportioned, and two faces joyned one to an other... and betwene the two heades, he had a thirde heade, whiche exceeded not the length of an eare.... [After he died] he was made a present to one of the kyng of Spaynes lieutenants, gouverning that countrey, so he thoughte it good to have him ripped and his bellie opened, and intrailes seen, which being done... he had two livers, two milts, and but one heart.... (Fenton)[37]

Cephalothoracopagus janiceps asymmetros conjoined twins.

1541a

A weaver's wife in St Francis Street, Freiburg:

[B]roughte forth a twin, joined together in the foreparts of the bodye, and imbracing one the other, the ninteenth of the Calendes of Februarie [14

221

January], There followed a sodaine cheapnesse of corne upon a great dearth. (Batman)[38]

Thoraco/omphalopagus conjoined twins.

1541b

In the Dukedom of Wittenberg 'there was borne a twinne having their bodies knit together as far as the Navil'.[39]

Thoraco/omphalopagus conjoined twins.

1542a

In Pilsen (Czech Republic):

A child was born who was the image of Christ our Saviour crucified, as when the Blessed Virgin held him at the deposition from the Cross: the feet were bent inwards one over the other, and if moved they immediately sprang back to their place, and the neck was also bent, so that it was difficult to put food in the mouth. For a time it lived in Vienna, Austria.[40]

Possibly arthrogryposis.

1542b

Germany: an anonymous broadside showing male parapagus dicephalus dibrachius dipus twins.[41]

1543a

[T]wo infants were born, joined laterally, with two heads, four arms and the same number of legs, a single umbilicus and of the female sex; of these one died at birth, the other lived for a while and presently died. (Rueff)

The eight of the Ides of Februarie [6 February] at five a clocke in the morning at Caffehuse [Schaffhausen] in Switzerland two women children were borne with two heds, foure armes, and so manye feete severall, but with one massie or whole bodye from the necke to the Navil, the string of the Navil hanging downe underneath. (Batman)[42]

Thoracopagus conjoined twins.

1543b

In the village of Rinach [Reinach] not far from Basil [Basel] a woman brought forth a twin, having both bodyes joined together over the Navil, with 4 armes, yet from the loynes he had two feete, he was a male, heis

222

trimely set out by Sebastian Munster in his Cosmography, from whence also Stomphius hath taken him into his worke of Chronicles.[43]

Parapagus tetrabrachius dipus conjoined twins.

1544a

Born in January in Milan, a female child with two heads, two breasts, four hands, two thighs, two feet, one belly; one body from the navel downwards, 'well formed' and 'corpulent', which died at birth. The surgeon Gabriel Cuneus made an anatomy:

> [H]e found a double wombe, all the intestines double... two livers, and so almost all the other partes, reserving the heart, which was single: the which moveth us to think (sayth Cardan) that Nature wold haue created two, saving that by some defecte she imperfected the whole. (Fenton)[44]

Parapagus tetrabrachius dipus conjoined twins.

1544b

At He[i]delberg standing by the river Neccarus [Neckar], on Whitson Sonday was borne two boyes joyned together, having two bodies closed by the belly part, two heades, foure handes and feete, whose mother was called Catherine: and Gasper Besler sayth they were christened, one called John and the other Jerome and lived a day and a halfe: when they were dead they found in the belly but one hart. (Batman)[45]

Thoracopagus rather than omphalopagus – the former usually have a common heart.[46]

1544c

The fift of the Kalends of September [28 August], at Strausburg [Strasbourg] the mother Citie of Alsatia, there was borne a woman childe with a horrible and monstrous heade, and wide open in the uppermost part, with a brode mouth, with Oxe eyes, and Eagles nostrils. (Batman)[47]

Anencephalic.

1545a

In Saxony in the moneth of Februarie a childe was born with a grisly looke, having a whole body and well compacte, but all his limes were brused, torne and loose, saving that his head was copped like a Sugerlofe, and as it were set out with a Turkish cap. (Batman)[48]

Possibly macerated, with moulding of the head.

1545b

In Acken [Achern] a towne of Saxony by the river Albis two children were seene… together by their hippes on one side, where the Hippes are fastened to the huckle bone in such sort that the right arme overcompasseth the left, as if they had embraced ech other. (Batman)[49]

Pygopagus with posterolateral union. The huckle bone may mean either the ischium or the whole innominate bone.

1546a

At Ploa [Plön] a towne of Witlande a monstrous childe was borne, for in him appeared neither back nor belly, saving that his entrails about his Brest hong farre down, he bent his feete towards his heade, he had his nauill in the hamme of the lefte legge, and he hadde a pointed head like a Sugerlofe.'(Batman)[50]

Probably macerated.

1546b

Paris:

[A] woman who was six months pregnant gave birth to a child having two heads, two arms, and four legs, which I opened; and I found inside it only one heart (which monster is in my house and I keep it as a monstrous thing), as a result of which one can say that it is only one child.[51]

Thoracopagus conjoined twins.

1547a

Born at Louvain, Maunday Thursday (7 April); twins, depicted as one male, one female: 'with two bodies under one head, four arms, four legs and with two hearts'.[52]

At Lovaine the 7 of the Ides of Aprill a twin was borne, having two severall bodies, but joyned together in one heade: of these maketh mention Gaspar Pucerus. (Batman)[53]

Cephalopagus conjoined twins.

1547b

On the feast of the conversion of St Paul (25 January):

> At Kraków a very curious monster was born, and lived for three days: the head was not unlike that of a human, but it had blazing eyes and a long, hooked nose like a flute. At the joints of its members, the elbors and knees, heads stood out resembling a dog, the hands and feet were like those of a goose, two eyes above the umbilicus. A tail an ell long curled back at the end like a fishhook. The sex was male. It is said that this monster was caused of God's making; nonetheless, through the sin of Sodomy, this detestable monster was of our own making [it lived for four hours and spoke thus]: 'Watch! For the Lord our God comes.' (Rueff)

> In Flanders upō the day of the conversion of S. Paule, (although there is some which write at Cracovie) there was borne a childe of honest and gentle parentes, verye hedious and horrible to behold, with flaming and sparkling eyes, having a mouth and Nostrels standing out with the forme of a horn, a back rough with dogs haires, Apes faces appearing in his breastes where his dugges should stand, Cats eyes under the navel, cruel, and currish dogs heades at both elbowes and knees, looking foreward, the forme of To[a]d[e]s feete, a tayle bending upward and turning againe crooked at the end an ell long: he is said to have lived foure houres after he was borne, and at length (after he had uttered these wordes, Vigilate, dominus deus vester adventat, that is, Watche, youre Lorde is a coming) to have dyed. Gasperus Pucer and Munster in his Cosmography. (Batman)[54]

Multiple congenital malformations.

1548a

> The 18 of the Kalendes of Maye [14 April] betweene sixe and seven a clock, at Mysena [Meißen], a childe was borne with the skul devided in the forehead, wt. one thigh, without lippes, having in the place of his mouth a little hole, and maimed in the reste of his bodye.' (Batman)[55]

The division of the skull suggests amniotic bands, and possible maceration. The illustration shows a siren with absent upper limbs.

1548b

Germany: a male child having the head divided from the body, one lower limb only, and no upper limbs; attributed to 'want or default in the seede'.[56]

1550a

Modena: An embalmed male baby with 'two child's faces, and for the rest a single body, very beautiful to see'.[57]

Diprosopus.

1550b

The third of August in the Dominion of the Abot of Urcium in the village of Rieden, 3 miles from Knafburin in Swedon, a Smith's wife brought forth a twin in all parts perfite, but joyned together in the bellye as far as the neck, which after they were borne, were longer than three quarters of the Sweadon elle.[58]

Thoracopagus conjoined twins.

1550c

In the Lordship or Domynyon of the prince Elector, in the day of the visitation of Mary [2 July] in the Village of Zelliu, a woman Childe was borne monstrous to behold withoute eyes and eares having a broade and open mouth, a bodye torne and wounded everye where, in many of his members like to one that were fleane [flayed]. (Batman)[59]

Macerated, perhaps an intra-uterine death due to holoprosencephaly.

1551a

At Damenwald a manour house in Marchia near Wodstocke a farmers wife brought forth a monster which Fincelius discribeth. Al the childs body was of a bright Bay, his heade had hornes, his eyes were greate and hanging out, he had no nose, his mouth broade a span long, amid whiche appeared a white tong and foure square, he had no neck, for his head grew close to hys shoulders, all his body was puffed up, and full of wrinckles, hys armes did sticke in his loynes, his feete were slender, and from his Navill there hung down to his feete a kinde of loose bowel. (Batman)[60]

Macerated: a span is some twenty centimetres, the crown-heel length of a nineteen-week gestation foetus. The reddish-brown colour, abdominal wall defect and skin slippage suggest intra-uterine death of several days' standing.

1551b

Pfedelbach, Germany, February:

[T]his monster was born of a sheapheardes wife, a boy without a mannes face, in place thereof he had smooth fleshe, saving that he had two great eyes unlike one the other standing out, not placed in the holes, horrible to beholde: in the place of his forehead, a point of flesh hanging out which stoode upright... neither was he christned, but forthwith buried.'[61]

Holoprosencephaly.

1551c

Breslau (Poland), December, a woman delivered:

[A] mass of living flesh the upper end of which terminated in a huge mouth like that of a tench. It wriggled about for some moments and then it perished like a fish out of water.[62]

Fetus amorphus.

1552a

The thirde of August, was borne a marvelous straunge Monster, At a place called Middleton eleaven miles from Oxford a woman brought forth a chlde, which had two perfecte bodies from the Navill upwarde, and were joined togither at the Navill, that when they were layde in length, the one heade and bodye was Eastward, and the other weaste, the legges for bothe bodyes grewe out at the middest where the bodies joined, and had but one issue for the excrement of both the bodies: they lived eighteen dayes, and when they were opened, it appeared they were women children. (Batman)

In England, not far from Oxford, we are informed that a certain birth occurred with two heads, four arms and hands, one belly and a single set of female genitals. From one side two feet came out sideways, and from the other side, a single, or more correctly a double foot, having ten digits. At the second hour of the fifteenth day first one then the other died. They had rarely cried. One had a cheerful demeanour, while the other was sleepy and sad. The twenty transverse digits were the same length and breadth precisely. (Rueff)

They were baptised John and Joanne.[63]
Thoracopagus conjoined twins.

1552b

Born at Windensbach near Schlensing, Germany, a monster:

[L]ike a childe, without feete, in a place whereof it had a poynte coming downwarde, and from the thyghs also, it had sharpe poynts standing out. (Batman)[64]

Sirenomelia.

1552c

A child born at Witzenhausen, Hessen, Germany, the third day after the feast of the Three Kings (9 January) with two heads and necks, the rest complete.[65]

Parapagus dibrachius dipus conjoined twins.

1553a

At Luneberg [Germany] a chylde was borne with awrie mouth, from whence came a cloven or double tong, the like monster was borne the yeare before. (Batman)[66]

1553b

At Herbesleb [Herbsleben, Germany]… the twentith of Marche, a twinne was borne with throe [*sic*] bellies together, and as it were bounde in one with a fleshye swadlebande imbracing one another aboute the myddle. They were Christened and two houres after gave uppe theyr Ghoste to God. (Batman)[67]

Possibly thoraco/omphalopagus conjoined twins.

1553c

19 June at Zichist, in Meißen: 'a Child was borne with two heads, having all his lims perfect.' (Batman)[68]

Parapagus dibrachius dipus conjoined twins.

1554a

At Stetin [Szczecin, Poland] a Monster was borne having thys forme: in the place of his head was a deformed lumpe moveable, as the entrails of a sheepe, in the place of one of his eares stoode an arme, in the place of the face, curled locks like to Cattes haire, and sticking thereon like the spaune of a Pike, throughe which beneath there appeared glassie brighte little eyes, his mouthe was a very smal hole without lippes, his nose little, and without a necke: the other arme grew out of his side, but ther was no likenesse of breast nor of backe, he was of no kind, his armes and long feete had house [hoofs], whole bone through, without ioyntes, elbowes, and hams, his handes and feete tender, and hanging down as it were twice brocken, like unto crooked and bending clawes. This monster describeth Iob Fincelius. (Batman)

[H]e had a great mass of flesh in place of a head, and where one of his ears should have been, came out an arm and a hand. He had upon his face writhen hairs like the whiskers of a cat. The other arm appeared out of one side. Neither the body nor the back was properly formed, and there was a line along his back. There could not be discerned any or either sex, the arms and legs consisted of a single bone without joints, knees, or elbows. The hands and feet were soft and hung down as if they were broken, like the curved claws of an otter. His mother gave birth to him dead, although he had lived in the womb. (Liceti)[69]

1554b

At Meißen: 'a chyld was borne without a head, having the forme of eyes standing in his brest.'[70]

A traditional Blemmye, possibly corresponding to iniencephaly.

1555a

At Geneva, a monster: 'utriusque generis, and that of the one side a male and the other a female'. Two faces 'as... Janus hadde', 'two greate pocketts hangyng upon hys backe, wherein were hys bowelles'. 'Also he was so huge above order, that it was impossible to draw him whole from the bellie of his mother.' (Fenton)

[T]he thighs which were apart were broken and pulled from the Mother when she was in travaile. (Batman)

Conrad Lycosthenes wrote, that in Geneva there was born a monster like the one shown here to a certain woman from Gaul living in Geneva. This monster was evidence of a lack of material: it had two faces; that is to say, like Janus was painted in olden times: on both sides the skin ballooned out, the intestines were protruding from the back, and also from the lower part of the belly hung down the liver, prolapsed through the vulva. This monster was of both sexes: on the right it was a man and on the left it was a woman. The painter Gaspar Maserius, who saw it along with many other people, made a picture of it from life. (Liceti)

As a matter of fact the painter Gaspar Masserius, who had arrived along with many other people, made a careful pencil drawing of the whole thing. (Aldrovandi)[71]

Cephalothoracopagus janiceps conjoined twins (Figure 6.2).

1555b

Born 27 September: 'in Freywerk [Freiburg], a town near Vogtland was born an infant with two heads… the sex was indifferent… its mother was the wife of a blacksmith'. (Liceti)[72]

Thoracopagus conjoined twins.

1556a

Leipzig:

> [A] chylde was borne with two heades, 4 hands, and so many feete but with one body alone' (Batman); 'utroque sexu' [Sexually indifferent]. (Liceti)[73]

Thoraco/omphalopagus conjoined twins.

1556b

At Basill [Basel] a Boye was borne hideous to beholde, having a bodye well enough compacte, but he had a rough hearye heade, more like unto a Dogge, a Catte, or an Ape, than a manne, he lived aboute an houre and a halfe. (Batman)[74]

Possibly anencephaly.

1556c

'At Basill was seene a man having on both handes five fingers.' (Batman)[75]

Polydactyly.

1556d

The firste daye of November at Tundorfe [Tundorf, Czech Republic], aboute foure a clocke in the Morning a potters wife was delivered of a horrible Monster: from the crowne of the head to the midrife, he was like a man but his mouth stoode out like a dogges, he hadde a frowning face, but from the Navill downwarde, he was destitute of the other partes of mannes bodye, he descended downwarde in forme of Piramides, in the poynte having the likenesse of the wrinckled tail of a Sowe, but on his backe bone there was the forme of a Navill standing out as it were a Tayle: the sexe of this monster did not appeare.[76]

Sirenomelia. The structure resembling a tail is probably a rudimentary penis:[77] the mouth like a dog could be an anteriorly displaced bilateral cleft lip.[78]

1556e

Born at Basel, 4 December, a male child:

> [W]ithoute anye eares, in whose place he had onelye two holes, whiche notwithstanding were so shutte uppe, that he could heare nothing, the Chylde lived sickelye till the moneth of August, at whose beginning he dyed with many griefes. (Batman)[79]

Absent pinnae and atresia of the ear canals is unusual as an isolated phenomenon.

1557a

> At Basill [Basel] about the feast of Easter a childe was borne with suche cloven and open Nostrels, that his braine was very easily sene from thence. (Batman)[80]

Probably severe facial clefts.

1557b

> The seventh of the Ides of August [7 August], with us at Basil [Basel], a man chylde was borne with a bodye well enough framed or compact, but withoute a necke, having his eyes of no common greatnesse, as they were placed in his foreheade, and he wanted the uppermoste parte of his heade: behinde his heade he hadde a bigge hole, out of the which hole there ran oute some blood, whereupon immediatelye after he was borne, he ended his life.'(Batman)[81]

Anencephalic.

1560

A double monster, born 21 April, shown in an anonymous German broadside.[82]

Possibly cephalothoracopagus janiceps.

1561a

Johannes Wynistorff and Magdalene Rudolfs of Stockholm, both without arms, were shown in broadsides of this date performing a variety of tasks with their feet.[83]

1561b

A child born in July: 'On each foot there were seven digits (the great toe, for instance, was double on each foot). On each hand there were six digits'. (Schenck)[84]

1561c

Germany: an anonymous broadside showing a male infant with ears like those of an animal, limb deformities and a hole in the suprapubic area.[85]

1562a

Born 24 May at Chichester:

> The father hereof is one Vyncent, a boutcher, bothe he and hys wife being of honest quiet conversation. They having had children before, in natural proportion: and went with this her full tyme. (Jhon D)

> ...the heade, armes, and legs, like unto an Anatomy the brest and belly monstrous bigge, from the Navil, as it were along string hanging about the necke, a greate coller of fleshe and skinne growing like to the ruffe of a shirt or neckercheffe coming up aboute the eares playting or foulding. (Batman)[86]

A morphologically normal macerated male infant. Drawn actual size, so some seventeen weeks gestation, and as she went to her full time the child had been dead for more than twenty weeks.

1562b

Born 1 November at in Villefranche-du-Queyran in the department of Lot-et-Garonne[87] in Gascony, a monster without a head. The illustration was given to Paré by Monsieur Hautin (Johannes Altinus), doctor of the faculty of medicine in Paris.

> Ambroise Pare acknowledges that in the town of Franca in Vasconia there was a girl without a head, having ears behind her shoulder-blades, a nose between them on her spine resembling a little proboscis, eyes in her shoulders, looking backwards, and a strange, high, tongue where the throat ought to have been, a portrait of which monster came from Fontano Agenesi, physician, who himself will dogmatically claim to have seen it. (Liceti)

Schenck described the same case from an illustration:

> [A]round the neck region was a subcutaneous swelling. At the rear of the body was a single rudimentary stalk like a nipple, coming out from the spiral line [it is unclear what structure is meant here], and depending from the

middle of the rostral end was something not unlike a copy of an elephant's curved proboscis... the head was entirely absent.

Probably anencephaly. The description is a typical 'blemmye' and probably stereotypical.[88]

1562c

On Tuysday being the xxi day of Apryll, in this yeare of our Lorde God [1562], there was borne a man-childe of this maymed forme at Muche Horkesley in Essex, a village about thre myles from Colchester, betwene a naturall father and a naturall mother, having neither hande, foote, legge, nor arme, but on the left syde it hath a stumpe growynge out of the shoulder, and the end thereof is rounde, and not so long as it should go to the elbowe; and on the right syde no mencion of any thing where the arm should be, but a litel stumpe of one ynche in length; also on the left buttocke there is a stumpe coming out of the length of the thygh almost to the knee, and rounde at the ende, and groweth something overthwart towardes the place where the right legge should be, that is no mencion of anye legge or stumpe. Also it hath a codde and stones, but no yearde, but a lytell hole for water to issue out. Finallye, it hath by estimation no tongue, by reason whereof it sucketh not, but is succoured wyth liquide substance put into the mouth by droppes, and nowe begynneth to feede wyth pappe, beyng very well favoured, and of good and chearefull face.

The aforesayde Anthony Smyth of Much Horkesley, husbandman, and his wyfe, were both maryed to others before, and have dyvers chyldren, but this deformed childe is the fyrst that the sayd Anthony and his wyfe had betweene them two; it is a man chylde. This chylde was begot out of matrimony, but borne in matrimonye; and at the making hereof was living, and like to continue.[89]

Tetradysmelia, absent penis and 'absent' (short?) tongue. Anderson made a diagnosis of Hanhart complex (oromandibular limb hypogenesis).[90]

1563

Born at Strasbourg; male twins joined at their heads posteriorly. An illustration shows them alive.[91]

Craniopagus.

1564

Born on the Isle of Wight, October, a monster 'with a cluster of long heare about the Navell, the fathers name is James Johnsun, in the parys of Freswater.'

> No caruer can, nor paynter then,
> The shape more ugly make,
> As itselfe dothe declare the truthe;
> A syghte to make vs quake![92]

Fetus amorphus (Figure 2.2).

1565a

Stony Stratford, Northamptonshire:

> This childe was borne on Fryday, being the xxvi daye of January, betwixt vi and vii of the clocke in the morninge, and lyved two howres, and was christened by the Mydwyfe, and are both Women Chyldren, having two bodies, joining togither. With iiii armes, and iiii legges perfecte, & from the Navell upward one Face, two Eyes, one Nose, and one Mouth, and three Eares, one beinge upon the backe side of the Head, a little above the nape of the Necke, having heare growynge upon the Head. Whyche Chylde was borne out of Wedlocke. The Fathers name is Rychard Sotherne, who is now fled And the Mother is yet lyvying in the same Towne. And this Childe was brought up to London, wheare it was seene of dyvers worshipfull men and women of the Cytie. And also of the Countrey.[93]

Cephalothoracopagus janiceps asymmetros conjoined twins.

1565b

Born at Herne in Kent. Two monstrous children of unspecified type.[94]

1565c

Born at Schmelz, 16 May 1565, a 'headless' infant; 'he had a mouth on the left shoulder and an ear on the right shoulder, his skin was black and his body without bones.'[95]

Blemmye (traditional).

1565d

Germany: an anonymous broadside showing parapagus tribrachius dipus twins.[96]

1566a

Born at Swanburne, Buckinghamshire, 4 April 1566:

[T]wo children having both their belies fast joined together, and imbracyng one an other with their armes: which children wer both a lyve by the space of half an hower, and wer baptized, and named the one John, and the other Joan.[97]

Thoracopagus conjoined twins (Figure 2.1).

1566b

Born at Micheham, Surrey, a child with:

[F]leshy skin behinde like unto a neckerchef growing from the veines of the back up unto the neck, as it were with many ruffes set one after another, and beeing as it were something gathered, every ruf about an inch brode, having here growing on the edges of the same, and so with ruffes coming over the shoulders and covering some part of the armes, proceding up unto the nape of the neck behinde, and almoste round about the neck, like a many womens gownes be.[98]

The illustration does not resemble skin slippage occurring owing to maceration. It may be an example of gyrate skin, a congenital anomaly typically involving the vertex of the skull,[99] but it must be admitted that this explanation is perhaps a little far fetched. Another possibility, suggested to me by Dr Elizabeth Gray, is cystic hygroma.

1566c

An adult male with a parasitic twin fused at the xiphisternum, complete except for the head.[100]

1566d

Germany: an anonymous broadside showing a male anencephalic.[101]

1567

[B]etweene Antwerpe[n] and Macline [Mechelen], in a village called Ubalen, a Chylde was borne whiche hadde two heades and four armes: it seemed two maydes joined togither and yet hadde but two legges.[102]

Parapagus tetrabrachius dipus conjoined twins.

1568a

'[At] Arles, was a strange child hairy, having the Navill where the nose should stande, and his eyes in the place of the mouth in the chinne.' The mother was one Jeanne Verdiere, the father Pierre Conlion, a tailor. (Batman)

[It] wandered besides thorow Fraunce... betweene the which [eyes] was a certaine opening: hys eares stode on either side the chinne, and his mouthe at the ende of the same. (Fenton)[103]

Cyclopia (lanugo hair?).

1568b

At Maydstone in Kent there was one Marget Mere, daughter to Richard Mere, of the sayd towne of Maydstone, who, being unmaryed, played the naughty packe, and was gotten with childe, being delivered of the same childe the xxiiij daye of October last past, in the yeare of our Lorde 1568, at vij of the clocke in the afternoone... which child, being a man-child, had first the mouth slitted on the right side, like a libardes mouth, terrible to beholde, the left arme lying upon the brest, fast thereto joyned, having as it were stumps on the handes, the left leg growing upward toward the head, and the ryght leg bending toward the left leg, the foote thereof growing into the buttocke of the sayd left leg. In the middest of the back there was a broade lump of flesh, in fashion like a rose, in the myddest whereof was a hole, which voyded like an issue. The sayd childe was borne alyve, and lyved xxiiij howres, and then departed this lyfe, – which may be a terror as well to all such workers of filthiness and iniquity.[104]

There are features of arthrogryposis multiplex congenita or Larsen syndrome,[105] although Trisomy 13 would be a more commonly occurring alternative (Figure 2.4).[106]

1569a

Born at Tours:

[T]win children having only one head, which were embracing each other; and they were given to me dry and dissected by master René Ciret, master barber and surgeon, whose renown is widespread enough throughout the country of Touraine... (These last two monsters are in the possession of the author). (Paré)

[O]ne heart was found. (Liceti)

Cephalothoracopagus conjoined twins. It is noteworthy that even after dissection (and presumably without having been reconstructed) the specimen was a valuable addition to Paré's collection.[107]

1569b

Germany: an anonymous broadside showing an infant with a swelling in front of the head.

Possibly teratoma/frontal encephalocoele.[108]

1569c

Born Germany, 10 June: female thoraco/omphalopagus twins.[109]

1570a

In Germany, conjoined twins, with ten toes on the shared foot: 'two children fused at the perineum and buttocks, with a common umbilicus.'[110]

Ischiopagus tripus.

1570b

Born in Paris, 20 July, Rue des Gravelliers, at the sign of the Bell:

> They were noted by the surgeons to be male and female and were baptized at St. Nicholas des Champs and named Louis and Louise. Their father's name was Pierre Germain, called Petit-Dieu, a mason's aid by trade, and their mother's name was Matthée Pernelle. (Paré)

Ischiopagus conjoined twins. The illustration does not show external genitalia and it is not clear how their sex was determined.[111]

1571a

Born in Gascoigne [Gascogne] nr Beaumont de Lomaigne, France, a boy with a parasitic twin attached at the upper chest by the head, with a dependent body. It was described by Seignior Camboline, doctor and 'consul', and also seen by M. Arnault Sylle, doctor of medicine and Jean Torneil, apothecary. The mother, aged 35, and the father, 40, were poor peasants.[112]

Thoracopagus parasite.

1571b

Antwerp:

> [T]he wife of a companion printer named Michel living at the home of Jean Mollin, a sculptor at the sign of the Golden Foot, on Camerstrate, on a proper day of St Thomas, about ten o'clock in the morning, gave birth to a

monster representing the shape of a real dog, except that he had a very short neck, and the head more or less like a fowl, except without hair; and it had no life at all, because said woman delivered before term.[113]

1572a

Born at Viabon on the road from Paris to Chartres, at the place of the Petites Bordes, to a woman named Cypriane Girande, wife of Jacques Marchant, a farmer, twins joined at the buttocks... the third leg was monstrous. (Liceti)

They had one umbilicus, two chests, four arms and three legs. An illustration shows them with only one set of female external genitalia (Paré); they lived until the following Sunday.[114]

Ischiopagus tripus conjoined twins.

1572b

10 July at Pont de Cé near Angers

[T]here were born two female children who lived for half an hour and received baptism; and they were well-formed, except that one left hand had only four fingers, and they were joined together by the anterior parts, to wit, from the chin to the umbilicus, and had only one navel, and a single heart, the liver being divided into four lobes.[115]

Thoracopagus conjoined twins. The brief description of the autopsy mentions only two organs, heart and liver, both associated with individuality, suggesting that the aim was to determine whether the twins were one or two.

1573

I saw in Paris, at the door of Saint Andrew of the Arts, a child about nine years old, a native of Parpeville, a village 3 leagues from Guise; its father was named Pierre Renard and the mother who bore it Marquette. The monster had only two fingers on its right hand, and the arm was rather well formed from the shoulder to the elbow, but from the elbow to the two fingers was very deformed. It was without legs, and yet there issued from his right buttock the incomplete form of a foot, appearing to have four toes; from the left buttock there issued from the middle two toes, one of which resembled, almost, the male rod. Which is shown to you just as it was through this present picture.

The phrase 'just as it was' is perhaps meant to imply that the picture, unlike others in Paré, is intended as an accurate representation.[116]

Delaunay offered a diagnosis of caudal regression syndrome, with which P.D. Pallister concurred.[117] Pallister writes that the ears are abnormal, though the illustration does not seem to me to show this. Walton *et al.* suggest femur-fibuloulna dysostosis.[118]

1575a

Germany, May: 'A two-headed child was born.' (Schott)[119]
Ischiopagus tetrapus conjoined twins.

1575b

Born 12 November at Arnhem; a monster that 'ranne under the bed'.

> [B]eing seen of many both men and women: a rough bodie hairie and blacke, except his belly which was like a swan, the two feete like Peacockes, clawed, his eyes shined like fire… a mouth like to a Storke… a tayle like an Oxe, two bending hornes on his heade, in steade of handes clawes… among them it was smothered to deathe betweene two beddes. (Batman)[120]

A sooterkin, resembling traditional images of devils.

1576a

Born at Taunton, England, 9 November:

> [A] man Childe with one heade, unto whiche was joined from the Navil downewarde, two bodies, that is, foure buttocks thighs and legs. (Batman)[121]

Cephalopagus conjoined twins.

1576b

A double monster with two heads, four arms and four legs but one trunk and abdomen with two umbilici and two nipples.[122]
Probably omphalopagus.

1577a

> We saw a youth, born without arms and hunchbacked, who nevertheless could write with his toes.[123]

1577b

Born in Germany, a male infant with bilateral cleft lip, frontal encephalocoele and talipes equinovarus.[124]

1578a

An anonymous German broadside, depicting cephalothoracopagus janiceps asymmetros twins with one cyclopic face. The illustration shows an abdominal swelling or hernia sac.[125]

1578b

Born 10 January at Piedmont in the town of Chieri:

> [T]he face being well-proportioned in all its parts... was found to be monstrous on the rest of the head, in that five horns approximating to those of a ram came out of it, the horns being arranged one against the other on the top of the forehead and at the rear a long piece of flesh hanging along the back, like a maiden's hood. It had around its neck a flap of double-layered flesh like a shirt collar all of one piece, the extremities of the fingers resembling the talons of some bird of prey, its knees like hams. The foot and right leg were an intense red colour. The remainder of the body was a smoky grey colour. (Paré).

> [A] hideous monster the length of a mans arme from the middle, all of dark greene colour except the right legge that was of redde colour, behind the head hong downie a long piece of fleshe to the Buttockes like a bagge, about his neck the fashion of a Friers cowle, on the head five hornes, each somewhat longer than foure fingers, the legges standing the contrarye waye with the knees backwarde, the handes and feete as clawes, this was born of parents well thought of, the Father a Doctour. (Batman)

Possible Meckel-Gruber syndrome, combining occipital encephalocoele with malformations of the hands and lower limbs. For an alternative diagnosis of neurofibromatosis, mosaic or diffuse, see Ruggieri and Polizzi, and Zanca.[126]

1578c

Born 25 September at Clodiae (Chioggia, Venice):

> [T]he mother felt the pains of labour in the third month.... Master John Baptiste Aquistapace Vincentino, doctor of medicine, dissected the girl. A large fleshy excrescence at the front was found to cover almost the entire face. (Schenck)[127]

Frontal encephalocoele.

1578d

A child born in Mecklenburg:

On whose head a fleshy excrescence was seen, covered by a membrane, which hung down in front, hiding the whole face, but the hidden human face is represented in the picture because it has been pulled upwards like a headdress such as is shown in images of Turks. All the bones of the head and cranium were absent, from which it is reasonable to infer that the brain was absent also. It also lacked ears, which could be distinguished by a protuberance of skin. The skin of the face had been peeled off, even of the open mouth, which was open as if it were screaming, and looked horrible. No tongue could be discovered. Sometimes when it opened, blood glittered like fire; certainly a frightening thing to look at. The eyes were always open and had no pupils. Blood came from a hole in the throat.... Its nose was wrinkled like that of a hound, the neck was very long and feeble.[128]

Possibly anencephalic, although it is not clear why absence of the brain would have had to be inferred. Acalvaria is another possibility.

1579a

Born dead at Aberwick, Northumberland, 5 January to John and Elinor Urine, aged 26 and 28:

[A] monstrous child having two heades, and two eares like a horse, joined together in the hinder parte of the two faces, a double body, that is two joined in one, two armes, two legs. The Fathers name John Urine a lewde Minstrell or Idle vagabonde, the child was borne dead. (Batman)[129]

Parapagus diprosopus conjoined twins.

1579b

Born at Lützow, Germany, 1 July:

The one chyldes head was copped like a Bishoppes mytre, the rest of the body in good proportion, saving where the hands should be, grew forth of the right arme the shape of a sworde, and forth of the lefte hande the forme of a rodde, of blackishe colour, it lived the space of three dayes.

1579c

The seconde chylde had two heades on one perfect body, the one head swarte coloured, the other naturall. This... childe lived also three dayes, it did continually crye: the Father of these children hadde to name Baltus Maler, and the mother Katherine, fortye yeares of age.[130]

Parapagus conjoined twins.

1579d

Born Tuesday 4 August, at Manchester, a child 'without a head, and the belly open, so that the bowels might be seene.'[131]
Anencephaly with gastroschisis, or omphalocoele, or maceration.

1579e

Born at Angers, France: 'brought forth by a whore, with seven heads, eared like a dogge, footed like a Toade'. (Batman).[132]

1579f

In an obscure lake-island, called Ferrières, came forth a monstrous female with a single head, from the occiput of which a large piece of flesh hung down: in the mouth two tongues.[133]

Posterior encephalocoele, possibly with the 'lobulated' tongue of Meckel syndrome.[134]

1579g

Born 24 July, Germany, female cephalothoracopagus, possibly janiceps twins.[135]

*c.*1580

Thomas Schweicker, a man without arms, is shown writing 'Deus est mirabilis in operibus suis' with his feet.[136] Examples of his writing were preserved until the eighteenth century.[137]
Amelia.

1580a

The XVII day of June last past... in the parish of Blamsdon, in Yorkshire, after a great tempest of lightning and thunder, a woman of foure score years old named Ales Perin, was delivered of a straunge and hideous Monster, whose heade was like unto a sallet or heade-peece.... Which Monster brought into the world no other news, but an admiration of the devine works of God. (Stow)

[W]as delivered an aged womam... Alice Perin of the yeres of 60... of a strange monster: whose head was like a sallet or head piece ['a light globular head-piece' – OED], the face somewhat formall, onely the mouth as long as a Rat, the fore part of the body like unto a man, having eight legges, and the one not like the other, a taile in length half a yard, like to the tayle of a Rat. (Batman)

Sooterkin (traditional).[138]

1580b

Born at Fennestanton in Huntingtonshire, 23 September: a 'strange monster' with 'a face blacke, mouth and eyes like a lyon, and both male and female.'[139]

1580c

Born near Chichester, Sussex, 1 February:

[A] monstrous chylde of little shape of body, trussed together, the head verye great, bigger than the body, the body in compasse 9 inches, the arme an inch long, and two inches about the face, of indifferent favour, on the cheeke and chin the likenesse of a blacke beard, the legs wanted thighs, the toes crooked. The mother of this misshapen child an adulteresse named Annis Figge.[140]

Possibly Roberts syndrome but there is insufficient detail for diagnosis.

1581

An anonymous German broadside showing a female dicephalus, born 15 April.[141]

1585a

At Rome, a man aged 32 with a parasitic twin:

[A] man was seen in his thirty-second year with the hips, legs and feet of an infant in his buttock region; the size was unequal; above the organ of generation a large mass was present.[142]

Ischiopagus parasite.

1585b

A young adult male exhibited in Rome. The rest of his body was well formed but without legs or thighs.[143]

Lower limb amelia.

1588

Born Brussels: thoraco/omphalopagus twins, one male, one female, shown in an anonymous German broadside.[144]

1591

Born November, Frankfurt, a male child:

> [I]t had a huge head; the eyes, ears, nose, chin and mouth, cranium and forehead were absent. Beneath this huge head the arms, hands, legs, feet and all its members were well proportioned. This child was seen, dead, by many, and was buried in St Peter's cemetery.[145]

1593a

On 6 October at:

> Monasterii Wolwerstalt [Wolwega?]… a woman gave birth to a girl with two heads, which, though dead, Valentinus Wager depicted in the colours of life.[146]

1593b

Born at Konigsberg: 'a boy with the ears of a rabbit, with a piece of flesh like a felt cap.'[147]

1596a

Born in Germany: a child with all limbs absent except the left leg.[148]

1596b

A broadside showing Magdalena of Mohre, an adult woman without arms.[149]

1597a

Born 29 May near Tübingen, Germany: a child with two heads and necks, ambiguous genitalia:

> [T]he head was not much different from the skull of a dead man... a double heart and lungs [four lungs?] and a double liver with a single stomach and intestine. [150]

Parapagus dibrachius dipus conjoined twins.

1597b

A woman born in England who in 1613 was seen in Strasbourg: her whole body was well-formed, except the feet. The right leg was three times bigger than the body and weighed 'fifty-two' (pounds?); the left, similarly, weighed twenty-two. On one foot there were six digits and on the other three.[151]

The limb swelling is probably acquired lymphoedema, the oligo- and polydactyly incidental.

1598

Born between Angera and Tortona, 26 October:

[A] human monster with two heads and a tail, two legs and four arms, two of which were in their proper places, the other two arose from the back between the two heads. The tail was two finger breadths above the anus, a span long, and it covered the anus, as the tails of quadrupeds do... No virile member or scrotum was apparent, and it was therefore regarded as female. (Schott)[152]

Parapagus tetrabrachius dipus.

1599a

Born near Brussels, August: a male child with two heads, the rest well formed, and a rudimentary wolf's tail:

[T]his went to full term in the uterus, it came from a farmhouse, the birth was troubled with much pain and the land where it died was immediately seized with trembling... for both heads had faces like apes: the rest of the girl was well-formed... the feet were like the feet of an ape. [153]

Parapagus dibrachius dipus conjoined twins.

1599b

Born 6 January, England: 'a monstrous deformed infant'. It was baptised 'What Godwill' and died on the third day.[154]

1600

A child of uncertain sex, born in Herefordshire, 5 January. It died on the third day and was said not to have slept because 'it had no eyelids'. The original description by Jones (1600) is quoted at length by Turnpenny and Hole, who suggested a diagnosis of Bartsocas-Papas syndrome.[155]

1605

'Eight-month female twins' born in Paris: 'The sternum and belly as far as the umbilicus were one... on dissection a single heart and liver were found.' (See Figure 3.2)[156]

Thoracopagus twins.

1606a

Seen at Haguenau in Alsace:

> [T]he body of a child the first day after its death, as it was first formed from its mother's womb: in the region of the umbilicus was a round, gaping hole, opening a way to the inner viscera of the belly, as though it had been pierced with a dagger, and through which food and excrement together came out. The body was opened and all the parts were complete, except the bladder, which was absent, and the anus, which was imperforate.[157]

Caudal regression sequence.

1606b

An anonymous German broadside showing cephalothoracopagus janiceps asymmetros twins.[158]

1608a

Born 27 November at Modbury, Devonshire: a female child without eyes, nose or ears, the body scored full of red strokes. Where the ribs met there was a 'seam' of flesh.[159]

Possibly macerated, or an harlequin foetus (congenital ichthyosis).

1608b

A male child, born 3 December at Plymouth to Susan, wife of Andrew White, a butcher. Above the forehead was a broad, misshapen bone growing out of the skull, covered with flesh. It also had a misshapen mouth and a 'pipe' growing out of the pit of its throat.[160]

1608c

Born at Haguenau, Alsace, September:

> [B]etween the upper lip and the nose was a mass of flesh, like a proboscis, like the mouth of a sheep, with the tongue thrust out as though it were bleating. This monstrous excrescence did not exceed the size of the nose, while the rest of the upper lip had broad fissures on both sides, that when the boy cries, or opens his mouth to suck, was an amazing sight to see. In addition a small mass of flesh was connected firmly with the nose and pulled downwards: for this reason air was not strongly drawn in that way, similarly eating and drinking was no less impaired. The boy was called John James, and has been alive for a long time.[161]

Bilateral cleft lip.

*c.*1609

A child born at Old Sandwich, Kent:

[I]t had no head... there onely appeared as it were two faces, the one visibly to be seene, directly placed in the breast, where it had a nose, and a mouth, and two holes for two eyes, but no eyes, all which seemed ugly... the other face was not perfectly to be seene, but retained a proportion of flesh in a great round lump, like unto a face quite disfigured. The face, mouth, eyes, nose, and breast, being thus framed together like a deformed peece of flesh... a caios of confusion, a mixture of things without any discription, from the breast downeward to the bowels it was smooth and straight... the armes grew out at the toppe of the shoulders, having neither joynt nor elbow, but round and fleshy, at the end of which armes, grew two hands, with fifteene fingers, the one hand had eight, the other seaven, of a contrarie shape, not like to the naturall fingers of new borne children: also it had foureteene toes, of each foote seaven, beeing as it were like unto geese or ducks feete [webbed?]. The wast and middle as I said before, was straight and without joynts, but the lower parts were al in a lump of flesh, like unto a lambs paunch... and withall the legges so short, that they seemed to have no proportion.

It was born dead and smelled 'earthly'.[162] The degree of maceration accounts for the absence of the eyes from their sockets. There may have been syndactyly or webbing as well as polydactyly. Meckel-Gruber is one of many possibilities here.

1610

In March 1610 at Mens in Pistoriensi [Pistoia] the wife of a charcoal burner gave birth to children joined around the pudenda and buttocks, of similar appearance, though it was not possible to tell their sexes however they looked female.[163]

Ischiopagus conjoined twins.

1613

Born 17 April at Standish, Lancaster: conjoined twins, '[t]estified by the reverend divine, Mr W. Leigh, bachelor of divinitie.'[164]

Rachipagus are shown, but probably pygopagus.

1614

Born 3 June in Villa Porcetti near Cologny (Switzerland) of 'rustic' parents: conjoined twins joined at the abdomen. One a well-formed male, the other malformed, with one lower limb and of indistinct sex: 'They died at birth. Within two hours illustrations were made.'[165]

Thoracopagus or omphalopagus conjoined twins.

1616

Germany: a young girl with upper limb amelia.[166]

1617a

Born 19 March, Genoa: Lazarus and John-Baptiste Colloredo.[167] This description is by a student of Wittenberg University – the Colloredo twins had visited the town in 1645:

> In public memory the well-known Lazarus Colredo of Genoa came to Wittenberg on 15 May 1645. Of good stature, his appearance was not unbecoming, with nothing whatsoever to suggest the presence of any deformity. The homunculus that he called his brother was towards his left side: he was called John Baptiste. Thus they had been born togeteher, formed in the same womb and there joined together: twins, after a fashion. John had a head, arms, chest and one foot. His hands were imperfect, with three digits, while his feet had four. His head and chest hung backwards, as though he were lying back and admiring his brother. He was congested with mucus, which poured from his nose. His eyes were closed as if half asleep, and he never moved his feet. His small lips were graceful and when they parted his front teeth could be seen. He never used these teeth because he never took food, being nourished through his brother. He had a proper beating heart, and breathed, and retained the vestiges of his faculties. But his belly never digested food, he never drank, being somehow a part of another.[168]

1617b

Born in Kent Street, London, to the wife of John Ladyman, after a long labour, on 21 August:

> [A] female child with a halfe forehead, without any scull... its mouth and eyes... neere upon the breast... the eyes being very bigge... brought forth alive.[169]

Anencephalic or iniencephalic.

1617c

At Venice, to a Hebrew mother: twins joined at the buttocks, 'utroque sexu'.[170]

Probably ischiopagus conjoined twins.

1617d

Born February, Berlin: a female child with two noses:

> ...three deformed mouths, three chins, two small, distorted eyes set close together, on the skin of the top of the head was a little net of hair, & the face red and horrible, almost the colour of blood.[171]

1620a

Male conjoined twins.[172]

Parapagus tetrabrachius tripus.

1620b

Born 14 August at Marck, Hungary: a child with a parasitic head.[173]

Craniopagus parasiticus.

1624

12 July at Fermo, Italy:

> [A] girl was born whose whole body was well formed except the head, which had a most horrible appearance: a secret eye was present in the back of the head; the other eye was in the head above the future crown. This slightly larger, human eye had neither lids nor lashes.

'Fortunately', it died almost at once. The prefect of Genoa had the body exhumed but the face had decomposed. A painter who had seen the child alive and after death made an engraving which was owned by Cardinal Barberini. Liceti's illustration, presumably adapted from this, appears very detailed, down to the absent philtrum.[174]

Cyclopia (Figure 6.1).

1628

Holland: Thoracopagus conjoined twins depicted in life and after autopsy in a painting by Everardt Crynz van der Maes (1577–1656).[175] There was a common heart.

1631

Gossau, Switzerland: 'a child was born with three arms and the like number of feet'.[176]

Parapagus tribrachius tripus conjoined twins.

1635

20 October, Plymouth, to Mrs John Persons, wife of a fisherman, a stillbirth with:

> Two heads, and neckes, two backes, and sets of ribbes, foure armes and hands, foure thighes and legges: in a word... two compleat and perfect bodies, but concorporate and ioyned together from breast to belly, two in one.[177]

Thoracopagus conjoined twins.

1638

At Leiden, a peasant woman delivered a foetus with 'the head of a cat'.[178]
Probable cleft lip/palate.

1640a

> [At] Bononia [Bologna] a 16-year-old youth... whose right arm ended at the elbow, where rudimentary fingers and nails were evident... and at the same place on 28 June... the wife of a carpenter was delivered of a boy intact in all his members save for the left arm, which ended at the elbow, where similar disordered rudiments of fingers and nails were visible.[179]

1640b

Born 4 September 1640 at Stuttgart: a child with iniencephaly or perhaps cranioschisis as Holländer suggests.[180]

1642

Born at Mears Ashby, Northamptonshire: 'A child without a head'.[181]
Possibly anencephaly, but perhaps an obstetric mishap is referred to.

1644

Born 28 November in Saxony: a boy with 'the heart and other viscera outside the thoracic cavity'.[182]
Ectopia cordis.

1645

Born Tuesday 16 September, Shoe Lane, London: two children, one arising from the 'upper part' of the other. The first had neither head nor feet but stumps for legs and branches for arms without hands. The nails grew out of the hips on each side. There arose from the neck a hollow lump of flesh, and from there a perfect man-child. The other appeared destined to be female.[183]

Parasitic twin or *fetus in fetu*.

1646

Stillborn 9 March 1646 at Nuremberg to Anna Maria, wife of Joh. George Pruckner Bamberg, a soldier: the rest of the child was well-formed but the head was monstrous. The face resembled a dog, with pendulous ears and the eyes were large. An autopsy was performed.[184]

Anencephalic.

1654

Cheapside, London:

> [A] child that was born without Armes, and had two little hands, which it could move, standing out of its shoulders, a poore woman had the child in her armes, begging with it. [185]

Phocomelia.

1655

Born 1 December, Yorkshire were 'two Children... Joyned together', one female, one a 'supposed manchild' with a 'lump... on the backe partes'.[186]

Thoraco/omphalopagus conjoined twins, possibly with a teratoma.

*c.*1656

A monster 'with foure hands and 4 heeles, 2 heads, 2 bodyes, two mouthes, 4 eyes and 4 eares.'[187]

Thoracopagus or omphalopagus conjoined twins.

*c.*1657

A male foetus was delivered by a 30-year-old peasant woman in 'Züllichau' (Sulechów, Poland): 'It had four perfect eyes, two noses and foreheads... two chins and a short neck... one head'. A 'shapeless mass' was present on the 'dorsal spine'. One explanation, 'if the mother were to blame', is that 'impurities in the uterus impeded it, for to some degree the lochia before the dead foetus was passed had been retained, and was disposed to putrefaction, and in this way the contagious rotteness impeded the second foetus and cheated it of perfection.'[188]

Diprosopus twins, perhaps with an additional neural tube defect.

1658a

A female child with two heads, born 13 November at the seventh hour in the evening at 'Broden' (Brodten, Germany) to Martha, the wife of Hansen Jahns, a peasant:

> [A] liveborn girl with two heads, two arms and two legs, who had two
> distinct chests, two hearts – this was decided because the chest pulsated in
> two places.... In the posterior part an excrescence protruded, not straight out,
> as the image shows, but sloping to one side.[189]

Parapagus tribrachius dipus conjoined twins. The excrescence is the third arm.

1658b

Conjoined twins with 'two heads, two necks, four arms', born to a soldier's wife at 'Werted' near Ardemburg, The Netherlands.[190]

1659

Born Smithfield, London: a male infant with two tongues.[191]

1660

A child with two hearts and 'two' (pairs of?) lungs born at Bologna in April 1660: 'but it did not extend the double principle to life, dying a few hours after her birth.'[192]

1661

Born at Woodbridge, England, 23 October 1661: 'a twobodyed one headed daughter or daughters'. See Chapter 4, 100–1.

Cephalothoracopagus conjoined twins.

1664a

Vienna, a monster born in March:

> It had two heads, but joined in one, the *crania* still distinct; all the organs of
> the head were double, with two ventricles, all the membranes, veins and
> arteries doubled, two nerve origins, two tongues, two mouths, four eyes, two
> noses together, except for the ears, of which there were only two. Two arms,
> neck, thorax and chest and all their organs were simple, and the heart
> likewise, but big... there was one stomach and one intestine. The body was

all one until the lumbar region, where it divided into two again with two spines... and the intestine duplicated.... Four kidneys, two uteri... two bladders and four feet. The body was put in balsam, after which it was kept at the house of an important man. (Greisel)[193]

Parapagus conjoined twins.

1664b

Born 26 October near Salisbury, conjoined twins: 'They were baptized at 3 a clock the same Morning... *Martin* and *Mary*.... It was dissected, and there were found two Hearts, two Livers, and all the inward parts complete, as the outward to the Navel, except only that it had but two Kidneys.' The dissector wrote to the Royal society, see Chapter 4:

> About three months ago, near the town of Salisbury, the wife of a Palefrenier [stableman] was delivered, after a labour of an hour, of a baby girl, a child who had two heads diametrically opposite, four arms and hands, one belly and two legs. They pondered for a long time how to baptise this creature, but at length they decided that it was double, and they baptised it with the names of Martha and Mary. It took nourishment from both heads, and passed excrement in the usual way. One of its two faces was much more cheerful than the other. This monster lived for about two days. Martha, who had always appeared less lively than Mary, died first, and Mary followed after a quarter of an hour. Both were opened by a medical man, who found the heads and chests all perfect, but not so the belly. The intestines were joined as far as the ductus communis, and they had one caecum, one bladder, and one uterus. But they had two livers, two spleens and two stomachs. The monster was embalmed, and it was carefully done. (Rollins)[194]

Ischiopagus tetrabrachius dipus conjoined twins.

1665

A child born with neither cranium nor neck, only a mass of flesh in their place. The child came into the world alive, but soon died.[195]

Anencephaly.

1666a

A female child born dead 15 February 1666:

> [E]xhibited... near the house of Peter Burdelot, Parisian physician and physician to Queen Christina and acknowledged by many very distinguished colleagues and most learned men of high honour, a girl recently born dead...

a mass of black and red flesh protruded from the head... the upper cranium was totally absent.[196]

A monster in the form of an ape was exhibited in the house of M. Bourdelot. Born after 5 months gestation: 'having all over its shoulders, almost to his Middle, a Mass of Flesh that came from the hinder part of the head... the Woman which brought it forth had seen on the Stage an Ape so clothed...'.[197]

Anencephaly with anterior neural tube defect.

1666b

Born 26 October 1666 at Thorn, The Netherlands: 'A hydropic little girl that neither internal nor external medicaments would make small, that after some days died of hydrops.'[198]

1666c

A hydrocephalic boy of the age of one year, dissected in the public anatomy theatre at Leiden.[199] Probably not congenital.

c.1667

A monster:

> [H]aving instead of a Head and Brains, a Mass of flesh like any Liver; and was found to move. And this Foetus occasioned a Question for the Cartesians, how the motion could be performed, and yet the Glandula pinealis, or Conarium be wanting; nor any nerves visible, which come from the Brain?[200]

Anencephaly.

1668a

6 August 1668 at Öls in Prussia (now Olesnica, Poland), a double monster stillborn after a labour of twenty-four hours. The text draws attention to a malformed auricle in one of the twins and a toe like 'the spur of a cock' on the third leg, which had seven toes besides. There was an autopsy, but the findings are not described.[201]

Parapagus tetrabrachius tripus male conjoined twins.

1668b

Born at Grasby, Nottinghamshire: 'Its head was long and sharp, proportioned after the fashion of a Sugar loaf [moulding].' It had no nose, eyes like a fish, eight fingers upon each hand, webbed like a goose, ears hanging down like the ears of a hound, and long black hair down its neck.[202]

1668c

Born in June, a child with cleft lip and palate: 'God be thanked, death supervened'.[203]

1669a

Born 5 January 1669, to an honest woman, the wife of a merchant: 'a girl with two heads, three arms, and two feet. I was called to this spectacle along with Dr Maximil. Ehrenreich Zollighoffer and a surgeon, and I opened the body by the wish of the parents.' There was one liver and two gall-bladders and pancreata. One stomach, two duodena and jejuna, one ilium, caecum, colon and rectum. Two kidneys, the left 'well-formed' and the right 'duplex, but with a single pelvis'. Double venae cavae that joined near the sacrum, 'two perfect hearts', the spine was double to the sacrum, the third arm hung down from the back.[204]

Parapagus tribrachius dipus.

1669b

A child born dead 13 October 1669 at Brandenburg. The left arm tapered to a point without hand or digits, there was a large left-sided abdominal wall defect with a hernial sac (omphalocoele?) and a tail.[205]

*c.*1670a

Venice:

> Having been honour'd here with the place of Publick Anatomist of Venice... I lighted upon two odd Births... one was of Twin-Females, very handsom, but so fastn'd together by the breast, that there was not discern'd but one only Trunk of the body; which having their Chin united together, seemed to kiss one another.

An autopsy showed one heart 'though greater and rounder than ordinary; so that Nature seemed to have united the Matter of two into one'; two lungs, and an intestinal tract single as far as the pylorus. There was a single liver, four kidneys, two spleens and two sets of female internal genitalia. (Grandi)

Thoracopagus conjoined twins.

*c.*1670b

[A] Boy, terrible to behold, born with his Breast open, the Bowels out of the Belly, the Leggs distorted, the Bladder in the place of the Fundament; in the Genitals, besides that the *Testiculi* were close to the Kidneys, there was nothing but a membranous expansion, wherein the Spermatick vessels were lost.

An autopsy was 'made in the presence of many Noblemen and Physitians'.[206]

1670a

Conjoined twins fastened together at the breast, born 22 October to Grace Battered of Plymouth, a woman 'of honest repute' and mother of five children. The ribs were united without a sternum, to give a common chest cavity. The twins weighed $8^{1}/_{4}$ lbs, crown-heel length $18^{1}/_{2}$". At autopsy there was found to be a single liver and gall-bladder, four kidneys, two bladders, a common intestinal tract as far as the rectum and two oesophagi, one communicating with the stomach and one blind-ending. Lungs were not identified, there was a single malformed heart, double aortic arches and two sets of female internal genitalia.[207]
Thoracopagus.

1670b

Born 4 March at Bad Waltersdorf, Austria. The father was one Michael Lauter and the mother, Dorothy: 'Above the chin, there was a small opening, from which a monstrous tongue protruded. Above this there was no trace of a nose, but a single eye... with two pupils'.[208] An autopsy was performed.
Cyclopia with encephalocoele.

1671

A male infant born 25 March at Eisenberg, Germany:

Between the mouth and the nose it had the tip of a virile member, the size of a walnut... there was a deep wound in the palate all the way down to the gullet... it ate nothing because it was unable to swallow... and it shortly died. I desired a post-mortem.[209]

Bilateral cleft lip and palate.

1672

A male child born with a large 'hydrocephalic' head, low-set, abnormal, forward-facing ears, bilateral cleft lip and facial clefts. There were no thumbs, and only three fingers each hand, the third finger on the right small. There were four toes on each foot, short limbs, micrognathia, absent radii and no femora or leg bones – the feet were attached to the pelvis directly. An autopsy was performed and it was exhibited after death.[210]

Roberts syndrome, see Chapter 7, 186–9 (Figure 7.2).

c.1672a

Born at Framlingham, Suffolk, in the month of January to Elizabeth, wife of Thomas Welles, barber, a child with no distinct sex and multiple defects: no ears, no skull only a membrane through which the brain was visible, a distorted fractured arm and a right-sided defect through which the viscera herniated.[211]

Maceration seems the most likely explanation, with separation of the skull bones, though acalvaria is possible.

c.1672b

A prodigious infant born in the village of (le) Mans, with a beard and 'other parts like a man of thirty years of age'. The child lived three and a half years, and his body was three feet long at the time of death.[212]

c.1673

I was called to a sick woman [in Paris], brought to bed the very day I went to see her... I asked for the child, which died, I heard, as soon as 'twas born.... The Body of it appeared outwardly well formed and very fat; but the head was so deformed, that it frighted all that were present. It had no front; the two eyes were on the top of the face, very big, and almost without an orbite to lodge them in. The upper part of the head was red like coagulated blood... I had it opened every way, but I found no hollowness nor brains in it.[213]

Anencephaly.

1674a

A peasant woman in Saxe-Gotha gave birth to a male foetus:

[T]he chest bulging, in place of the abdomen a membranous sac, transparent, monstrous, and hanging down to the feet, in which the intestines and other viscera of the belly were contained and which could be seen with singular clarity. From the back of the head hung a shapeless mass of tapering flesh. Dr Johann Andreas Bechmann will still show its skeleton.

Posterior encephalocoele and a massive omphalocoele.[214]

1674b

Born at Köln, near Meissen: the wife of a peasant farmer and craftsman gave birth to:

> [A] two-headed girl, one head truly adorned with a ribbon like a girl, with four feet and two arms and hands, two bellies and the thorax from the level of the umbilicus upwards fused into one, and not even the eyes of a lynx could discern any difference between them.

The illustration shows two ears only posteriorly.[215]
Cephalothoracopagus janiceps asymmetros twins.

c.1674

A female child born dead, the bones of the skull 'separated', the head was 'totally devoid of brain'.[216]
Anencephaly or maceration.

1675a

Born 1 May, to the wife of a labourer aged 36, a child whose,

> whole abdomen was so transparent that the entire course of the intestine, with its proper coils protruding like a large hernia, was visible to the eye. Indeed, the anal opening was visible above the female parts.... Liquid green excrement was produced. The right foot had only two digits, and the thumb was horribly bent back to the wrist.[217]

1675b

Born at Schaffhausen, Switzerland; female twins: 'joined at the sacrum and obscene parts... each had a uterus and vagina, but a common vulva; also two recta, but one anus.'[218]
Pygopagus conjoined twins.

c.1677

> [A] woman gave birth to a monster entirely lacking a head, with a bag filled with congealed blood in its place. The face was depressed and it appeared to have no neck, but the vertebrae of the neck rose up in a lump above the level of the ears. The skin of the back was open and appeared lacerated, exposing the muscles of the back to view... the hands and feet were very distorted.

An anencephalic child, attributed to maternal imagination.[219]

1677a

Twin female infants united below the diaphragm, stillborn 20 December at Petworth in Sussex to Joan Peto: 'the Left Head was the bigger, and stayed longer in the Bearing. The Right Head was perceived to breath, but not heard to cry. Betwixt the heads was a protuberance like another Shoulder.' There were two upper and two lower limbs. An autopsy showed that the spine was double to the loins; there were two hearts, the left bigger, two pairs of lungs, and a Y-shaped inferior vena cava. The two stomachs contained 'Meconium, as is usual in Children newly born.' There was a single liver, spleen and uterus.[220]

Parapagus conjoined twins.

1677b

At Brescia, Italy; a man aged about 20 years: 'on whose chest was implanted another head, a little different from the true one, but almost complete'.[221]

1678

Born at Ratisbon:

> This man was a Tall and well Shaped man, att his Navel came out of his Body a head and neck Down to the Breast, the face Perfectly well Shaped with Eyes nose mouth chin forehead and ears, all well Shaped and a Live but Could not Speak Eat nor Drink nor open its Eyes though he had two Eyes and Showed no sign of Life it had a good Colour and two Long Locks of hair on its head, of a Black Colour, and a Downy Beard it had Teeth wee Could not see if it had a Toung for it did not Speak. Its brother was born so and in all other respects a perfect man of Good Sence and Understanding Healthe and Strong Eat and Drank very Hartily, Spoke and Rit Several Languages as Latin, French, Italian High Dutch, and Pritty good English. He was Born about the Year 1678, near Ratisbonn in Germany and was seen by me James Paris in London in the Year 1698, in the Mounth of December.[222]

Parasitic twin attached at the epigastrium.

c.1679a

A woman of 'our city' gave birth to a dead foetus with a 'deformed body... the belly was first opened [and the uterus found] the neck and thorax were not distinct'.[223]

Iniencephalic with ?posterior encephalocoele.

*c.*1679b

A foetus of nine months gestation with a 'monstrous' head.[224]

1680a

Born at Ebeleben, Germany, 1 May 1680; conjoined twins.[225]

Cephalothoracopagus, shown with two fused faces and three eyes.

1680b

Born 19 May 1680 (to a mother of five previous children), female conjoined twins, joined from breast to navel, baptised Aquila and Priscilla: 'they suck and cry heartily, exonerate apart freely, and are likely to live, if the Multitudes that come to see them (sometimes 500 in a Day) do not occasion the shortening of their Lives.' A similar case had occurred some forty years previously in Wales: 'the Children lived so long as to be able to talk to one another, and that in Tears, when the one thought what the other should do when either should happen to die; and that both died together.'[226]

Thoraco/omphalopagus conjoined twins.

*c.*1681

A well-formed child with an extra head like the head of a cat. M. Vescher, who preserved it in his cabinet, said that he had seen it alive.[227]

Dicephalus with one anencephalic head.

1682

7 May (old style):

> A monstrous birth, of two female children joyned together at the crowne of their heads as in the figure. They are both liveing sometimes one sleeps whilst the other wakes, Cryes or Eats &ct... they are both baptised.... That they are distinct in life, soul and brains appear plainly from the actions which they have... many people come daily to see them, and give 3 stivers apiece: their parents are offered a great sum of money for them to be carried about.[228]

Craniopagus conjoined twins.

1684a

Friday 29 February 1684 near Haldensleben in Germany: a soldier's wife gave birth to a child which died immediately. There were fleshy excrescences on the legs, six toes on the right foot, a tail 'a quarter of a Zealandish ell' long and excrescences on the forehead resembling 'artificial laces: which the Painter, who 3 Days after it was dead, did draw the Scheme, testifieth to have been almost spoiled or rotten by the touching of so many Hundreds of

People that went to see this Creature. But before, when the Head of the Child was turned against the Light of the Sun, these physical Laces seemed to be very artificially done.' It had a hood, 'as women wear'.[229]

1684b

Twins born in Normandy, 20 July. They had seperate brains in a common head. See Chapter 7, 180.[230]

Diprosopus.

c.1685

I saw here twelve years ago an infant with two heads, on one of which there was a kind of pocket resembling the hood of a Benedictine and which was attached like a collar to the length of the other head. Monsieur Pierre surgeon juror opened it in the presence of Monsieur Bayle, doctor of medicine and professor of arts, and of Monsieur Carboneau, surgeon juror. Water ran out.[231]

The infant lived fifteen days.

Parapagus twins.

1685

Born at Hagenhausen (Germany), January: 'female twins... joined at the thorax'. They had one liver and small intestine, but the rest of the organs, including the rectum, were double. The two hearts were joined. They were liveborn and baptised but died soon afterwards.[232]

Thoracopagus conjoined twins.

c.1686

An infant was sent into the world without nostrils, which the author explains on the grounds that a foetus in the belly of its mother breathes and takes nourishment via the mouth.[233]

Probably holoprosencephaly.

1686a

James Poro born at Jena, Germany. He had a parasitic head attached just below the xiphisternum. He exhibited in London.[234]

1686b

[T]wo perfectly form'd Children above and below the belly, having two heads, four arms and four legs, only the two arms which stood next other were not perfectly form'd into hands and fingers, the breasts beginning to joyn thereabouts; there was but one belly, tho' somewhat bigger than ordinary, one Navel and Navel-string tyed to one afterbirth.... It is thought they might have been brought forth alive, but that they stayed so long in the Birth; for that both heads presenting together, the Midwife thought they had been Twins, and thrust one of them always back.[235]

Thoraco/omphalopagus conjoined twins.

1686c

A child normal except for:

[I]t having two heads, the one standing behind the other, the foremost less than the due proportion... the other bigger than ordinary, standing somewhat higher, having no face.[236]

Probably an encephalocoele.

1686d

A female infant born 19 December near 'Ultenthann' (possibly Ultental, South Tyrol) and baptised before death. A mass of flesh and bone, arising from the middle of the palate, resembled a 'rudimentary head'.[237]

Congenital teratoma.

c.1687

Born at Berenstadt, Germany: a child with the umbilicus open and the intestines hanging outside the body.

Umbilical hernia/gastroschisis.[238]

1687

A child with two heads, attributed in general terms in this very short article to the 'vehement terrors of the imagination of women'.[239]

Parapagus conjoined twins.

1688a

Born 7 November at Stuttgart: a woman aged 21 gave birth to a boy with 'double hare-lip' and a depression in the top of the head. It died shortly after. The second day the dead body was opened.[240]

Cleft lip.

1688b

Born 5 June in Endenburg, Germany: A girl with a large 'tumour' arising next to the anus (the illustration shows a tumour approximately as large as the child). The tumour was amputated and shown to contain structures resembling bones, but the child died.[241]

Sacral teratoma.

c.1689

In Hüttlingen, Germany, a woman called Clementia Meyerin gave birth to twins baptised Elizabeth and Catharine. They were joined (*invicem adnatorum*) by 'cartilage' in the region of the umbilicus. They were separated by placing a tight ligature around the bridge, which was then cut.[242]

Xiphopagus conjoined twins (Figure 7-1).

1689a

A Man with very Flat Leggs…. This Man was a very poor Man, who begged his Bread about London Streets his two Leggs were as flat as an Inch Board att the Calf of his Leggs joyned together in the Manner of a Taylors Leggs and foalded under him But Could not be parted nor Extended. He was born thus in Sussex in the Year 1689 and I James Paris have seen him many Times in London.[243]

1689b

A male infant born 10 May near Stuttgart 'with a good colour', and baptised. The angles of the mouth extended too far laterally, especially to the left. 'It breathed well, ate, drank, and excreted'.[244]

1689c

Born 10 May at Wangen (Bavaria): a male child without limbs, baptised with the father's name. At 14 days it was living and a drawing was made; at 17 it was dead.[245]

Tetra-amelia.

c.1690a

Born at Holzhausen: a child with a large 'swelling' in the abdomen, which was covered by a thin, transparent membrane through which the intestines could be seen. It died on the third day.

Possible 'prune belly' syndrome.

*c.*1690b

A second 'horrible' case, also illustrated, born dead at Arnstadt, Germany, the head ornamented by a crest like a cockerel's, the intestines hanging out, a fleshy sac hanging from the occiput, prominent eyes, hare-lip, cleft palate and right side of nose, a small round hole in the chest through which the heart hung out, naked and bifid, mutilated digits. Unlike the first, this underwent an autopsy.[246]

Posterior encephalocoele, a large abdominal wall defect with the liver, stomach and intestines exteriorised, right-sided cleft lip and mutilated digits.

*c.*1690c

A 45-year-old frenchwoman who had had her first baby five years previously had felt foetal movements until nine days before term in her second pregnancy. The child was stillborn, and was about a foot long. It was not possible to distinguish the sex. The eyes were prominent and the back of the head flat and dark, like a cow. 'Such a great deformity of the head cast doubt upon the conformation of the brain, which is the seat of the soul. Had the infant been born alive, the difficulty would have been whether to baptise it. Several ecclesiastics who I consulted agreed that it would have been proper to give it *sub conditione.*' It was attributed to maternal impressions: 'this woman had, some months previously, lost a cow with a black poll, and she had been much affected by this loss.'[247]

Anencephaly.

c.1690d

A woman aged 47 gave birth to 'a vague, rough mass... neither head, arms, or legs could be distinguished, but a trunk only, carelessly put together'. It had a heart, lungs and liver.[248]

Fetus amorphus.

1690a

Born dead 13 February at Pressburg, Germany (now Slovakia): a female infant with a hare-lip and nasal clefts, with a round fleshy mass arising from the occiput.

Encephalocoele and bilateral cleft lip (Figure 4.1).[249]

1690b

Born 25 October, Magdeburg:

'Two hours after [the birth of the monster], she first produced a well formed but weak premature girl'. The head was absent and the upper limbs were short and deformed; the right hand had only two digits. The chest and abdomen were opened and 'the heart and lungs were absent'.[250]

Fetus amorphus.

1691a

Born 8 December, Passau, Germany a male monster with two heads, four arms and two legs. 'The foetus, expelled alive, was soon dead, though happily fortified with baptism.'[251]

Parapagus conjoined twins.

1691b

A child born 14/15 of November with 'a single foot with a toe resembling a hoof reversed, no ankle, a single metatarsal bone, two joints, a very broad, flat femur'. The anus was imperforate. A detailed autopsy was performed: 'The meticulous surgeon Mr Wagner, who preserved the monster in balsam, presented it to our museum.' The abnormality was attributed to maternal impressions.[252]

Sirenomelia.

1692a

A child with right-sided cleft lip and palate, born 28 February among the Jews of Rome.[253]

1692b

Male conjoined twins born 10 July.[254] An autopsy was performed and showed no shared organs except the liver.

Omphalopagus conjoined twins.

1694

A girl born in France 22 July 1694 with:

> [A] bony cap, which adhered to the bones of the superior jaw... there was not the least bit of it [the brain], no more than of the cerebellum.... According to Descartes, this child, who had as fine a face, as any new-born child I ever saw, could not be a reasonable human creature; for as she wanted the glandula pinealis, which according to him, is the seat of the soul, she could have no soul at all.[255]

Anencephaly.

1695

3 April 1695, a woman aged 28 gave birth to 'a male child, that lived half an Hour, and received Baptism... all the Parts of the Baby well proportioned, except the Head, the hinder part whereof was flat, as if it had been taken off with the Stroke of some Weapon'. It was dissected under the direction of M. du Verney.[256]

Anencephaly.

c.1697a

An infant whose skull was 'depressed'. It was dissected, but 'I had not an opportunity of fully satisfying myself, the Child being to be Buried presently... I opened the cranium'. The brain 'might be included in a Walnut-shell'.[257]

c.1697b

'[A] newborn term male infant on whom there was no trace of the occipital, parietal, or the greater part of the frontal bones above the superior orbital ridges.' The eyes resembled the horns of a newborn calf. The infant lived four or five days.[258]

Anencephaly.

1698

A French woman living at 'Dung-hill' gave birth to:

[A] Boy... without the least mark of Corruption, except that his Eyes did look as though they had been placed at the top of the Forehead; the skull was unequal, the skin whereof, though full of Hair, was a little redder than the rest of the Body. The Midwife said, the Child came alive out of the Uterus; but tho' we cannot trust such Report... I was sent for to open this Child's head.[259]

Anencephaly.

1699

London: a monstrous child with one body and belly, otherwise two children.[260]

Thoraco/omphalopagus conjoined twins.

*c.*1700

Born dead to a woman aged 26 her first child, with a 'beautiful' face and 'a monstrous inferior excrescence, like a tail... It looked like pictures of Sirens.' A detailed autopsy was performed and it was found to be 'sexless'.[261]
Sirenomelia.

1700

A child born 7 May, France: 'there was no more of the skull, than is generally left on, when it is sawed off, to shew the brain'.[262]
Anencephalic.

Notes

1. In Hassia infans quidam foeminei sexus bene distinctis mébris natus est, nisi quod auribus, oculis & naribus in vniuersum careret, & in facie solum os haberet: J. Rueff, *De Conceptu et Generatione Hominis ...* (Basel: C. Waldkirch, 1586), I, 382; F. Liceti, *De Monstris: Ex Recensione Gerardi Blasii...* (Amsterdam: A. Fris, 1665), 55, 57.

2. Anon., *Monstrificus Puer...* (1511), see E. Holländer, *Wunder Wundergeburt und Wundergestalt...* (Stuttgart: F. Enke, 1921), 343.

3. Anon., *Zu Wissen: Ein Wunderlichs von Erschrockenlich Ding* (n.p: W. Traut, 1511), see Holländer, *op. cit.* (note 2), 77.

4. *Ravennae monstrum natum est, quod habebat cornu in capite, alas duas, brachia nulla, pedem unum ut avis rapax, oculum in genu, sexum utrunq; in medio pectore ypsilon & crucis effigie.* Rueff, *op. cit.* (note 1), I, 384; A. Paré (ed. and transl. J.L. Pallister), *On Monsters and Marvels* (Chicago and London: University of Chicago Press, 1982), 6–7; L.G. Gerlin, *Disputatio Philosophica de Monstris* (Wittenberg: C. Tham, 1624), 8. Broadsides describing the monster are reproduced in I. Ewinkel, *De Monstris: Deutung und Funktion von Wundergeburten auf Flugblättern im Deutschland des 16 Jahrhunderts* (Tübingen: Niemeyer, 1995), 326–8. J. Céard, *La Nature et les Prodiges* (Geneva: Droz, 1977), 154–5, considers various illustrations.

5. M.T. Walton *et al.*, 'Of Monsters and Prodigies: The Interpretation of Birth Defects in the Sixteenth Century', *American Journal of Medical Genetics*, xlvii (1993), 7–13: 12; but see M.-L. Martinez-Frias, 'Another Way to Interpret the Description of the Monster of Ravenna of the Sixteenth Century', *American Journal of Medical Genetics*, il (1994), 362.

6. Holländer, *op. cit.* (note 2), 66–8; J. Bondeson, *The Two-Headed Boy, and Other Medical Marvels* (Ithaca: Cornell University Press, 2000), 166.

7. L. Landucci, quoted by L. Daston and K. Park, *Wonders and the Order of Nature, 1150–1750* (New York: Zone Books, 1998), 190, their translation.

8. *[Ex] cujus pectore aliud integri hominis, ejusdemque sexus corpus omnibus*

membris absolutum ad genua usque propendebat, solo capite in alio corpore infixo: Liceti, *op. cit.* (note 1), 81.

9. Fuit autem infans biceps... In capitibus crines aliquanto longiores, ac nigricantes. Inter utrumque caput ex collimito humerorum tertia porrigebatur manus, sed quae aures longitudine non excederet, nec integra visebatur omnio. Reliquum corpus prorsus bene compactum, ac citra ullam maculae foedit atem: C. Schott, *Physica Curiosa...* (Würtzburg: J. Hertz for J.A. Endter and Wolff, 1662), I, 660.

10. Cardinalis de Grassis tunc Bononiae Episcopus coelesti lavacro expiavit, & Mariam appellavit; sed vitam ad quartum tantum diem protraxit...: *Ibid.*, I, 675.

11. ...oculis prorsus et naribus carentem, memorat Cornelius Gemma in Cosmocrit. delata fuit puella ignoti cuiusdam civis Bononiensis, ad D. Petri templum, ut baptismi sacramento renasceretur...: Schott, *op. cit.* (note 9), I, 675; C. Gemma, *De Naturae Divinis...* (Antwerp: C. Plantin, 1575), I, 94.

12. J. Rueff, *De Conceptu et Generatione Hominis...* (Zurich: C. Froschauer, 1554), 44; C. Lycosthenes, *Prodigiorum ac Ostentorum Chronicon...* (Basel: H. Petri, 1557), 521; Paré, *op. cit.* (note 4), 21. In Germania visus est justae vir aetatis, cui aliud caput ex umbilico exertum prominebat; quod in morem superioris etiam cibum assumebat: Hujus meminerunt itidem Jacobus Rueffus: Liceti, *op. cit.* (note 1), 81; U. Aldrovandi, *Monstrorum Historia...* (Bononia: N. Tebaldini, 1642), 410–13; J.G. Schenck, *Observationum Medicarum Rariorum...* (Leyden: J.-A. Huguetan, 1644), 7; Schott, *op. cit.* (note 9), I, 663. J.F. Malgaigne (ed. and transl. W.B. Hamby), *Surgery and Ambroise Paré* (Norman: University of Oklahoma Press, 1965), considered it imaginary.

13. S.K. Biswas *et al.*, 'An Unusual Case of Heteropagous Twinning', *Journal of Pediatric Surgery*, xxvii (1992), 96–7.

14. Anon., *Diss Künd ist Geboren Worden zu Tettnang* (Munich: H. Burgkmair, 1516), reproduced in Ewinkel, *op. cit.* (note 4), 345 and Daston and Park, *op. cit.* (note 7), 186.

15. Schenck, *op. cit.* (note 12), 8; Paré, *op. cit.* (note 4), 41–2.

16. Anon., *Im XXIIIII Tag des Mai, also am Sankt-Urbans-Tag, Zwischen Fünf und Sechs Vormittags, Hat Eine Siebenundzwanzigjährige Frau in der Stadt Landshut an der Donau in Bayern ...* [1517], reproduced in Holländer, *op. cit.* (note 2), 76; Ewinkel, *op. cit.* (note 4), 346; Bondeson, *op. cit.* (note 6), 167.

17. Anon., *Billich Verwundert Sich Jung und Alt* (Zurich: 1519). Tiguri Hermaphroditus vel androgynos natus est, supra umbilicum egregie formatus, sed circa umbilicum rubeam carnis massam habens, sub qua membrum muliebre, & infra hoc, loco conuenienti, virile quoque: Rueff, *op. cit.* (note 1), I, 382; Schenck, *op. cit.* (note 12), 501.

18. [C]aput hominis erat facies, longum porrectum nasum habeat, in vertice

glabrum & depile instar rasi monachi, & coronam velut in monachis conspicitur, collumq[ue]; gruis: brachia, femora, pedes, manusq[ue], prorsus humanos habebat, distentum & rotundum ventrem, brachiis alatum erat, & plumis femora vestita fuerunt…: Gerlin, *op. cit.* (note 4), 8.

19. Anon., *Im Fünffzehenhunderten und Dreyundzweintzigsten Jaren* (n.p: H. Sebald Beham, 1523).

20. *Alius Wittembergae sine capite ortus*: Schenck, *op. cit.* (note 12), 7.

21. *Puellus alibi postea exoritur, qui brachiis penitus orbatus, reliqua corporis forma rectissima fruebatur; pedibus, quum ad vigesimum aetatis annum pervenisset, vice manuum mire utebatur, accipiendo, fecando, ori inferendo, nec non etiam alea, & chartis colludeno*: Schenck, *op. cit.* (note 12), 629; Schott, *op. cit.* (note 9), I, 678; Liceti, *op. cit.* (note 1), 55.

22. *[In] quodam Hercyniae syluae superioris pago infans natus est, & in instae staturae virum excrenit, vniuersa corporis figura mas recte habens, nisi quod vbera haberet, & exipsius pectore corpus alterius proponderet, sine capite & humeris, brachiorum informem figuram protendens, manibus plus ad pedum quam manuum formam accedentibus*: Rueff, *op. cit.* (note 1), I, 382; *[In] cuius corpusculo circa pectus aliud praeterea corpus membris omnibus absolutis propendebat ad genua usque, solo capite in alio corpore recto. Pervenit hoc monstrum ad virilem aetatem pererrans orbem*: Liceti, *op. cit.* (note 1), 83.

23. Schott, *op. cit.* (note 9), I, 683; Liceti, *op. cit.* (note 1), 83, dates them 1531. Paré's illustration is fanciful, as is his attribution of the report to Giovanni Pontano, who died in 1503. Perhaps the same as the male twins with a single head shown in Anon., *An Dem Achte Tag des Octobers* (n.p., 1524).

24. *[O]bscoeno vulto… in frontem & occipite massam carnosam duram et prominens*: Schenck, *op. cit.* (note 12), 12. Schott *op. cit.* (note 9), I, 673 places the birth in 1550.

25. *[Et} dit on qu'il auoit esté engender de quelque femme perdue, qui se prostituoit à tout le monde indifferemment*: P. Boaistuau, *Histoires Prodigieuses* (Paris: J. de Bordeaux, 1571), fo. 82v. E. Fenton, *Certaine Secrete Wonders of Nature…* (London: H. Bynneman, 1569), fo. 69r, has a similar illustration, but less skilfully drawn; Paré, *op. cit.* (note 4), 10, locates him in Paris.

26. S. Batman, *The Doome Warning All Men to the Judgement…* (London: R. Nubery, 1581), 315; Schott *op. cit.* (note 9), I, 660, has 29 August.

27. Anon., *Anzeygung Wunderbarlicher Geschichten* (n.p.: E. Schoen, 1531); *mulier peperit primo caput humanum membranis involutum, secundo bipedem serpentem, cui lucij caput, corpus ranae & pedes, cauda lacertae, Tertio porcum omnibus partibus integrum*: C. Peucer, *Commentarius de Præcipuis Divinationum Generibus…* (Wittenberg, 1553), 326.

28. *[C]onjunctis lateribus, qui propter matris graviter parturientis augustias nimium compressi, fere oppressi non diu vixerunt*: Liceti, *op. cit.* (note 1), 83.

29. *Bremopyrgi Marchiae urbe, notante Fincelio, natus est infans ita in corpore circumflua, & laxa carnis mole, ut militari sago Germanico indutus appareret. ibid.*

30. Batman, *op. cit.* (note 26), 328; Aldrovandi, *op. cit.* (note 12), 406; Schott, *op. cit.* (note 9), I, 660; Liceti, *op. cit.* (note 1), 83. Probably this is the 'infans biceps' referred to by Gemma, *op. cit.* (note 11), I, 92, where it is located at Louvain and illustrated as hermaphroditic parapagus tetrabrachius dipus conjoined twins, and by Schenck, *op. cit.* (note 12), 7.

31. *[I]nfans tria habens capita, tria pectora, sex brachia, totidemque; pedes, natus est, qui ex triplicis capitis ore & lac fugebat & vagiebat. Tres habuisse animas id monstrum ex triplici pectore, ex quo triplex cor infertur...*: Gerlin, *op. cit.* (note 4), 8.

32. Benedetto Varchi (1548), cited in Z. Hanafi, *The Monster in the Machine...* (Durham: Duke University Press, 2000), 18, 21.

33. Schott, *op. cit.* (note 9), I, 678.

34. Batman, *op. cit.* (note 26), 330; Paré, *op. cit.* (note 4), 30; Schenck, *op. cit.* (note 12), 7. Schott, *op. cit.* (note 9), I, 661 is a translation of Batman.

35. Batman, *op, cit.* (note 26), 330; Paré, *op. cit.* (note 4), 8. Schenck, *op. cit.* (note 12), 7 writes that she was seen in 1541.

36. Batman, *op. cit.* (note 26), 332; Schott, *op. cit.* (note 9), I, 661; Liceti, *op. cit.* (note 1), 85.

37. Fenton, *op. cit.* (note 25), ff. 98v–99r, incorrectly illustrates a parapagus; Paré, *op. cit.* (note 4), 19, has the same case, also shown as dicephalus. See also C.J.S. Thompson, *The Mystery and Lore of Monsters* (London: Williams and Norgate, 1930), 41. A single heart is uncommon but other examples have been reported: see T.H. Grundfest and S. Weisenfeld, 'A Case of Cephalothoracopagus', *New York State Medical Journal*, l (1950), 576–9.

38. Peucer, *op. cit.* (note 27), 328; Batman *op. cit.* (note 26), 334; Liceti, *op. cit.* (note 1), 85.

39. Batman *op. cit.* (note 26), 334.

40. C. Bauhin, *Hermaphroditorum Monstrosorumque...*(Frankfurt: M. Becker, 1600), 119; see also Peucer, *op. cit.* (note 27), 329; Schenck, *op. cit.* (note 12), 9.

41. Anon., *Eine Wuenderliche Geburt eines Zweykoepffigen Kindes* (n.p., B.W., 1542).

42. Anon., *Anno a Christo Nato 1543...* (Zurich, E. Froschauer, 1543) see Ewinkel, *op. cit.* (note 4), 337; *Scashusiae Helveticorum anno 1543 infante duo nati sunt, conjuncto altero latere, capitibus duobus, brachiis quatuor, totidemq: pedibus, umbilico uno, foeminei sexus uterq. Ex his alter mortuus in lucem prodijt, alter vero viuus prodiens, continuo expiravit.* Rueff, *op. cit.* (note 12), 381; Batman, *op. cit.* (note 26), 335, places the birth on 8 February;

Liceti, *op. cit.* (note 1), 85.

43. Batman, *op. cit.* (note 26), 336.

44. Fenton, *op. cit.* (note 25), fo. 36r–v, based on J. Cardan, *De Rerum Varietate...* (Basel: S.H. Petri, 1581), book 14, ch. 77. See also Batman, *op. cit.* (note 26), 338; Schott, *op. cit.* (note 9), I, 661.

45. Anon., *Warhafftige Contrafractur einer Wunder Geburt* (Frankfurt: H. Gülfferich, 1544), reproduced in Holländer, *op. cit.* (note 2), 345; Batman, *op. cit.* (note 26), 338; Schenck, *op. cit.* (note 12), 7; Liceti, *op. cit.* (note 1), 86.

46. See L.M. Gerlis *et al.*, 'Morphology of the Cardiovascular System in Conjoined Twins: Spatial and Sequential Segmental Arrangements in 36 Cases', *Teratology*, xlvii (1993), 91–108.

47. Batman, *op. cit.* (note 26), 339; Schenck, *op. cit.* (note 12), 9.

48. Batman, *op. cit.* (note 26), 339; Liceti, *op. cit.* (note 1), 141. Gerlin, *op. cit.* (note 4), gives 1544; Peucer, *op. cit.* (note 27), 329, has 1546. Possibly related to Paré's undated monster born in Saxony having the hands and feet of an ox: *op. cit.* (note 4), 40.

49. Batman, *op. cit.* (note 26), 342; Liceti, *op. cit.* (note 1), 86.

50. Batman, *op. cit.* (note 26), 345; Schott, *op. cit.* (note 9), I, 687, gives 1547, as does Liceti, *op. cit.* (note 1), 129.

51. Paré, *op. cit.* (note 4), 13–14.

52. Anon., *Diese Gegenwertig Wunderberlich Kindszgepurt*, see I. Blickstein, 'The Conjoined Twins of Löwen', *Twin Research*, iii (2000), 185–8. Gemma, *op. cit.* (note 11), 91, illustrates female twins.

53. Batman, *op. cit.* (note 26), 345; Liceti, *op. cit.* (note 1), 87.

54. Anon., *Anno Tausendt Fünffhundert Viertzig und Drey Jar* (n.p., n.d.); see Ewinkel, *op. cit.* (note 4), 329. *Cracoviae mirabile sane monstrum natum est, quod & triduo vixit. Caput erat humanae formae non absimile, nisi quod flammescerent oculi, nasus vero longus & aduncus tibiae instar existeret. In membrorum iuncturis, ad vlnas, cubitos & genua, canina eminebant capita, manus pedesq[ue]; anserinus pedibus similes, oculi supra vmbilicū duo. Cauda pecuina à tergo, hamum extremitate referens. Sexu erat masculus. Informis ante huius monstri causas soli Deo transcribimus, & tamen pro nostre rationis captu Sodomiae quoq; peccatum hoc monstro detestatum colligimus.* Rueff, *op. cit.* (note 1), I, 383; Gemma, *op. cit.* (note 11), 173–4; Peucer, *op. cit.* (note 27), 326; Batman, *op. cit.* (note 26), 337, has 1543; Aldrovandi, *op. cit.* (note 12), 373.

55. Batman, *op. cit.* (note 26), 348; Schott, *op. cit.* (note 9), I, 678, is a translation of this.

56. Fenton, *op. cit.* (note 25), fo. 140v.

57. Daston and Park, *op. cit.* (note 7), 191.

58. Batman, *op. cit.* (note 26), 351.
59. Batman, *op. cit.* (note 26), 354 [352]; Liceti, *op. cit.* (note 1), 57, gives the date as 1552.
60. Batman, *op. cit.* (note 26), 356; Schenck, *op. cit.* (note 12), 13; Schott, *op. cit.* (note 9), I, 668, is a translation of Batman.
61. Batman, *op. cit.* (note 26), 371–2.
62. Anon., *Ware Abcontractur und Bericht eines Kindes* (Breslau: 1551), see Holländer, *op. cit.* (note 2), 162; Ewinkel, *op. cit.* (note 4), 344; P. Salmuth, *Observationum Medicarum Centuriae Tres Posthumae* (Brunswick: G. Muller, 1648), quoted by J.B. Salgues, *Des Erreurs et des Préjugés Répandus dans la Société* (Paris: F. Buisson, 1810–13), 116.
63. Anon., *Thou Shalte Understande, Chrysten Reader...* (London, 1552): two handwritten annotations in the BL copy, one in German and one in Latin, record that one child died on 17 August and the other the next day; Peucer, *op. cit.* (note 27), 327; Schenck, *op. cit.* (note 12), 7; Liceti, *op. cit.* (note 1), 57. E. Howes, *Annales, or, a Generall Chronicle of England / Begun by John Stow...* (London: A. Mathewes, 1631), 1026; *in Anglia non procul ab Oxonia informis quidam partus natus est, capitis duobus, brachijs quatuor, manib. totidem, ventre vno, membro muliebri, sede vna. Ex vna parte pedes transuersi duo erant, ex altero vnus tantum, rite exporrectus, forma duorum pedum, digitos habens decem. Horum alter diebus quindecim, alter vero vno superuixit. Lachrymarunt hoc tempore raro. Alter ex his laetus ad modum, alter vero somniculosus & tristis extitit. Viginti digitos transuersos erat longitudo & latitudo ipsorum:* Rueff, *op. cit.* (note 1), I, 382; Fenton, *op. cit.* (note 25), fo. 141r, Batman, *op. cit.* (note 26), 358; Schott, *op. cit.* (note 9), I, 661. Batman's illustration is accurate according to Rueff's description, rather than his own.
64. J. Fincelius, *De Miraculis Nostri Temporis*, cited in Batman, *op. cit.* (note 26), 360; Schott, *op. cit.* (note 9), I, 678; Liceti, *op. cit.* (note 1), 57.
65. Schenck, *op. cit.* (note 12), 7; Schott, *op. cit.* (note 9), I, 661.
66. Batman, *op. cit.* (note 26), 362; Liceti, *op. cit.* (note 1), 130 gives 1550 as the date of the earlier monster.
67. Batman, *op. cit.* (note 26), 363; Liceti , *op. cit.* (note 1), 89.
68. Batman, *op. cit.* (note 26), 365; Schenck, *op. cit.* (note 12), 7; Liceti, *op. cit.* (note 1), 89.
69. *...cui capitis loco massa informis erat, mobilis, ut exta ovilla; loco unius auriculae brachium stabat; loco faciei cincinnus similis pilis felinis; & lupi piscis ova, per quae inferius lucebant ocelli vitrei, & renidentes; os contractissimo erat foramine, sine labiis, nasus quoque minutissimus erat; absque collo; alterum brachium e latere prominebat: sed neque pectoris, neque dorsi effigies aderat; lineola solum notabatur rachi; nullus erat omnino sexus: brachia, & longa crura continuo rigebant osse sine juncturis, cubitis, & poplitibus: manus, & imi pedes*

erant molles, & penduli tanquam bis fracti, similes unguibus curvis, & aduncis Lutrae: mortuum mater peperit, licet in utero viveret. Liceti, *op. cit.* (note 1), 130.

70. J. Fincelius, *De Miraculis Nostri Temporis,* cited by Batman, *op. cit.* (note 26), 370. Schenck, *op. cit.* (note 12), 7, 143; Liceti, *op. cit.* (note 1), 58 and Schott, *op. cit.* (note 9), I, 657, all have 1544.

71. Fenton, *op. cit.* (note 25), fo. 142v; Batman *op. cit.* (note 26), 373 [374]; *Etenim Gaspar Masserius pictor, qui una cum multis aliis ibidem aderat, penicillo diligenter cuncta delineavit.* Aldrovandi, *op. cit.* (note 12), 408–9; *Conradi Lycosthenis testimonio, Geneuae apud Allobroges, monstrum, quale hic subiectum vides, ex Galla quadam muliere, Geneuae tunc habitante, natum est: quod materiae reductantis indicium fuit: Id monstrum binas habuit facies, hoc est bifrous erat, qualem Ianum pinxit antiquitas: quod utrimque pendet inflatum, intestina sunt ex dorso prodeuntia: quod autem ex ventris inferiore parte pendet, id iecur est, ex feminae vulva prolapsum: monstrum hoc utrumque habet sexum, ad dextram mas est, ad laevam femina: ad viuum expressit Gaspar Maserius pictor, qui tum ibidem cum multis aliis aderat.* F. Liceti, *De Monstrorum Caussis, Natura, & Differentiis* (Padua: P. Frambott, 1634), 88; Schott, *op. cit.* (note 9), I, 673.

72. Aldrovandi, *op. cit.* (note 12), 408, has 7 September; Schott, *op. cit.* (note 9), I, 662; *In pago Freywerck, non procul ab Adorffio Voitlandiae oppido, natus est infans biceps... sed carens utroque sexu; in cuius loco umbilicum habebat: mater illi fuit uxor fabriferrarii:* Liceti, *op. cit.* (note 1), 111.

73. Batman, *op. cit.* (note 26), 375; Liceti, *op. cit.* (note 1), 111.

74. Batman, *op. cit.* (note 26), 377; Schenck *op. cit.* (note 12), 9; Schott, *op. cit.* (note 9), I, 668.

75. Batman, *op. cit.* (note 26), 379; Schott, *op. cit.* (note 9), I, 686.

76. Batman, *op. cit.* (note 26), 379.

77. See E. Gilbert-Barness, *Potter's Pathology of the Fetus and Infant* (St Louis: Mosby, 1997), I, 77

78. Sirenomelia and cleft lip are associated: see Rodriguez *et al.,* 'Sirenomelia and Anencephaly', *American Journal of Medical Genetics,* xxxix (1991), 25–7.

79. Batman, *op. cit.* (note 26), 380, Liceti, *op. cit.* (note 1), 58; Schott, *op. cit.* (note 9), I, 674.

80. Batman, *op. cit.* (note 26), 380; Liceti, *op. cit.* (note 1), 58–9; Schott, *op. cit.* (note 9), I, 674, gives 1556.

81. Batman, *op. cit.* (note 26), 381; Schenck, *op. cit.* (note 12), 9; Schott, *op. cit.* (note 9), I, 674 gives 1556.

82. Anon., *Warhaffte Abconterfectur der Erschrocklichen Wundergeburt* (Augsburg: P. Ulhart, 1560), reproduced in Holländer, *op. cit.* (note 2), 62.

83. See Holländer, *op. cit.* (note 2), 118–20.

84. *[I]n utroque pede septem inerant digiti (pollex namque, pede in vtroque duplex erat) & in utraque manu digiti sex. In sinistra vero manu annularis & medius coniuncti absque ullo interstitio erant. Pedes vero admodum latos, perinde atque manus, puer habebat.* Schenck, *op. cit.* (note 12), 636; Schott, *op. cit.* (note 9), I, 686; originally from F. Valleriola's (1504–80) *Observationem Medicinalium* (Lyons, A. Gryphius, 1605), book 4, obs. 2.

85. Anon., *Ein Wunderbarliche Seltzame Erschroeckliche Geburt* (Augsburg: M.M. Brieffmaler, 1561).

86. J.D., *A Discription of a Monstrous Chylde* (1562), see Philobiblon Society (eds), *Ancient Ballads & Broadsides Published in England...* (London: Whittingham & Wilkins Society, 1867), 299; Howes, *op. cit.* (note 63), 1096. Batman, *op. cit.* (note 26), 390 perhaps conflates it with, or re-interprets it in the light of, *The True Discription of a Childe with Ruffes* (1566). It is also mentioned in Machyn's diary (ed. J.G. Nichols, 1848): 'ther was a chyld browth to the cowrte in a boxe, of a strange fegur, with a longe strynge commyng from the navyll, – browth from Chchester'.

87. Céard, *op. cit.* (note 4), 169.

88. Paré, *op. cit.* (note 4), 36, 190; Schott, *op. cit.* (note 9), I, 657; *Ambrosius Paraeus confiteur Villae Francae in Vasconia ortam esse puellam sine capite, habentem aures in scapulis retro, nasum inter eas in spina, qui proboscidem paruam referret; oculos in humeris retrorsum aspicientes; & linguam sursum externam, unde collum provenire debuisset: cuius monstri effigem a Fontano Agenesi Medico, qui se id vidisse sancta affirmabat...*: Liceti, *op. cit.* (note 1), 131; *[A]uersa corporis parte singulis scapulis rudimenta quaedam papillarum, ex spirali linea ductarum, apparent, ex quarum demissione regione media rostellum incuruum elephantis proboscidi haud absimile exprimitur... capite in uniuersum careat.* Schenck, *op. cit.* (note 12), 7. Anencephaly may be combined with cyclopia: see R.C. Gupta *et al.,* 'Human Cyclopia with Associated Microstoma and Anencephaly (A Case Report)', *Indian Journal of Ophthalmology,* xxix (1981), 121–3; but iniencephaly is another possibility. Iniencephalics are however well described elsewhere (1640b, *c.*1679a) and the true basis of the blemmyae depicted with a proboscis, eyes in the chest, and ears on the shoulders (1565c) is uncertain.

89. Anon., *The True Reporte...* [1562], see Philobiblon Society, *op. cit.* (note 86), 38–42.

90. T. Anderson, 'Artistic and Documentary Evidence for Tetradysmelia from Sixteenth-Century England', *American Journal of Medical Genetics,* lii (1994), 475–7.

91. *Warhafftige und Eigentliche...*(1563), see Holländer, *op. cit.* (note 2), 75.

92. J. Barkar, *The True Description of a Monsterous Chylde...* (London: W. Gryffith, 1564).

93. Anon., *The True Fourme and Shape of a Monsterous Chyld...* (London, 1565), reproduced in H.L. Collmann (ed.), *Ballads & Broadsides Chiefly of the Elizabethan Period...* (Oxford: Oxford University Press, 1912), 113.

94. Anon., *The True Discription of Two Monsterous Chyldren Borne at Herne in Kent...* (London: T. Colwell, 1565).

95. J. Wolff quoted by Salgues, *op. cit.* (note 62), 116: 'one may ask Jean Wolff how the little demon child could make a loud cry without a head'.

96. Anon., *Ein Neuwe Seltzame Warhafftige Wundergeburt* (Augsburg: H. Zimmerman, 1565).

97. J. Mellys, *The True Description of Two Monsterous Children...* (London: A. Lacy, 1566).

98. H.B., *The True Discription of a Childe with Ruffes...* (London: J. Allde, 1566), see Philobiblon Society, *op. cit.* (note 86), 360.

99. See Gilbert-Barness, *op. cit.* (note 77), II, 1361.

100. Anon., *Abconterfetung der Wunderbaren Gestalt / so Hans Kaltenbrunn...* (1566), reproduced in Holländer, *op. cit.* (note 2), 102.

101. Anon., *Ware Abcontrafactur einer Missgeburt* (Schmalkalden: M. Schmuck, 1566).

102. Batman, *op. cit.* (note 26), 393.

103. Fenton, *op. cit.* (note 25), fo. 146r; Batman, *op. cit.* (note 26), 395, has 1569.

104. Anon., *The Forme and Shape...* (London: J. Awdeley, 1568).

105. T. Anderson, 'Earliest Evidence for Arthrogryposis Multiplex Congenita or Larsen Syndrome?', *American Journal of Medical Genetics,* lxxi (1997), 127–9.

106. A.W. Bates, 'Birth Defects Described in Elizabethan Ballads', *Journal of the Royal Society of Medicine,* xciii (2000), 202–7.

107. *Cujus monstri cadaver quum dissecuisset, unicum cor reperit. Ex quo scire licet, unicum eum infantem extitisse:* Liceti, *op. cit.* (note 1), 118; Paré *op. cit.* (note 4), 15–16, 186.

108. Anon., *Ein Newe und Warhafftige Zeittung* (Strasburg: P. Hug, 1569).

109. Anon. *Warhafftige Beschreibung* (Augsburg: M. Manger, 1569).

110. *[N]atos esse ait duos infantes perineo ad nates conjunctos, communem umbilicum:* Liceti, *op. cit.* (note 1), 90.

111. Anon., *L'Androgyn Né a Paris...* (Lyon: M. Jove, 1570). Boiastuau's illustration shows them androgynous-looking, with only one cord: P. Boaistuau, *Histoires Prodigieuses...* (Anvers: G. Janssens, 1594), 471; also Paré, *op. cit.* (note 4), 17.

112. Boaistuau, *op. cit.* (note 111), 477.

113. Paré, *op. cit.* (note 4), 69.

114. *Viabani Paroecia, qua Carnutum Lutetia itur, in pagulo Parvarum Bordarum, Cyprianam Girandam Jacobi Mercatoris agricolae uxorem peperisse gemellas ad*

nates junctas... sed terna crura monstro. Liceti *op. cit.* (note 1), 90; Paré *op. cit.* (note 4), 21–2.

115. Paré, *op. cit.* (note 4), 18; Liceti, *op. cit.* (note 1), 111.
116. Paré, *op. cit.* (note 4), 33, 35; Schenck, *op. cit.* (note 12), 633; Schott, *op. cit.* (note 9), I, 686; Liceti, *op. cit.* (note 1), 59–60.
117. Paré, *op. cit.* (note 4), 178–9.
118. M.T. Walton *et al.*, *op. cit.* (note 5), 9. Cornelia de Lange syndrome also seems to me a possible diagnosis, though the lower limb defects are rather severe.
119. Anon., *Warhafftige und Erschroeckliche Geburt* (Heidelberg: M. Schirat, 1575); see Ewinkel, *op. cit.* (note 4), 349–50; Schott, *op. cit.* (note 9), I, 662. Could this be the same as the ischiopagus tetrapus twins described in the anonymous canards ...*Monstroso Nato in Ghetto...* and ...*Monstruoso Nato di una Hebrea...* both of 1575?
120. Batman, *op. cit.* (note 26), 401.
121. Anon., *The Discription and Figure of a Monstruous Childe Borne at Taunton the viij of November 1576* (London: H. Jackson, 1576); Batman, *op. cit.* (note 26), 402, appears to have used the ballad as a source.
122. They appear to have been drawn from life, but are not neonates; see Holländer, *op. cit.* (note 2), 78.
123. *Nos vidimus adolescentem, sine brachius natum ac gibbosum, qvi nihilominus pedum digitis ad scribendum*. J.C. Westphal, *Natura Peccans, Septenario Problematum Numero Proposita...* (Leipzig: C.G., 1687), sig. C2*v*.
124. D. Merula, *Ware/Eigentliche/ und Umbstendigliche Beschreibunge* (Frankfurt: J. Weissen, 1577).
125. Anon., *Newe Zeytung: Eine Erschreckliche Mißgeburt* (Nürnberg: M. Rauch, 1578), see Holländer, *op. cit.* (note 2), 353.
126. Anon., *Briefz Discours d'un Merveilleux Monstre Né a Eusrigo...* (Chambéry: F. Poumard, 1578); Anon., *Vray Pourtraict, et Sommaire Description d'un Horrible et Merveilleux Monstre, Né a Cher, Terre de Piedmond, le 10 de Janvier 1578...* (Chambéry: 1578); Anon., *Horribil Mostro, Nato in Cher* (n.p., 1578), see Ewinkel, *op. cit.* (note 4), 331, 333; Batman, *op. cit.* (note 26), 405; Paré, *op. cit.* (note 4), 10–11, puts the birth at 8pm on 17 January; Schott, *op. cit.* (note 9), I, 676, has 1577. See M. Ruggieri and A Polizzi, 'From Aldrovandi's "*Homuncio*" (1592) to Buffon's Girl (1749) and the "Wart Man" of Tilesius (1793): Antique Illustrations of Mosaicism in Neurofibromatosis?', *Journal of Medical Genetics*, xl (2003), 227–32 and A. Zanca, 'Iconografia Dermatological del XVI Secolo: Un Caso di Neurofibromatosi Multipla Illustrato da Ulisse Aldrovandi', *Arch Ital Dermatol Venereol Sessuol*, xl (1975), 119–23.
127. *[Q]uam mater, angina laborans mense 3 abortiuit, non sine magno vitae*

discrimine, divino tamen auxilio matrem curavi; puellam vero praesente Domino
Ioanne Baptista Aquistapace Vicentino medicinae Doctore dissecui, in cuius
fronte magnam carnis excrescentiam reperi, quae totam fere occupabat faciem,
collumque una cum malis suo colore tingens: Schenck, op. cit. (note 12), 12.

128. *Cuius capiti agnatum visum est carneum quasi & membranaceum
integumentum, quod ubi in anticam partem propendebat, faciem universam ita
obvelabat, atque obtegebat, ut obscuram hominis faciei imaginem repraesentaret,
quod a facie detractum & sursum tensum, tiaram quandam, aut totius Turcici
vel Ruthenici pilei imaginem praebebat: caput in universum ossibus & cranio
carebat, unde colligere licebat cerebro etiamnum caruisse. Sed & auribus quoque
destituebatur, quod ea parte integumentum enatum cerneretur. Velamen istud
facie abstractum & surrectum, una quoque oris rictus, instare clamantis, aut os
diducentis, horribili aspectu apparebat. In ore lingua nulla deprehensa. Quo
subinde patente, atque hiante, sanguine atque igne collucere, formidando sane
aspectu visebatur. Oculi semper aperti, sine pupilla ulla, cavi non minus atque
fauces apertae sanguineum... Nasus ei instar molossorum canum corrugatus.
Collo erat oblongo nimis, adeoque molli...: ibid., 12–13.*

129. Anon., *A True Report of a Straung...* (London: T. Gosson, 1580); Batman,
op. cit. (note 26), 408.

130. *Ibid.*

131. *Ibid.*, 407.

132. Anon., *Horibile et Marauiglioso Mostro Nato in Eusrigo Terra del Nouarese*
(n.p., 1578), see Ewinkel, *op. cit.* (note 4), 330, 333–6; Batman, *op. cit.*
(note 26), 407. Schott, *op. cit.* (note 9), I, 664 gives 1587.

133. In insula obscuri lacus, Ferrariensi ditione, ortum est ex muliere monstrum
uno capite, cui ad occipitum frustum grande carnis dependebat: in ore duae
linguae...: Liceti, *op. cit.* (note 1), 91; Schenck, *op. cit.* (note 12), 13.

134. See Moerman *et al.*, 'The Meckel Syndrome: Pathological and Cytogenetic
Observations in Eight Cases', *Human Genetics*, lxii (1982), 240–5.

135. Anon., *Ein Newe Wundergeburt* (n.p., 1579).

136. Holländer, *op. cit.* (note 2), 115; Schott, *op. cit.* (note 9), I, 680; Schenck,
op. cit. (note 12), 629.

137. Du Plessis, *A Short History of Human Prodigious & Monstrous Births...*
(1730), 215.

138. Batman, *op. cit.* (note 26), 412; C. Whitley, 'Chroniclers and Antiquaries', in
A.W. Ward and A.R. Waller (eds), *The Cambridge History of English and
American Literature* (New York: G.P. Putnam, 1907–21).

139. See Anon., *The Description of Monstrous Childe Borne at Ffenny Stanton in
Huntingdonshire* (London: H. Bynneman, 1580); Batman, *op. cit.* (note 26),
414; *Notes and Queries*, series 10, ix, 249.

140. Batman, *op. cit.* (note 26), 415. There are two extant ballads describing

monstrous births in Chichester, but neither corresponds to this case.

141. Anon., *Von einer Warhafftigen/ doch Erschrecklichen und Nicht Bald Erhoerten Misgeburt* (n.p., 1581).

142. *[V]isus est vir trigesimum secundum natus annum, coxis, & cruribus, pedibusque infantis nuper nati partes consimiles magnitudine non aequantibus, supernis membris debitam aetati molem obtinentibus:* Liceti, *op. cit.* (note 1), 58

143. See Holländer, *op. cit.* (note 2), 127

144. Anon., *Erschroeckliche und Warhafftige Contrafaytung* (Brüssel: J. Wollaert, 1588).

145. *Caput habens ingens & praeter modum magnum; oculis, auribus, naso, mento & ore, cranio & fronte carens; sub hoc tam monstroso capite humeri, manus, crura, pedes, aliaque membra naturalia, proportionibus suis fuere distincta: mortuus hic puer à multis conspiciebatur, & tandem in Caemiterio S. Petri, sepultus est:* Schenck, *op. cit.* (note 12), 9.

146. *[u]xor cujusdam cauponis puellam bicipitem peperit; quam mortuam Valentinus Wager vivis coloribus delineavit:* Schott, *op. cit.* (note 9), I, 662.

147. *[A]ure leporinâ, cum portione carnis instar pilei: ibid.,* I, 676.

148. Holländer, *op. cit.* (note 2), 124.

149. Anon., *Eine Rechte Warhaffte Abcontrofactur…1596…*(Prague, 1616). This resembles another case, *Abbildung einer Jungfrawen / so Nunmehr Etlick Jahr Alt / Aber ein Mikgeburt / so Auff einem Dorff…* (Jahr, 1616), see Holländer, *op. cit.* (note 2), 125–6.

150. *Capita a craniis defunctorum hominum non multum distabant, quorum singulae frontes in medio non aliter divisae apparebant, ac si essent discissae. Crura bina, una cum parvulis manibus, & pedibus macris, in angustum contractis, erant, ut solent in hujusmodi abortibus conspici…cor duplex, pulmo item & jecur duplex, in ventre inferiori stomachus simplex, & simplicia intestina:* Schott, *op. cit.* (note 9), I, 662.

151. Bauhin, *op. cit.* (note 40), 81.

152. *[M]onstrum humanum biceps cum cauda, duobus pedibus, & quatuor brachiis; quorum duo ritu humano proprium locum occupabant, alia duo juxta dorsum ex medio utriusque capitis ortum trahebant: cauda supra podicem spatio duorum digitorum erat, longitudine palmi, & excrementorum exitum tegebat, velut in quadrupedibus caudatis observatur; quae quidem juxta initium erat latitudinis digiti auricularis, & deinceps in acutum definebat. Nulla forma genitalis virilis & scroti apparebat, ideo foeminei sexus esse fuit creditum:* Schott, *op. cit.* (note 9), I, 663; Aldrovandi, *op. cit.* (note 12), 410–12.

153. *Haec absoluto gestationis uteri cursu, rure domum veniens, gravibus partus doloribus vexata, in terram cadens, extemplo epilepsia correpta est, & nocte adventante, foetum edidit, animamquae eadam nocte, post novem horarum paroxismum comitialis morbi, efflavit Infans autem fuit horrendi aspectus: nam*

duo capita simiarum facies aemulabantur; reliqua pars corporis puello bene constitutio similis erat, praeter brachia, quae aliqua ex parte manca videbantur; pedes formam potius pedem simiarum...: Aldrovandi, *op. cit.* (note 12), 410.

154. R.J., *A Most Strange and True Discourse...* (London, 1600).

155. P.D. Turnpenny and R. Hole, 'The First Description of Lethal Pterygium Syndrome with Facial Clefting (Bartsocas-Papas Syndrome) in 1600', *Journal of Medical Genetics*, xxxvii (2000), 314–15; see also R. Hole, 'Incest, Consanguinity and a Monstrous Birth in Rural England, January 1600', *Social History*, xxv (2000), 183–99.

156. J. Riolan, *De Monstro Nato Lutetiae Anno Domini 1605* (Paris: O. Varennaeum, 1605), fo. 1r–v; Liceti, *op. cit.* (note 1), 91, 115, 117.

157. *[C]adaver infantis primo statim die mortui, qui a prima in utero materno conformatione, umbilico tenus foramen rotundum, ac patulum, ad intima ventris viscera, aperta via, penetrans, quasi pugione confossum habebat; per quod & alimenta, & excrementa statim effluxerant. Cadavere aperto, caeteris partibus integris, corpus vesica destitutum, & anus imperforatus fuit inventus.* Schott, *op. cit.* (note 9), I, 687.

158. Anon., *Bildniß unnd Abcontrefeyung* (Strasbourg: J. Martin, 1606).

159. Anon., *Two Most Strange Births* (London: R.B., 1608); see also *Harleian Miscellany*, x, 462.

160. Anon., *ibid.*

161. *[Q]uod circa superioris labri & nasi interstitium monstrosa caro, veluti quaedam proboscis erat adnata, & referebat figuram oris ovini, exerta lingua tanquam balantis, & haec monstrosa caro spatium nasi non excedebat, reliquo superiori labro ad utrumque latus fisso. Qua propter puellus eiulans, diducto ore, & hiantibus alis superioris labri, admirandum vultum spectantibus exhibebat. Praeterea nasus huic carunculae prorsus connatus, impervius, & depressus fuit; ideoque ad aerem attrahendum nulla vi illi patebat; quemadmodum etiam ad hauriendum alimentum non parum erat impedimento. Puer fuit vocatus Joannes Jacobus, & diu vixit.* Schott, *op. cit.* (note 9), I, 676–7.

162. Anon., *Strange News out of Kent...* (1605).

163. *Deinde monstra dividi solent ratione sexus, ut si aliquid incerti nascitur sexus, & an mas and foemina sit dignosci nequit. Sic anno 1610 Mens. Martio in agro Pistoriensi ex conjugibus carbonariam factitantibus, nati sunt infantes pariter circa pudenda & nates adeo connexi, faciebus similiter oppositis, ut sexus distingui non posset, quamvis sexum potius foemineum participare viderentur.* J.C. Rausch, *Disputatio Physica de Monstris* (Jena: J.J. Bauhofer, 1665), sig. A5*v*.

164. W. Leigh, *Strange News of a Prodigious Monster...* (n.p.: J.P. &c, 1613).

165. *Obierunt à nativitate. Horum duorum monstrorum hae fuerunt imagines.* Liceti, *op. cit.* (note 1), 116.

166. *Abbildung einer Jungfrawen...* (n.p., 1616), see Holländer, *op. cit.* (note 2), 123.

167. This very well documented case is considered in Chapter 6, 150–1. See also M. Parker, *The Two Inseparable Brothers* (London: T. Lambert, 1637); T. Bartholin, *Historiarum Anatomicarum Rariorum Centuria I et II* (Amsterdam, J. Henrici, 1654), 117; Liceti, *op. cit.* (note 1), 114, 274; Bondeson, *op. cit.* (note 6), viii–xix.

168. *Indicit in animum ille Lazarus Colredo Genuensis Liguri Wittebergam venit anno 1645. die 15. Martii Statura bona, facies non indecora erat, neq: occurrebat quicquam, deformitatem quod obferret spectantibus. Sinistro lateri adnatus erat homunculo, quem fratrem suum appellabat, cuius nomen Johannes Baptista. Sic nati simul, simul in utero formati & concreti fuerunt, gemellorum in morem: Habebat Johannes caput, brachia, thoracem, & pedem unum. Manus erant imperfectae, trium digitorum, pes quatuor. Caput cum pectore vergebat deorsam, ita ut resupino vultu intueretur Lazarum. Muco praeterea refertum erat, qui & in nares profluebat. Oculi clausi erant, semisomnis, pedem movebat nonunquam. Labraminus decenti coitu conjuncta sed diducta quadantenus ut anteriores dentes conspicerentur. Quanquam nullus dentium usus. Cum ore cibum non caperet, sed è Lazaro traheret nutrimentum. Proprium cordis motum habebat, & respirationem, & reliqua facultatem vitalem attinentia. Sed nulla in ventriculo coctio, nulla in epate, aliqua incaeteris partibus.* C. Wallrich, *Disputatio Physica de Monstris quam Deo Juvante* (Wittenberg: J. Borckardt, 1655), sig. A2v.

169. Anon., *A Wonder Woorth the Reading...* (London: W. Jones, 1617).

170. Liceti, *op. cit.* (note 1), 113.

171. J.L. Gotfrid, *Historische Chronicle* part 8, 1184, quoted in Westphal, *op. cit.* (note 123), sig. C2*v*.

172. Anon., *Warhaffte unnd Eigentliche Contrafactur einer Selßamen Zwentopffigen Wunder Mickgeburt...* (Nürnburg: P. Isselburg, 1620), reproduced in Holländer, *op. cit.* (note 2), 82.

173. Anon., *Icon Sive Vera Repraesentatio* (Nürnberg: P. Isselburg, 1640); see Hollander, *op. cit.* (note 2), 285; J. Bondeson and E. Allen, 'Craniopagus Parasiticus: Everard Home's Two-Headed Boy of Bengal and Some Other Cases', *Surgical Neurology*, xxxi (1989), 426–34.

174. *[E]xorta est puella toto corpore bene organizata, excepto capite, quod est aspectu foedissimum; nam videtur in occipite velut oculus obscurus: alter oculus vis itus elatus in capite supra futuram coronalem, referens oculum humanum, & paulo majorem, sed sine palpebris, & absque ciliis, quorum sunt capilli capitis...*: Liceti, *op. cit.* (note 71), 132–3.

175. See G.T.Haneveld, 'Een Nederlands Schilderij van een Samengegroeide Tweeling (Thoracopagus) uit de 17e eeuw', *Nederlands Tijdschrift voor*

Geneeskunde, cxviii (1974), 801–5. The picture currently hangs in the Municipal Museum of The Hague.

176. Rausch, *op. cit.* (note 163), sig. B2r. This could be the same case as Anon., *Warhafftige Abbildung und Beschreibung* (Nürnberg: J. Hauer, 1631), see Ewinkel, *op. cit.* (note 4), 368.

177. T. Bedford, *A True and Certain Relation of a Strange Birth...* (London: A. Griffin, 1635), 4.

178. Westphal, *op. cit.* (note 123), sig. C2.

179. *[A]dhuc Bononiae adolescens annorum sexdecim, Thomas Bug Anellus nomine, cui brachium dexterum in cubito terminabatur, ubi rudimenta quaedam digitorum & unguium apparebant....eodemque in loco, die 28 Junii, uxor cuiusdam fabri lignarii enixa est puellum integris omnibus membris, praeter sinistrum brachium, quod in cubitum desinebat, ubi similiter rudimenta confusa digitorum & unguium conspiciebantur...*: Schott, *op. cit.* (note 9), I, 682

180. *Warhafftiges Abcontrant und Beschreibung...* (1640), reproduced in Holländer, *op. cit.* (note 2), 331.

181. J. Locke, *A Strange and Lamentable Accident...* (London: R. Harper and T. Wine, 1642).

182. F. Lachmund, 'Visceribus Sub Cute Prominentibus in Foetu', *Miscellanea Curiosa*, series 1, iii (1672), 166–7.

183. Anon., *The Most Strange and Wovnderfvll Apperation of Blood in a Poole at Garraton...* (London: I.H., 1645).

184. M. Hofmann, 'Anatome Partus Cerebro Carentis', *Miscellanea Curiosa*, series 1, ii (1671), 60–4.

185. J.B[ulwer], *Anthropometamorphosis...* (London: W. Hunt, 1653), 302.

186. D. Woodward, 'Some Difficult Confinements in Seventeenth-Century Yorkshire', *Medical History*, xviii (1974), 349–53.

187. Anon., *A Tempenie With Foure Hands and 4 Heeles, 2 Heads, 2 Bodyes, Two Mouthes, 4 Eyes and 4 Eares* (London: W. Gilbertson, 1656).

188. *[S]i culpa uxori tribuenda, impedevit illud impuritas uteri, qui aliquid de lochiis antea exclusi foetus mortui retinuit, ad putredinem disposuit, hacq; putredine contagium spirituosum ad alterius foetus perfectionem intendendam impediit & elusit...*: S. Ledel, 'De Foetu Monstroso', *Miscellanea Curiosa*, series 2, vi (1687), 152–3.

189. *[P]uellam vivam bicipitem, duobus brachiis & pedibus peperit, cui erant duo distincta pectora, cordaque duo, quod adstantes ex pulsatione cordium in utroque pectore manifesta & palpabili judicarunt...In posteriore parte prodibat excrescentia, non recta in altum diducta, uti effigies monstrat, sed ad latus vergens...*: M. Fribe, 'De Partu Monstroso Bicipiti', *Miscellanea Curiosa*, series 1, iii (1672), 254.

190. Anon., *Gods Judgement from Heaven; Or, A Very Strange Wonder to be*

Declared of a Monster in Flanders, at a Place Cal'd Sluce (1658) reprinted in
H.E. Rollins (ed.), *The Pack of Autolycus...* (Cambridge: Harvard University
Press, 1927), 139.

191. Anon., *The True and Most Miraculous Narrative...* (London: R. Harper,
1659).

192. Anon., 'Museo Cospiano Annesso a Quello del Famoso Ulisse Aldrovandi &
Donaro alla Sua Patria Dall' Illustrissimo Signore Ferdinando Cospi Patricio
di Bologna & Senatore &c Descrizzione di Lorenzo Legati Cremonese In fol
in Bologna', *Journal des Savans* (1678), 297–302 (book review).

193. G. Greisel, 'De Anatome Monstri Gemellorum Humanorum', *Miscellanea
Curiosa*, series 1, i (1670), 132–3.

194. Anon., *Nature's Wonder?...* (1664), quoted in Rollins, *op. cit.* (note 190),
140; Anon., 'Extrait d'une Lettre Escrite d'Oxfort, le 12 Novembre 1664',
Journal des Savans, i (1665), 11–12.

195. F. Mouriceau, 'Des Maladies des Femmes Grosses & Accouchées &c.',
Journal des Savans (1669), 8–11: 10–11.

196. C. Rayger, 'De Capite Monstro Sine Cranio et Cerebro', *Miscellanea Curiosa*,
series 1, iii (1672), 427.

197. Anon., 'Extract of a Letter, Written from Paris, Containing an Account of
Some Effects of the Transfusion of Bloud; and of Two Monstrous Births,
&c.', *Philosophical Transactions*, ii (1667), 479–80.

198. G. Seger, 'De Embryone Hydropico', *Miscellanea Curiosa*, series 1, i (1670),
114–15.

199. A.H. Cumm, 'De Hydrocephalo Dissecto', *Miscellanea Curiosa*, series 1, i
(1670), 120.

200. Anon., *op. cit.* (note 197).

201. H. Vollgnad, 'De Monstroso Foetu', *Miscellanea Curiosa*, series 1, iii (1672),
446–7.

202. Anon., *The Strange Monster...* (London: P. Lillicrap, 1668).

203. E. Gockel, 'Foetus Monstrosus cum Superiori Maxilla & Labio in Utroque
Latere Fisso', *Miscellanea Curiosa*, series 2, vii (1688), 237–8.

204. *[B]ina cernebantur corda*: C. Rayger, 'De Anatomia Monstri Bicipitis',
Miscellanea Curiosa, series 1, i (1670), 21–3.

205. J.S. Elsholt, 'De Conceptione Tubaria, qua Humani Foetus Extra Uterica
Vitatem in Tubis Quandoq; Concipiuntur: Itemque de Puella Monstroso,
Berolini Nuper Nata, Epistola ad Dn. D. Wolrathum Huxholtium Sereniss,
Principis Landgraviae Hessorum Regentis Archiatrum, &c.', *Miscellanea
Curiosa*, series 1, iv (1674), appendix.

206. J. Grandi, 'An Extract of an Italian Letter', *Philosophical Transactions*, v
(1670), 1188–9.

207. W. Durston, 'A Narrative of a Monstrous Birth in Plymouth, Octob. 22,

1670: Together with the Anatomical Observations, Taken Thereupon',
Philosophical Transactions, v (1670), 2096–7.

208. J. Jaenis, 'De Infante Sine Capite', *Miscellanea Curiosa*, series 1, iii (1672),
442–4.

209. J.J. Waldschmid, 'Monstrum Humanum Abominandum', *Miscellanea
Curiosa*, series 1, ii (1671), 313.

210. F. Bouchard, 'Infante Monstroso Lugduni in Viam Publicam die V Martii A.
MDCLXXI Exposito', *Miscellanea Curiosa*, series 1, iii (1672), 14–16.

211. H. Sampson, 'De Foetu Monstrosissimo', *Miscellanea Curiosa*, series 1, iii
(1672), 279.

212. L'Abbé de Claustre, *Table Générale des Matiéres Contenues dans le Journal des
Savans de l'Édition de Paris, Depuis l'Année 1665* (Paris: Briasson, 1753–64),
lists a letter from M. Gerberon, a physician (*Journal des Savans* 1672,
supplement, 8), concerning this case. I have yet to see the original.

213. 'An Extract of a Letter, Written by Monsieur Denys Novemb. 17 Last from
Paris, Concerning an Odd Foetus Lately Born There & English't out of
French', *Philosophical Transactions*, viii (1673), 6157.

214. *Pectus aliqualiter gibbosum: loco abdominis erat saccus membraneus, isq;
pellucidus, monstrosè ad pedes usque propendens, in quo intestina cum ceteris
infimi cerni poterant. Ex capite dorsum versùs dependebat informis massa
carnosa acuminata*: C.F. Paullin, 'Observationes Medico-Physicae, Selectae &
Curiosae, Variis Antiquitatibus Historico-Germanicis Bonâ Fide Interdum
Conspersae', *Miscellanea Curiosa*, series 2, vi (1687), appendix, 53–4.

215. J.M. Nester, 'De Foetu Monstroso', *Miscellanea Curiosa*, series 1, vi (1675),
60.

216. J. Schmidt, 'De Monstro Foeminini Sexus', *Miscellanea Curiosa*, series 1, iv
(1674), 27–9.

217. *[A]bdomen totum, pellucidum adeò, ut intestinorum, suo ordine convolutorum,
gyri oculis cerui possent, ingentis herniae instar prominebat; ani enim orificium
supra muliebria extabat, idque ad latus dextrum nonnihil declinans atque
prominulum, (unde ortum de sexu dubium) conspiciebatur, per quod excrementa
alvi liquida, colore subvirida, cum obscurâ flavedine, subinda prodibant. In
dextro pede duo omnino digiti desiderabantur, & pollux reflexus metacarpio
turpiter incumbedat…*: G.A. Mercklin, 'De Gravidae Imaginatione Foetui
Noxia', *Miscellanea Curiosa*, series 1, viii (1677), 73–5.

218. J.C. Peyer, 'De Gemellis Monstrosis, Coalitis Partibus Obscoenis',
Miscellanea Curiosa, series 2, ii (1683), 267.

219. A. Khon, 'Partu Monstroso Miranda Imaginationis vi Oborto', *Miscelanea
Curiosa*, series 1, ix (1678), 74.

220. S. Morris, 'A Relation of a Monstrous Birth… Sent to Dr Charles Goodall of
London, both of the College of Physicians', *Philosophical Transactions*, xii

(1678), 961–2.

221. Salgues, *op. cit.* (note 62), III, 127.

222. Du Plessis, *op. cit.* (note 137), 31–2; Bondeson, *op. cit.* (note 6), xvi.

223. G.C. Göller, 'Abortus Humani Monstrosi Hist. Anatom.', *Miscellanea Curiosa*, series 2, ii (1683), 311–18.

224. Anon., 'Extrait d'une Lettre Ecrite d'Allemagne à l'Auteur du Journal Continant Quelques Curiositez', *Journal des Savans* (1679), 144.

225. B. Scharf, 'Monstrum à Constricctione', *Miscellanea Curiosa*, series 2, ii, (1683), 254–6.

226. A.P., 'A Letter from Mr A.P. in Somersetshire, Giving an Account of a Strange Birth that in May Last Happened at Hillbrewers in that County', *Philosophical Collections*, ii (1681), 21–2; Anon., '*A True Relation of a Monstrous Female-Child...* (London, D. Mallet, *c.* 1680); see also J. Bondeson, 'The Isle-Brewers Conjoined Twins of 1680', *Journal of the Royal Society of Medicine*, lxxxvi (1993), 106–9.

227. Hansen, 'Extrait de Deux Lettres Ecrites à l'Auteur du Journal', *Journal des Savans* (1681), 46–7.

228. Anon., *A Letter from an Eminent Merchant in Ostend...* (n.d.). A high-quality engraving shows one awake and the other asleep.

229. C. Krahe, 'The Description of a Monstrous Child...', *Philosophical Transactions*, xiv (1684), 599–600.

230. Salgues, *op. cit.* (note 62), III, 118–19; see also J. Gélis, *History of Childbirth. Fertility, Pregnancy and Birth in Early Modern Europe* (Polity Press: Oxford, 1991), 268. Du Plessis, *op. cit.* (note 137), mentions an account from a French periodical 'le mercure sailant...January 1684', which I have yet to see.

231. Galliard, 'Observations Particulieres sur Differentes Maladies', *Journal des Savans* (1697), 338.

232. J.M. Hoffmann, 'De Monstro Gemello', *Miscellanea Curiosa*, series 2, iv (1685), 288–90. Plates show detailed dissections of their thoracic and abdominal viscera: fig. XXXVI (facing 289) is the earliest illustration I have seen where the intestines are arranged in a mirror-image fashion.

233. Vander Wiel, 'Extrait des Nouv. de la Rep. des Lettres', *Journal des Savans* (1686), 263–4.

234. Du Plessis, *op. cit.* (note 137); see Bondeson, *op. cit.* (note 6), xvi.

235. G. Garden, 'Two Monstrous Births in Scotland', *Philosophical Transactions*, xv (1686), 1156.

236. *Ibid.*

237. *[S]ed temporis brevitas & voluntas monstrosae puellae Patris obstabant, hic enim nec precibus nec nummis a philiatris oblatis se permoveri patiebatur, ut corpusculum defunctae cultro Anatomico subjici permitteret...*: J.M. Hoffmann,

'De Foetu Monstroso', *Miscellanea Curiosa*, series 2, vi (1687), 333–6.

238. E. Gockel, 'Infans ex Fortissima Matris Imaginatione, Monstrosa Umbilici Relaxatione, ac Intestinorum extra Corpus Propendentium Prolapsu, Natus', *Miscellanea Curiosa*, series 2, vi (1687), 263–4.

239. C.J. Myller, 'Foetus Quodammodo Monstrosus à Partu', *Miscellanea Curiosa*, series 2, vii (1688), 429.

240. S. Reisel, 'De Labiis Leporinis Geminis, Oculis Clausis & Coecis, & Fovea Cranii in Vertice', *Miscellanea Curiosa*, series 2, viii (1689), 135–6.

241. J.M. Hoffmann, 'Foetu Monstroso ex Imaginatione Matris', *Miscellanea Curiosa*, series 2, viii (1689), 483–5.

242. E. Konig, 'Gemelli Sibi Invicem Adnati Feliciter Separati', *Miscellanea Curiosa*, series 2, viii (1689), 305–7.

243. Du Plessis, *op. cit.* (note 137), 91.

244. S. Reisel, 'Infans Truncus Sine Artubus', *Miscellanea Curiosa*, series 2, viii (1689), 136–7.

245. *Ibid.*

246. J.A. Hünerwolff, 'De Foemellis Duabus Monstrosis', *Miscellanea Curiosa*, series 2, ix (1690), 170–1.

247. *[C]ette grande difformité de la teste fit douter la conformation du cerveau, qui est le siege de l'ame. Si l'enfant avoit eu vie, la difficluté auroit este plus grande pour lui donner le baptême. Quelques ecclesiastiques qui se trouverent présens, jugerent qu'il auroit fallu lui donner sous condition... Cette femme avoit perdu depuis quelque mois une vache de poil noir, & avoit senti cette perte avec beaucoup de douleur.* Le Prieur de Lugeris, 'Extrait d'une Lettre de Monsieur le Prieur de Lugeris en Champagne, Sur un Enfantement Arrivé au Mois de Mai Dernier', *Journal des Savans* (1690), 53–4.

248. J. Lanzoni, 'Partus Mirabilis Scandiani Editus 26 Maji A. 1690', *Miscellanea Curiosa*, Series 2, ix (1690), 73–6; M. Malpighi, *Opera Posthuma...Quibus Praefixa est Ejusdem Vita a Seipso Scripta* (London, A. and J. Churchill, 1697), 87.

249. A. Löw, 'Foetus, Quà Caput, Monstrosus', *Miscellanea Curiosa*, series 2, ix (1690), 200–2.

250. G.C. Scheihammer, 'Monstrum Acephalum', *Miscellanea* Curiosa, series 2, ix (1690), 258–9.

251. C.Patini, 'Monstrum Biceps Masculinum', *Miscellanea Curiosa*, series 2, x (1691), 72–3. An illustration shows them alive, standing and smiling.

252. P.J. Hartmann, 'Anatome Monstri', *Miscellanea Curiosa*, series 2, x (1691), 258–62.

253. J. Lanzoni, 'De Monstro Mentulato & Bicorpori', *Miscellanea Curiosa*, series 3, i (1692), 185–6.

254. *Ibid.*

255. La Motte (transl. T. Tomkyns), *A General Treatise of Midwifry...* (London, J. Waugh, 1746), 455–7.

256. C. Preston, 'An Account of a Child Born Without a Brain, and the Observables in it on Dissection', *Philosophical Transactions*, xix (1697), 457–67. Preston was lodged in Paris, 'for the Benefit of Accouch-mens... I carried the subject to Monsieur Du Verney, Professor of Anatomy in the Royal Garden at Paris, to have it more carefully examined'. He had seen 'several' foetuses 'dissected' in the 'private lectures' of du Verney.

257. E. Tyson, 'An Observation of an Infant, Where the Brain was Depressed into the Hollow of the Vertebrae of the Neck', *Philosophical Transactions*, xix (1697), 533-5.

258. Anon., 'Suite des Observations Faites a Toulouse', *Journal des Savans* (1697), 359–60.

259. Bussiere, 'An Anatomical Account of a Child's Head, Born Without a Brain in October last, 1698', *Philosophical Transactions*, xxi (1700), 141–4.

260. Anon., *By His Majesty's Authority: At the Sign of Charing-Cross, at Charing Cross, There is to be Seen a Strange and Monstrous Child...* (London, 1699).

261. J.H. Hottinger, 'Monstruo Humano Absque Sexu, Pedibus, &c in Excrescentiam Caudiformem Definente', *Miscellanea Curiosa*, series 3, ix (1700), 413–16.

262. La Motte, *op. cit.* (note 255), 457.

Bibliography

Primary Sources

1. Manuscripts

Du Plessis, [James Paris], *A Short History of Human Prodigious & Monstrous Births of Dwarfs, Sleepers, Giants, Strong Men, Hermaphrodies, Numerous Births, and Extream Old Age &c.* (1730) BL MS Sloane 5246.

Du Plessis, [James Paris], (1732) BL MS Sloane 3253.

2. Broadsides and Tracts – listed by date of publication

Anon., *Monstrificus Puer hic in Districtu Diocesis Argentinensis et Pago Witterswiler Prope Nuwiler Oppidum ex Paupercula Muliere His Menbris [sic] et Corporis Liniamentis, Undecima Die Marij Anno Undecimo Supra Millesimum & Quingentisimum In Lucem Editus Extitit* (n.p: Sebastian Brant, 1511).

Anon., *Zu Wissen: Ein Wunderlichs von Erschrockenlich Ding* (n.p: Wolf Traut, 1511).

Anon., *Disz Künd ist Geboren Worden zu Tettnang* (Munich: Hans Burgkmair, 1516).

Anon., *Am XXIIIII Tag des Mai, Also am Sankt-Urbans-Tag, Zwischen Fünf und Sechs Vormittags, Hat eine Siebenundzwanzigjährige Frau in der Stadt Landshut an der Donau in Bayern...* (n.p., 1517).

Anon., *Billich Verwundert Sich Jung und Alt* (Zürich, 1519).

Melanchthon, Philip and Martin Luther, *Deuttung der Zwo Grewlichen Figuren, Bapstesels zu Rom und Munchkalbs zu Freyburg in Meyssen Funden* (Wittenberg: N. Schirlentz, 1523).

Anon., *Im Fünffzehenhunderten und Dreyundzweintzigsten Jaren* (n.p: Hans Sebald Beham, 1523).

Anon., *An dem Achte Tag des Octobers* (n.p., 1524).

Anon., *Anzeygung Wunderbarlicher Geschichten* (n.p: Erhard Schoen, 1531).

Anon., *Eine Wuenderliche Geburt eines Zweykoepffigen Kindes* (n.p: B.W., 1542).

Anon., *Warhafftige Contrafractur einer Wunder Geburt* (Frankfurt: Herman Gülfferich, 1544).

Anon., *Thou Shalte Understande, Chrysten Reader, That the Thyrde Daye of August Last Past, Anno MCCCCCLII...in a Towne Called Myddleton stonye...at the In, Called the Sygne of the Egle, There the Good Wyfe of the Same, Was Deliuered of Thys Double Chylde, Begotten of her Late Housbande John Kenner...* (London, 1552).

Anon., *Warhaffte Abconterfectur der Erschrocklichen Wundergeburt* (Augsburg: Philipp Ulhart, 1560).

Anon., *Ein Wunderbarliche Seltzame Erschroeckliche Geburt* (Augsburg: Michel Moser Brieffmaler, 1561).

F[ulwood], W[illiam], *The Shape of ii Monsters, MDlxii* (London: John Alde, 1562).

Anon., *The Description of a Monstrous Pig, the Which was Farrowed at Hamsted Besyde London, the xvi Day of October This Present Yeare of Our Lord God MDLXII* (London: Alexander Lacy for Garat Dewes, 1562).

Anon., *The True Reporte of the Forme and Shape of a Monstrous Childe Borne at Muche Horkesley, a Village Three Myles from Colchester, in the Countye of Essex, the xxi Daye of Apryll in This Yeare* (London: Thomas Marshe, 1562).

D., Jhon, *A Discription of a Monstrous Chylde, Borne at Chychester in Sussex, the xxiiii Daye of May: This Being the Very Length, and Bygnes of the Same* (London: Leonard Askel for Fraunces Godlyf, 1562).

Anon., *Warhafftige und Eigentliche Contrafactur einer Wunderbarlichen Geburt* (Strasbourg: Thiebolt Berger, 1563).

Barkar, John, *The True Description of a Monsterous Chylde/ Borne in the Ile of Wight, in this Present Yeare of Oure Lord God, MDLXIIII the Month of October, After This Forme With a Cluster of Longe Heare About the Nauell, the Fathers Name is Iames Iohnson, in the Parys of Freswater* (London: Wylliam Gryffith, 1564).

Anon., *The True Fourme and Shape of a Monsterous Chyld, Whiche was Borne in Stony Stratforde, in North Hamptonshire: The Yeare of Our Lord, MCCCCCLXV* (London: Colwell, 1565).

Anon., *The True Discription of Two Monsterous Chyldren Borne at Herne in Kent: The xxvi Daie of Auguste In the Yere of Lorde MCCCCCLXV...* (London: T. Colwell, 1565).

Anon., *Ein Neuwe Seltzame Warhafftige Wundergeburt* (Augsburg: Hans Zimmerman, 1565).

Mellys, John, *The True Description of Two Monsterous Children, Laufully Begotten Between George Stevens and Margerie his Wyfe, and Borne in the Parish of Swanburne in Buckynghamshyre the iiij of Aprill Anno Domini 1566 the Two Children Hauing their Belies Fast Ioyned Together, and Imbracing One an Other with their Armes: which Children Wer Both a Lyue by the Space of Half an Hower, and Wer Baptized, and Named the One Iohn, and the Other Ioan* (London: Alexander Lacy, 1566).

B., H., *The True Discription of a Childe with Ruffes, Borne in the Parish of Micheham in the Coñtie of Surrey, in the Yeere of Our Lord MDLXVI* (London: John Allde, 1566).

Anon., *Ware Abcontrafactur einer Missgeburt* (Schmalkalden: Michel Schmuck, 1566).

Anon., *The Forme and Shape of a Monstrous Child, Borne at Maydstone in Kent, the xxiiij of October, 1568* (London: John Awdeley, 1568).

Anon., *Ein Newe und Warhafftige Zeittung* (Strasbourg: Peter Hug, 1569).

Anon., *Warhafftige Beschreibung* (Augsburg: Michael Manger, 1569).

Anon., *L'Androgyn Né a Paris, le xxi Juillet, MDLXX: Illustré des Vers Latins de Jean Dorat Poéte du Roy Tres-Chrestien, Contenans l'Interpretation de ce Monstre; Avec la Traduction d'Iceux en Nostre Vulgaire Français, Dediee à Monseigneur le President l'Archer* (Lyon: Michael Jove, 1570).

Anon., *Nova et Ridiculosa Expositione del Monstro Nato in Ghetto* (Venice, 1575).

Anon., *Discorso Sopra il Significato del Parto Monstruoso Nato di une Hebrea in Venetia* (Venice: Domenico Farri, 1575).

Anon., *Warhafftige unnd Erschroeckliche Geburt* (Heidelberg: Michael Schirat, 1575).

Anon., *The Discription and Figure of a Monstruous Childe Borne at Taunton the viij of November 1576* (London: Hugh Jackson, 1576).

Merula, Dietmar, *Ware/ Eigentliche/ und Umbstendigliche Beschreibunge* (Frankfurt: Jacob Weissen, 1577).

Anon., *Briefz Discours d'un Merveilleux Monstre Né a Eusrigo, Terre de Novarrez en Lombardie, au Moys de Janvier en la Presente Annee 1578: Avec le Vray Pourtraict d'Icelluy au Plus Prez du Naturel* (Chambéry: François Poumard, 1578).

Anon., *Vray Pourtraict, et Sommaire Description d'un Horrible et Merveilleux Monstre, Né a Cher, Terre de Piedmond, le 10 de Janvier 1578: A Huit Heaures du Soir, de la Femme d'un Docteur, Avec Sept Cornes, Celle Qui Pend Jusques a la Saincture et Celle qui est Autour du Col sont de Chair* (Chambéry: François Poumard, 1578).

Pauli, Simon, *Bildtnuß und Gestalt* (Rostock: Jacobus Lucius, 1578).

Anon., *Newe Zeytung: Eine Erschreckliche Mißgeburt* (Nürnberg: Matthäus Rauch, 1578).

Anon., *Warhaffte und Gewisse Abcontrafeytung einer Mißgeburt* (Nürnburg: Lucas Mayer Furmschneider, 1578).

Anon., *Ein newe Wundergeburt* (n.p., 1579).

Anon., *The Description of Monstrous Childe Borne at Ffenny Stanton in Huntingdonshire* (London: Henry Bynneman, 1580).

Anon., *A True Report of a Straung and Monsterous Child, Born at Aberwick, in the Parish of Eglingham, in the County of Northumberland, this Fifth of January* (London: Thomas Gosson, n.d.).

Anon., *Von einer Warhafftigen/ doch Erschrecklichen und Nicht Bald Erhoerten Misgeburt* (n.p., 1581).

Anon., *A Right Strange and Wonderful Example of the Handie Worke of a Mightie God, to Move Us Wretched Sinners to Amendement of Our Wicked Lyves, by This Lamentable Spectacle for Al Men & Women to Behold, of the Birth of Three Children Borne in the Parish of PASKEWET, in the County of Monmouth, on Thursday, the Third of February Last 1585 and Are at this Present to be Seene at London* (London: Richard Jones, 1585).

Anon., *Erschroeckliche und Warhafftige Contrafaytung* (Brüssel: Johann Wollaert, 1588).

J[ones], R[ichard], *A Most Strange and True Discourse of the Wonderfull Judgement of God, of a Monstrous Deformed Infant, Begotten by Incestuous Copulation, Between the Brother's Sonne, and the Sister's Daughter, Being Both Unmarried Persons: Which Child was Born at Colwall, in the County and Diocese of Hereford, upon the Feast of the Epiphany, Commonly Called Twelfth-Day, 1599; A Notable and Most Terrible Example of Incest and Whoredom* (London, 1600).

Anon., *Discours Prodigieux et Veritable, d'une Fille de Chambre, Laquelle a Produict un Monstre...* (Paris: F. Bourriquant, n.d.).

Anon., *Bildniß unnd Abcontrefeyung* (Strasbourg: Jost Martin, 1606).

Anon., *Two Most Strange Births* (London: R.B., 1608).

Anon., *Histoire Miraculeuse, Advenue dans la Ville de Geneve...* (Lyon: C. Farine, 1609).

Anon., *Strange Newes out of Kent, of a Monstrous and Misshapen Child, Borne in Olde Sandwitch, upon the 10 of Julie Last, the Like (for Strangeness) Hath Never Beene Seene* (London: T.C. for W. Barley, 1609).

Leigh, W., *Strange News of a Prodigious Monster Born on the Township of Adlington, in the Parish of Standish, in the County of Lancaster, the 17 Day of Aprill, 1613: Testified by the Reverend Divine, Mr W. Leigh, Bachelor of Divinitie, and Preacher of God's Word at Standish Aforesaid* (n.p: J.P. etc., 1613).

Anon., *A Wonder Woorth the Reading, or, A True and Faithfull Relation of a Woman, Now Dwelling in Kent Street, Who, Upon Thursday, Being the 21 of August Last, Was Deliuered of a Prodigious and Monstrous, Child, in the Presence of Diuers Honest, and Religious Women to their Wonderfull Feare and Astonishment* (London: William Jones, 1617).

B[edford], Th[omas], *A True and Certain Relation of a Strange Birth, Which Was Born at Stonehouse, in the Parish of Plimouth, the 20th of Oct. 1635; Together With the Notes of a Sermon Preached, Oct. 23d, in the Church of Plimouth, at the Intering of the Said Birth* (London: Anne Griffin, 1635).

Parker, Martin, *The Two Inseparable Brothers...* (London: Thomas Lambert, 1637).

Anon., *A Lamentable List, of Certaine Hidious, Frightfull, and Prodigious Signes...* (London: Tho. Lambert, 1638).

Anon., *A Certaine Relation of the Hog-Faced Gentlewoman...* (London: J.O., 1640).

Anon., *Icon Sive Vera Repraesentatio* (Nürnberg: Peter Isselburg, 1640).

Locke, John, *A Strange and Lamentable Accident that Happened Lately at Mears-Ashby in Northamptonshire 1642: Of One Mary Wilmore, Wife to John Wilmore, Rough Mason, Who Was Delivered of a Childe Without a Head, and Credibly Reported to Have a Firme Crosse on the Brest, as this Ensuing Story Shall Relate* (London: Richard Harper and Thomas Wine, 1642).

Anon., *The True Picture of a Female Monster Born Near Salisbury* (n.p., 1644).

Anon., *The Most Strange and Wovnderfvll Apperation of Blood in a Poole at Garraton...* (London: I.H., 1645).

Anon., *A Declaration of a Strange and Wonderfull Monster: Born in KIRKHAM Parish in LANCASHIRE (the Childe of Mrs. Haughton, a Popish Gentlewoman) the Face of it Upon the Breast, and Without a Head (After the Mother had Wished Rather to Bear a Childe Without a Head Than a Roundhead...* (London: Jane Coe, 1646).

Anon., *Strange News From Scotland...* (London: E.P. for W. Lee, 1647).

Anon., *The Ranters Monster: Being a True Relation of one Mary Adams, Living at Tillingham in Essex...With the Manner How She was Deliver'd of the Ugliest Ill-Shapen Monster That Ever Eyes Beheld...* (London: George Horton, 1652).

Anon., *A Tempenie With Foure Hands and 4 Heeles, 2 Heads, 2 Bodyes, Two Mouthes, 4 Eyes and 4 Eares* (London: Wm. Gilbertson, 1656).

Anon., *Gods Judgement from Heaven; Or, A Very Strange Wonder to be Declared of a Monster in Flanders, at a Place Cal'd Sluce* (n.p., 1658).

Anon., *The True and Most Miraculous Narrative, of a Child Born With Two Tongues, at the Lower End of East-Smithfeild [sic] in the Suburbs of London... who Thee Dayes After His Birth, Was Heard Plainly, Expresly to Cry Out, A King, A King, A King...* (London: R. Harper, 1659).

Anon., *Nature's Wonder? A True Account How the Wife of One John Waterman an Ostler in the Parish of Fisherton-Anger, Near Salisbury, was Delivered of a Strange Monster Upon the 26th of October 1664 Which Lived Untill the 27th of the Same Moneth: It Had Two Heads, Foure Armes, and Two Legs, The Heads Standing Contrary Each to the Other; and the Loines, Hipps, and Leggs Issuing Out of the Middle, Betwixt Both; They Were Bothe Perfect to the Navell, and There Joyned in One, Being but One Sex, Which Was the*

Female; She Had Another Child Born Before It (Of the Female Sex) Which is Yet Living, and is a Very Comely Child in All Proportions; This is Attested for Truth, by Several Persons Which Were Eye Witnesses (n.p., 1664).

Anon., *The Strange Monster or, True News from Nottingham-Shire of a Strange Monster Born at Grasly in Nottingham-Shire, Three Miles from Nottingham, With a Relation of His Strange and Wonderful Shape, the Time His Mother Was in Travail With Him, With Several Other Things of Note: Together With a Brief Relation of Several Monstrous and Prodigious Births Which Happened Heretofore in This Our Nation* (London: Peter Lillicrap, 1668).

L., T., *The Wonder of Wonders, or, the Strange Birth in Hampshire* (London: J. Hose and E. Oliver, n.d.).

Anon., *A True Relation of a Monstrous Female-Child, With Two Heads, Four Eyes, Four Ears, Two Noses, Two Mouths, and Four Arms, Four Legs, and All Things Else Proportionably, Fixed to One Body: Born About the 19 of May Last, at a Village Called Ill-Brewers Near Taunton Dean in Somerset-Shire; Likewise a True and Perfect Account of its Form so Prodigiously Strange...As It Was Faithfully Communicated in a Letter, by a Person of Worth, Living in Taunton-Dean, to a Gentleman Here in London...* (London: D. Mallet, n.d.).

Anon., *A Letter From an Eminent Merchant in Ostend...* (n.p., n.d.) BL N.TAB.2026/25.

Anon., *A Collection of 77 Advertisements, Relating to Dwarfs, Giants, and Other Monsters and Curiosities Exhibited for Public Inspection* [*c.*1680–*c.*1700] BL N.TAB.2026/25.

Anon., *The Wonder of this Present Age: or, An Account of a Monster Born in the Liberty of Westminster, on the 16th of this Instant September 1687: Having Two Heads, Four Arms and Hands; As Like-Wise Four Leggs and Feet, Yet But One Body From the Lower Parts to the Breast* (London: J. Deacon, 1687).

Anon., *The Cruel Midwife... A Most Sad and Lamentable DISCOVERY That Has Been Lately Made in the Village of POPLAR in the Parish of STEPNEY: At the House of One Madame Compton Alias Norman a Midwife, Wherein Has Been Discovered Many Children That Have Been Murdered; Particularly Two That Were Lately Found in a Hand-Basket on a Shelf in the Sellar, Whose Skins, Eyes, and Part of Their Flesh Were Eaten by Vermin; The Skelliton of Six Others That Were Found Buried in the Sellar; With the Design of Digging for Others in the Garden* (London: R. Wier, 1693).

Anon., *By his Majesty's Authority: At the Sign of Charing-Cross, at Charing Cross, There is to be Seen a Strange and Monstrous Child, With One Body and One Belly, and Yet Otherwise it Hath all the Proporsions of Two Children...* (n.p., 1699) BL N. TAB. 2026/25.

W., L., *True Wonders, and Strange News from Rumsey in Hampshire...* (n.p., n.d.).

3. Books and Contributions to Journals

Primary Sources

Aldrovandi, Ulysse, *Monstrorum Historia...* (Bononia: N. Tebaldini, 1642).

Anon., 'Extrait d'une Lettre Escrite d'Oxfort, le 12 Novembre 1664', *Journal des Savans* (1665), 11–12.

Anon., 'Extract of a Letter, Written from Paris, Containing an Account of Some Effects of the Transfusion of Bloud; and of Two Monstrous Births, &c, A Monstrous Birth Like a Monkey, at Paris', *Philosophical Transactions*, ii (1667), 479–80.

Anon., 'Extrait d'une Lettre Ecrite d'Allemagne à l'Auteur du Journal Continant Quelques Curiositez', *Journal des Savans* (1679), 144.

Anon., 'Suite des Observations Faites a Toulouse', *Journal des Savans* (1697), 359–60.

Bacon, Francis, 'The Great Instauration', in James Spedding, Robert Leslie Ellis and Douglas Dendon Heath (eds), *The Works of Francis Bacon* (London: Longman, 1857–74).

Bartholin, Thomas, *Historiarum Anatomicarum Rariorum Centuria I et II* (Amsterdam: Joann Henrici, 1654).

Bartholin, Thomas, 'De Sirene Danica', *Miscellanea Curiosa*, series 1, i (1670), 73–7.

Batman, Stephen, *The Doome Warning All Men to the Judgement: Wherein...* (London: Ralphe Nubery, 1581).

Bauhin, Caspar, *Hermaphroditorum Monstrosorumque Partuum Natura ex Theologorum, Jureconsultorum, Medicorum, Philosophorum, & Rabbinorum* (Frankfurt: Mathaeus Becker, 1600).

Bayle, 'Dissertationes Physicae in Quibus Principia Proprietatum in Mixtis, Aeconomia in Plantis & Animalibus, Causa & Signa Propensionum in Homine &c Demonstrantur', *Journal des Savans* (1677), 161–3.

[Blondel, James], *The Strength of the Imagination in Pregnant Women Examined* (London: J. Peale, 1727).

Boaistuau, Pierre, *Histoires Prodigieuses les Plus Memorables Qui Ayent Esté Obseruées, Depuis la Natiuité de Iesus Christ, Iusques à Nostre Siecle: Extraictes de Plusieurs Fameux Autheurs, Grecz, & Latins, Sacrez & Prophanes* (Paris: Vincent Sentenas, 1560).

Boaistuau, Pierre, *Histoires Prodigieuses... Divisees en Deux Tomes* (Paris: Jean de Bordeaux, 1571).

Boaistuau, Pierre, *Histoires Prodigieuses les Plus Memorables Qui Ayent Esté Obseruées, Depuis la Natiuité de Iesus Christ, Iusques à Nostre Siecle: Extraictes de Plusieurs Fameux Autheurs, Grecz, & Latins, Sacrez & Prophanes: Mises en Nostre Langue Par P. Boaistuau... Avec les Pourtraictz & Figures* (Anvers: G. Ianssens, 1594).

Boaistuau, Pierre (ed. Stephen Bamforth), *Histoires Prodigieuses: MS 136 Wellcome Library* (Milan: Franco Maria Ricci, 2000).

Boorde, Andrew, *The Breviary of Helthe, for All Maner of Syckenesses and Diseases the Whiche May be in Man, or Woman doth Folowe / Expressynge the Obscure Termes of Greke, Araby, Latyn, and Barbary in to Englysh Concerning Phisicke and Chierurgye* (London: W. Middleton, 1547).

Bouchard, François, 'Infante Monstroso Lugduni in Viam Publicam Die V Martii A. MDCLXXI Exposito', *Miscellanea Curiosa*, series 1, iii (1672), 14–16.

Bracesco da Iorci Novi, Giovanni, *La Espositione de Geber Philosopho* (Venice: G. Giolito, 1544).

Bridoul, Toussaint, *The School of the Eucharist* (London: Randall Taylor, 1687).

Browne, Thomas, *Pseudodoxia Epidemica, Or, Enquiries Into Very Many Received Tenents, and Commonly Presumed Truths* (London: T.H. for E. Dod, 1646).

Browne, Thomas, *Religio Medici* (London: Andrew Crooke, 1642).

Browne, Thomas (ed. Jean-Jaques Denonain) *Religio Medici* (Cambridge: Cambridge University Press, 1953).

B[ulwer], J[ames], *Anthropometamorphosis: Man Transform'd; or, the Artificial Changeling; Historically Presented, in the Mad and Cruel Gallantry, Foolish Bravery, Ridiculous Beauty, Filthy Finenesse, and Loathsome Lovelinesse of Most Nations, Fashioning and Altering their Bodies from the Mould Intended by Nature; With a Vindication of the Regular Beauty and Honesty of Nature; and an Appendix of the Pedigree of the English Gallant* (London: William Hunt, 1653).

Bussiere, 'An Anatomical Account of a Child's Head, Born Without a Brain in October Last, 1698', *Philosophical Transactions*, xxi (1700), 141–4.

Cardan, Jerome, *De Rerum Varietate...* (Basel: Sebastian Henri Petri, 1581).

Castiglione, Baldassare (transl. Charles Singleton), *Book of the Courtier* (New York: Anchor Books, 1959).

Claustre, Abbé de, *Table Générale des Matières Contenues dans le Journal des Savans de l'Édition de Paris, Depuis l'Année 1665* (Paris: Briasson, 1753–64).

Cleveland, John, *A Character of a Diurnal-Maker* (London: W.S., 1651).

Cumm, Alard Hermann, 'De Hydrocephalo Dissecto', *Miscellanea Curiosa*, series 1, i (1670), 120.

Dareste, Camille, 'Recherches sur les Conditions Organiques des Hétérotaxies', *Comptes Rendus Séances de la Societe de Biologie et de ses Filiales*, series 3, i (1859), 8–11.

Dareste, Camille, *Recherches sur la Production Artificielle des Monstruosités ou Essais de Tératogénie Expérimentale* (Paris: C. Reinwald, 1877).

Day, John, *The Parliament of Bees* (London: William Lee, 1641).

Denys, 'An Extract of a Letter, Written by Monsieur Denys Novemb. 17 Last From Paris, Concerning an Odd Foetus Lately Born There & English't out of French', *Philosophical Transactions*, viii (1673), 6157.

Durston, William, 'A Narrative of a Monstrous Birth in Plymouth, Octob. 22 1670; Together With the Anatomical Observations, Taken Thereupon', *Philosophical Transactions*, v (1670), 2096–7.

Elsholt, Joan. Sigism., 'De Conceptione Tubaria, Qua Humani Foetus Extra Uterica Vitatem in Tubis Quandoq[ue] Concipiuntur: Itemque de Puella Monstroso, Berolini Nuper Nata, Epistola ad Dn. D. Wolrathum

Huxholtium Sereniss. Principis Landgraviae Hessorum Regentis Archiatrum, &c.', *Miscellanea Curiosa*, series 1, iv (1674), appendix.

Evelyn, John (ed. Guy De La Bédoyère), *The Diary of John Evelyn* (Woodbridge: Boydell, 1995).

Fenton, Edward, *Certaine Secrete Wonders of Nature, Containing a Descriptiõ of Sundry Strange Things, Seming Monstrous...Gathered out of Divers Learned Authors as well Greeke as Latine, etc.* (London: H. Bynneman, 1569).

Fontenelle, Bernard de, *Histoire du Renouvellement de l'Académie Royale des Sciences...* (Amsterdam: Pierre de Coup, 1709).

Galliard, 'Observations Particulieres sur Differentes Maladies', *Journal des Savans* (1697), 338–40.

Garden, Geo[rge], 'Two Monstrous Births in Scotland', *Philosophical Transactions*, xv (1686), 1156.

Gemma, Corn[elius], *De Naturae Divinis...* (Antwerp: Christopher Plantin, 1575).

Gerlin, Laurent Gualther, *Disputatio Philosophica de Monstris* (Wittenberg: Christian Tham, 1624).

Gockel, Eberhard, 'Foetus Monstrosus cum Superiori Maxilla & Labio in Utroque Latere Fisso', *Miscellanea Curiosa*, series 2, vii (1688), 237–8.

Göller, Georg. Christoph., 'Abortus Humani Monstrosi Hist. Anatom.', *Miscellanea Curiosa*, series 2, ii (1683), 311–18.

Grandi, Jacomo, 'An Extract of an Italian Letter...', *Philosophical Transactions*, v (1670), 1188–9.

Greisel, Georg, 'De Anatome Monstri Gemellorum Humanorum', *Miscellanea Curiosa*, series 1, i (1670), 132–3.

Guazzo, Francesco Maria (ed. Montague Summers), *Compendium Maleficarum* (Secaucus, NJ: University Books, 1974).

Hakluyt, Richard, *The Principal Navigations, Voyages, Traffiques and Discoveries of the English Nation...* (Glasgow: Maclehose, 1903–5).

Hall, A. Rupert and Marie Boas Hall (eds and transl.), *The Correspondence of Henry Oldenburg* (Madison: University of Wisconsin Press, 1965–77).

Hansen, [Untitled letter from Oxford], *Journal des Savans* (1681), 46–7.

Hartmann, Philipp Jacob, 'Anatome Monstri', *Miscellanea Curiosa*, series 2, x (1691), 258–62.

Harvey, William (ed. and transl. C.D. O'Malley, F.N.L. Poynter and K.F. Russell), *Lectures on the Whole of Anatomy: An Annotated Translation of Prelectiones Anatomiae Universalis* (Berkeley: University of California Press, 1961).

Havers, G. (transl.), *A General Collection of Discourses of the Virtuosi of France…* (London: Thomas Dring and John Starkey, 1664).

Hermann, Paul, *Catologus Musei Indici: Continens Varia Exotica, tum Animalia, tum Vegetabilia, Nativam Figuram Servantia, Singula in Liquore Balsamico Asservata; ut & varia Arida Curiosa, Insecta, Mineralia, Lapides, Radices Medicinales, Ligna, Semina, & Fructus: Quin etiam Elegantissimam Collectionem Concharum, Conchyliorum, Corallorum & Plurimorum Marinorum &c. Quae Magno Labore, Industria ac Sumtubus Collecta Sunt, A Celeberrimo Doctissimoque Viro Paulo Hermanno, dum Viveret, Med. ac Botanices in Academia Lugduno Batava Professore* (Leiden: Joh. du Virie, 1711).

Hoffmann, Johann Maurice, 'De Monstro Gemello', *Miscellanea Curiosa*, series 2, iv (1685), 288–90.

Hoffmann, Johann Maurice, 'De Foetu Monstroso', *Miscellanea Curiosa*, series 2, vi (1687), 333–6.

Hofmann, Maurice, 'Anatome Partus Cerebro Carentis', *Miscellanea Curiosa*, series 1, ii (1671), 60–4.

Hottinger, Johann Henri, 'Monstruo Humano Absque Sexu, Pedibus, &c. In Excrescentiam Caudiformem Definente', *Miscellanea Curiosa*, series 3, ix (1700), 413–16.

H[owell], J[ames], *Epistolae Ho Elianae… Familiar Letters Domestic and Forren; Divided into Six Sections: Partly Historicall, Politicall, Philosophicall, upon Emergent Occasions* (London: H. Moseley, 1645).

Howes, Edmund, *Annales, or, a Generall Chronicle of England / Begun by John Stow: Continved and Augmented with Matters Forraigne and Domestique, Ancient and Moderne, Vnto the End of This Present Yeere, 1631* (London: A. Mathewes, 1631).

Hünerwolff, Jacob August, 'De Fœmellis Duabus Monstrosis', *Miscellanea Curiosa*, series 2, ix (1690), 170–1.

Jaenis, Johann, 'De Infante Sine Capite', *Miscellanea Curiosa*, series 1, iii (1672), 442–4.

Josselin, Ralph (ed. E. Hockliffe), *The Diary of the Rev. Ralph Josselin, 1616–1683* (London: Camden Society, 1908).

Khon, Alphons, 'Partu Monstroso Miranda Imaginationis vi Oborto', *Miscelanea Curiosa*, series 1, ix (1678), 74.

König, Emanuel, 'Gemelli Sibi Invicem Adnati Feliciter Separati', *Miscellanea Curiosa* series 2, viii (1689), 305–7.

Krahe, Christopher, 'The Description of a Monstrous Child, Born Friday the 29th of February 1684 at a Village Called Heisagger, Distant About 4 English Miles From Hattersleben, a Town in South-Jutland, Under the King of Denmark's Dominion', *Philosophical Transactions*, xiv (1684), 599–600.

Kramer, Heinrich, and James Sprenger (ed. and transl. Montague Summers), *Malleus Maleficarum* (London: John Rodker, 1928).

La Motte, [Guillaume Mauquest de] (transl. Thomas Tomkyns), *A General Treatise of Midwifry: Illustrated with Upwards of Four Hundred Curious Observations and Reflexions Concerning that Art* (London: James Waugh, 1746).

Lanzoni, Joseph, 'Partus Mirabilis Scandiani Editus 26 Maji A. 1690', *Miscellanea Curiosa*, series 2, ix (1690), 73–6.

Lehmann, Abraham, *De Monstris* (Wittenberg: Georgii Müller, 1634).

Lemne, Levin (transl. J[acques] G[ohorry]), *Les Occultes Merveilles et Secretz de Nature avec Plvsievrs Enseignemens des Choses Diuerses, tant par Raison Probable, que par Coniecture Artificielle: Exposées en Deux Liures, de non Moindre Plaisir que Profit au Lecteur Studieux* (Paris: Galiot du Pré, 1574).

Liceti, Fortunio, *De Monstrorum Caussis, Natura, et Differentiis* (Padua: Casparem Crivellarium, 1616).

Liceti, Fortunio, *De Monstrorum Caussis, Natura, & Differentiis* (Padua: Paul Frambott, 1634).

Liceti, Fortunio, *De monstris: Ex Recensione Gerardi Blasii…qui Monstra Quaedam Nova & Rariora ex Recentiorum Scriptis Addidit* (Amsterdam: Andre Fris, 1665).

Löw, Andreae, 'Foetus, Quà Caput, Monstrosus', *Miscellanea Curiosa*, series 2, ix (1690), 200–2.

Lowthorp, John (ed.) *The Philosophical Transactions and Collections, to the End of the Year MDCC, Abridged and Disposed under General Heads* (London: W. Innys *et al.*, 1749).

Lugeris, le Prieur de, 'Extrait d'une Lettre de Monsieur le Prieur de Lugeris en Champagne, Sur un Enfantemant Arrivé au Mois de Mai Dernier', *Journal des Savans*, (1690), 53–4.

Lycosthenes, Conrad, *Prodigiorum ac Ostentorum Chronicon, Quae Praeter Naturae Ordinem...* (Basel: H. Petri, 1557).

Maier, Michael, *Symbola Aureae Mensae Duodecim Nationum: Hoc est, Hermaea seu Mercurii Festa ab Heroibus Duodenis Selectis, Artis Chymicae Usu, Saientia et Authoritate Paribus Celebrata, ad Pyrgopolynicen seu Adversarium Illum tot Annis Iactabundum, Virgini Chemiae Iniuriam Argumentis tam Vitiosis, quam Convitiis Argutis Inferentem, Confundendum et Exarmandum...* (Frankfurt: Lucae Jennis, 1617).

Maier, Michael, *Atlanta Fugiens, Hoc est Emblemata Nova de Secretis Naturae Chymica: Accommodata Partim Oculis & Intellectui, Figuris Cupro Incisis, Adjectisque Sententiis, Epigrammatis & Notis, Partim Auribus & Recreationi Animi Plus Minus 50 Fugis Musicalibus Trium Vocum, Quarum Duae ad Unam Simplicem Melodiam Distichis Canendis Peraptam, Correspondeant...* (Oppenheim: Theodor de Bry, 1618).

Malpighi, Marcello, *Opera Posthuma...Quibus Praefixa est Ejusdem Vita a Seipso Scripta* (London: A. and J. Churchill, 1697).

Massaeus, Christian, *Chronicorum Multiplicis Historiae Utriusque Testamenti...* (Antwerp: Johannes Crinitus, 1540).

Maubray, John, *The Female Physician, Containing All the Diseases Incident to that Sex... To Which is Added, the Whole Art of New Improv'd Midwifery... Together with the Diet and Regimen of Both the Mother and Child* (London: J. Holland, 1724).

McNair, John R. (ed.), *The Doome Warning All Men to the Judgement (1581)* (New York: Scholars' Facsimiles and Reprints, 1984).

Mercklin, Georg Abraham, 'De Gravidae Imaginatione Foetui Noxia', *Miscellanea Curiosa*, series 1, viii (1677), 73–5.

Montaigne, Michel de (transl. John Florio), *The Essays* (London: M. Bradwood, 1613).

Montaigne, Michel de (transl. G.B. Ives), *The Essays of Montaigne* (Cambridge: Cambridge University Press, 1925).

Morris, S., 'A Relation of a Monstrous Birth... Sent to Dr Charles Goodall of London, Both of the College of Physicians', *Philosophical Transactions*, xii (1678), 961–2.

Mouriceau, François, 'Des Maladies des Femmes Grosses & Accouchées &c.', *Journal des Savans* (1669), 8–11.

Musche de Moschau, Johan Ignatius, 'Ala Locustae Literis Hebraicis Decorata', *Miscellanea Curiosa*, series 2, ix (1690), 204–11.

Nester, Johann Matthias, 'De Foetu Monstroso', *Miscellanea Curiosa*, series 1, vi (1675), 60.

Nigrisoli, Francesco Maria, *Considerazioni Intorno alla Generazione de' Viventi* (Ferrara: B. Barbieri, 1712).

Obsequens, Julius (ed. Conrad Lycosthenes), *Prodigiorum Liber...* (Basel: J. Oporini, 1552).

P., A., 'A Letter From Mr A.P. in Somersetshire, Giving an Account of a Strange Birth that in May Last Happened at Hillbrewers in that County', *Philosophical Collections*, ii (1681), 21–2.

Paré, Ambroise, *Les Oevres d'Ambroise Paré... Diuisees en Vingt Sept Liures, Auec les Figures et Portraicts, tant de l'Anatomie que des Instruments de Chirurgie, et de Plusieurs Monstres* (Paris: G. Buon, 1575).

Paré, Ambroise (ed. and transl. Janis L. Pallister), *On Monsters and Marvels* (Chicago and London: University of Chicago Press, 1982).

Patini, Carol, 'Monstrum Biceps Masculinum', *Miscellanea Curiosa*, series 2, x (1691), 72–3.

Paullin, Christian Francis, 'Observationes Medico-Physicae, Selectae & Curiosae, Variis Antiquitatibus Historico-Germanicis Bonâ Fide Interdum Conspersae', *Miscellanea Curiosa*, series 2, vi (1687), appendix, 53–4.

Peucer, Caspar, *Commentarius de Præcipuis Divinationum Generibus...* (Wittenberg: Johannes Lufft, 1553).

Peucer, Caspar, *Commentarius de Praecipuis Divinationum Generibus, in quo a Prophetiis Autoritate Divina Traditis et a Physicis Conjecturis, Discernuntur Artes et Imposturae Diabolicae, atque Observationes Natae ex Superstitione et cum hac Conjunctae: Et Monstrantur Fontes et Causae Physicarum*

Praedictionum; Diabolicae Vero ac Superstitiosae Confutatae Damnantur; Recens Editus & Auctus Accessione Multiplici (Wittenberg: I. Crato, 1560).

Peyer, Joh. Conrad, 'De Gemellis Monstrosis, Coalitis Partibus Obscoenis', *Miscellanea Curiosa*, series 2, ii (1683), 267.

Philalethes, *The Sooterkin Dissected* (London: A. Moore, 1726).

Philobiblon Society (eds), *Ancient Ballads & Broadsides Published in England in the Sixteenth Century, Chiefly in the Earlier Years of the Reign of Queen Elizabeth* (London: Whittingham and Wilkins, 1867).

Porta, Giovanni Battista della, *Natural Magick... in Twenty Bookes* (London: T. Young and S. Speed, 1658).

Posner, Caspar, *De Monstris* (Jena: Stanno Steinmanniano, 1652).

Preston, Charles, 'An Account of a Child Born Without a Brain, and the Observables in it on Dissection', *Philosophical Transactions*, xix (1697), 457–67.

Rausch, Johann Caspar, *Disputatio Physica de Monstris* (Jena: Johann Jacob Bauhofer, 1665).

Rayger, Carol, 'De Anatomia Monstri Bicipitis', *Miscellanea Curiosa*, series 1, i (1670), 21–3.

Reisel, Salomon, 'De Labiis Leporinis Geminis, Oculis Clausis & Coecis, & Fovea Cranii in Vertice', *Miscellanea Curiosa*, series 2, viii (1689), 135–6.

Reisel, Solomon, 'Infans Truncus Sine Artubus', *Miscellanea Curiosa*, series 2, viii (1689), 136–7.

Remy, Nicholas (ed. Montague Summers, transl. E.A. Ashwin), *Demonolatry* (Secaucus, NJ: University Books, 1974).

Renaudot, Theophraste (ed. and transl. G. Havers), *A General Collection of Discourses of the Virtuosi of France, Upon Questions of All Sorts of Philosophy, and Other Natural Knowledge: Made in the Assembly of the Beaux Esprits at Paris by the Most Ingenious Persons of that Nation* (London: Thomas Dring and John Starkey, 1664).

Rhodiginus, Caelius, *Antiquarum Lectionum...*(Venice: Aldus, 1516).

Riolan, Jean, *De Monstro Nato Lutetiae Anno Domini 1605: Disputatio Philosophica* (Paris: Olivarum Varennaeum, 1605).

Robbins, Robin (ed.), *Sir Thomas Browne's* Pseudodoxia Epidemica (Oxford: Clarendon Press, 1981).

Rollins, H.E. (ed.), *The Pack of Autolycus; or, Strange and Terrible News of Ghosts, Apparitions, Monstrous Births, Showers of Wheat, Judgments of God, and Other Prodigious and Fearful Happenings As Told in Broadside Ballads of the Years, 1624–1693* (Cambridge, MA: Harvard University Press, 1927).

Rueff, Jacob, *De Conceptu et Genratione Hominis, et iis quae Circa hec Potissimum Consysderantur* (Zürich: Christopher Froschauer, 1554).

Rueff, Jacob, *De Conceptu et Generatione Hominis, et iis qvae Circa haec Potissimum Considerantvr* (Basel: Conrad Waldkirch, 1586).

Rueff, James, *The Expert Midwife, or An Excellent and Most Necessary Treatise of the Generation and Birth of Man...* (London: E.G. for S.E., 1637).

Ruysch, Frederic, *Observationum Anatomico-Chirurgicarum Centuria, Accedit Catalogus Rariorum, Quae in Museo Ruyschiano Asservantur* (Amsterdam: Henricum & Theodori Boom, 1691).

Ruysch, Frederic, *Catalogus Musaei Ruyschiani, sive Permagnae, Elegantissimae, Nitidissimae, Incomparabilis, & Vere Regiae Collectionis; Praeparatorum Anatomicorum, Variorum Animalium, Plantarum, Aliarumque Rerum Naturalium, quas Maximo Labore, Studio, Sumtu, Singulari Artificio & Industria Collegit, Praeparavit, & Conservavit, dum Viveret, Vir Summus & Celeberrimus Fredericus Ruyschius* (Amsterdam: Jausson Waesberg, 1731).

Sampson, Henric, 'De Foetu Monstrosissimo', *Miscellanea Curiosa*, series 1, iii (1672), 279.

Scharf, Benjamin, 'Monstrum à Constricctione', *Miscellanea Curiosa*, series 2, ii, (1683), 254–6.

Scheihammer, Günther Christophor, 'Monstrum Acephalum', *Miscellanea Curiosa*, series 2, ix (1960), 258–9.

Schenck, Johann Georg., *Observationum Medicarum Rariorum...* (Leyden: Joan-Antoni Huguetan, 1644).

Schlüter, Christophor, *De Monstris* (Wittenberg: Georg Muller, 1634).

Schmidt, Johann, 'De Monstro Foeminini Sexus', *Miscellanea Curiosa*, series 1, iv (1674), 27–9.

Schott, Caspar, *Physica Curiosa, Sive Mirabilia Naturae Et Artis Libris XII Comprehensa, Quibus pleraq[ue] quae de Angelis, Daemonibus, Hominibus, Spectris, Energumenis, Monstris, Potentis, Animalibus, Meteoris, etc., Rara*

Arcana Curiosaque Circumferuntur, ad Veritatis Trutinam Expenduntur, Variis ex Historia ac Philosophia Petitis Disquisitionibus Excutiuntur, et Innumeris Exemplis Illustrantur (Würtzburg: Jobus Hertz for Johann A. Endter and Wolff, 1662).

Schuyl, Francis, *A Catalogue of All the Chiefest Rarities in the Publick Anatomie-Hall, of the University of Leyden* (Leyden: Diewertje vander Boxe, 1723).

Seger, Georg, 'De Phthisici Pueri Anatome', *Miscellanea Curiosa*, series 1, i (1670), 53–6.

Seger, Georg, 'De Embryone Hydropico', *Miscellanea Curiosa*, series 1, i (1670), 114–15.

Seneca (transl. M. Winterbottom), *Controversiae* (Cambridge: Loeb Classical Library, 1974).

Senguerd, Arnold, *Continens Quaestiones de Monstris* (Utrecht: Petrum Danielis Sloot, 1645).

Sharp, Jane, *The Midwives Book: Or the Whole ART of Midwifry Discovered* (London: Simon Miller, 1671).

Sinistrari, Lodovico Maria (ed. and transl. Montague Summers), *Demoniality* (London: The Fortune Press, 1927).

Sorbin, Arnaud, *Tractatus de Monstris, quae a Temporibus Constantini Hucusque Ortum Habuerunt, ac iis, quae Circa Eorum Tempora Misere Acciderunt, ex Historiarum, cum Graecarum, tum Latinarum Testimoniis...* (Paris: Hieronymum de Marnef and Gulielmum Cavellat, 1570).

Sperling, Paulus, *Disputatio Philosophica de Monstris* (Wittenberg: Christian Tham, 1624).

Stricer, Johann, *Disputatio Physica de Monstro* (Wittenberg: Joh. Röhner, 1665).

Topsell, Edward, *The History of Four-Footed Beasts and Serpents...* (London: E. Cotes, 1658).

Turner, Daniel, *The Force of the Mother's Imagination upon the Foetus in Utero... by way of Reply to Dr. Blondell's Book* (London: J. Walthoe, 1730).

Tyson, Edward, 'An Observation of an Infant, Where the Brain was Depressed into the Hollow of the Vertebrae of the Neck', *Philosophical Transactions*, xix (1697), 533–5.

Valleriola, François, *Observationum Medicinalium* (Lyons, A. Gryphius, 1605).

Vander Wiel, 'Extrait des Nouv. de la Rep. des Lettres', *Journal des Savans* (1686), 263–4.

Vanini, Julius Caesar, *De Admirandis Naturae Reginae, Deaeque Mortalium Arcanis* (Paris: Adrien Perrier, 1616).

Vanini, Julius Caesar (ed. Pierre Bayle), *The Life of L… Vanini… With an Abstract of his Writings… With a Confutation of the Same, and Mr. Bayle's Arguments in Behalf of Vaninus… Answered* (London: W. Meadows, 1730).

Volgnad, Henric, 'De Monstroso Foetu', Miscellanea Curiosa, series 1, iii (1672), 446–7.

Vreeswijck, Goossen van, *De Goude Leeuw, of den Asijn der Wysen…* (Amsterdam: Johannes Janssonius van Waesberge, 1675).

Waldschmid, Joh. Jacob, 'Monstrum Humanum Abominandum', *Miscellanea Curiosa*, series 1, ii (1671), 313.

Wallrich, Christophor, *Disputatio Physica de Monstris quam Deo Juvante* (Wittenberg: Johann Borckardt, 1655).

Wepfer, Johann Jacob, 'De Puella Sine Cerebro Nata, Historia', *Miscellanea Curiosa*, iii (1672), 175–203.

Westphal, Joach. Christian, *Natura Peccans, Septenario Problematum Numero Proposita, de qua… Disputabit* (Leipsig: Christian G., 1687).

Worm, Olao, *Museum Wormianum Seu Historia Rerum Rariorum, tam Naturalium, quam Artificialium, tam Domesticarum, quam Exoticarum, quae Hafniae Danorum in Aedibus Authoris Servantur* (Amsterdam: Ludovic and Daniel Elzevir, 1655).

Secondary Sources

Allen, Eric W., 'International Origins of the Newspaper: the Establishment of Periodicity in Print', *Journalism Quarterly*, vii (1930), 307–19.

Altick, Richard D., *The Shows of London* (Cambridge: The Belknap Press of Harvard University Press, 1978).

Anderson, T., 'Artistic and Documentary Evidence for Tetradysmelia from Sixteenth-Century England', *American Journal of Medical Genetics*, lii (1994), 475–7.

Anderson, T., 'Earliest Evidence for Arthrogryposis Multiplex Congenita or Larsen Syndrome?', *American Journal of Medical Genetics*, lxxi (1997), 127–9.

Anderson, T., 'Documentary and Artistic Evidence for Conjoined Twins from Sixteenth-Century England', *American Journal of Medical Genetics*, cix (2002), 155–9.

Arber, Agnes, *Herbals: Their Origin and Evolution, a Chapter in the History of Botany, 1470–1670* (Cambridge: Cambridge University Press, 1986).

Arrizabalaga, J., 'Problematizing Retrospective Diagnosis in the History of Disease', *Asclepio*, liv (2002), 51–70.

Ashworth, William B., Jr., 'Emblematic Natural History of the Renaissance', in N. Jardine, J.A. Secord and E.C. Spary (eds), *Cultures of Natural History* (Cambridge: Cambridge University Press, 1996), 17–37.

Baljet, B., and R.-J. Oostra, 'Historical Aspects of the Study of Malformations in The Netherlands', *American Journal of Medical Genetics*, lxxvii (1998), 91–9.

Ballantyne, J.W., 'The Teratological Records of Chaldea', *Teratologia*, i (1894), 127–42.

Ballantyne, J.W., 'Preauricular Appendages', *Teratologia*, ii (1895), 18–36.

Ballantyne, J.W., 'Antenatal Pathology and Heredity in the Hippocratic Writings', *Teratologia*, ii (1895), 275–87.

Ballantyne, J.W., 'The Biddenden Maids – The Mediaeval Pygopagous Twins', *Teratologia*, ii (1895), 268–74.

Balme, D.M., '"Ἄνθρωπος ἄνθρωπον γεννᾷ: Human is Generated by Human', in G.R. Dunstan (ed.), *The Human Embryo: Aristotle and the Arabic and European Traditions* (Exeter: University of Exeter Press, 1990), 20–31.

Bates, A.W., 'Cures at Newnham Regis Spa, 1579', *Warwickshire History*, x (1996), 19–25.

Bates, A.W., 'Birth Defects Described in Elizabethan Ballads', *Journal of the Royal Society of Medicine*, xciii (2000), 202–7.

Bates, A.W., 'The *De Monstrorum* of Fortunio Liceti: A Landmark of Descriptive Teratology', *Journal of Medical Biography*, ix (2001), 49–54.

Bates, A.W., 'A Case of Roberts Syndrome Described in 1737', *Journal of Medical Genetics*, xxxviii (2001), 565–7.

Bates, A.W., 'Conjoined Twins in the Sixteenth Century', *Twin Research*, v (2002), 521–8.

Bates, A.W., 'Autopsy on a Case of Roberts Syndrome Reported in 1672: The Earliest Description?', *American Journal of Medical Genetics*, cxvii A (2003), 92–6.

Bates, A.W., 'The Sooterkin Dissected: The Theoretical Basis of Animal Births to Human Mothers in Early Modern Europe', *Vesalius*, ix (2003), 6–14.

Bates, A.W., and S.M. Dodd, 'Anomalies in Cephalothoracopagus Synotus Twins and their Implications for Morphogenesis in Conjoined Twins', *Pediatric and Developmental Pathology*, ii (1999), 464–72.

Bath, Michael, 'Recent Developments in Emblem Studies', *Bulletin of the Society for Renaissance Studies*, vi (1998), 15–20.

Beirne, P., 'The Law is an Ass: Reading E.P. Evans' *The Medieval Prosecution and Capital Punishment of Animals*', URL: www.colchsfc.ac.uk/english/barnes10.htm, viewed 19 April 2002.

Berg, J.M. and M. Korossy, 'Down Syndrome Before Down: A Retrospect', *American Journal of Medical Genetics*, vol. cii (2001), 205–21.

Biagioli, Mario, 'Galileo the Emblem Maker' *Isis*, lxxxi (1990), 230–58.

Birch, Thomas, *The History of the Royal Society of London for Improving of Natural Knowledge, From its First Rise* (London: A. Millar, 1756–7).

Biswas, S.K., A.N. Gangopadhyay, B.D. Bhatia, D. Bandopadhyay and S. Khanna, 'An Unusual Case of Heteropagus Twinning', *Journal of Pediatric Surgery*, xxvii (1992), 96–7.

Blickstein, Isaac, 'The Conjoined Twins of Löwen', *Twin Research*, iii (2000), 185–8.

Bondeson, Jan, 'The Biddenden Maids: A Curious Chapter in the History of Conjoined Twins', *Journal of the Royal Society of Medicine*, lxxxv (1992), 217–21.

Bondeson, Jan, 'The Isle-Brewers Conjoined Twins of 1680', *Journal of the Royal Society of Medicine*, lxxxvi (1993), 106–9.

Bondeson, Jan, *A Cabinet of Medical Curiosities* (London: I B Tauris, 1997).

Bondeson, Jan, *The Feejee Mermaid and Other Essays in Natural and Unnatural History* (Ithaca: Cornell University Press, 1999).

Bondeson, Jan, *The Two-Headed Boy, and Other Medical Marvels* (Ithaca: Cornell University Press, 2000).

Bondeson, J., and E. Allen, 'Craniopagus Parasiticus: Everard Home's Two-Headed Boy of Bengal and Some Other Cases', *Surgical Neurology*, xxxi (1989), 426–34.

Bondeson, J., and A. Molenkamp, 'The Countess Margaret of Henneberg and Her 365 Children', *Journal of the Royal Society of Medicine*, lxxxix (1996), 711–6.

Boorstin, Daniel J., *The Discoverers* (New York: Random House, 1983).

Bos, C.A., and B. Baljet, 'Cynocephali en Blemmyae: Aangeboren Afwijkingen en Middeleeuwse Wonderbaarlijke Rassen', *Nederlands Tijdschrift voor Geneeskunde*, cxliii (1999), 2580–5.

Bothe, H.W., W. Bodsch and K.A. Hossmann, 'Relationship Between Specific Gravity, Water Content, and Serum Protein Extravasation in Various Types of Vasogenic Brain Edema', *Acta Neuropathologica (Berlin)*, lxiv (1984), 37–42.

Bovey, Alixe, *Monsters and Grotesques in Medieval Manuscripts* (London: British Library, 2002).

Britto, J.A., R.H. Ragoowansi and B.C. Sommerlad, 'Double Tongue, Intraoral Anomalies, and Cleft Palate – Case Reports and a Discussion of Developmental Pathology', *The Cleft Palate-Craniofacial Journal*, xxxvii (2000), 410–15.

Brown, Harcourt, 'History and the Learned Journal', *Journal of the History of Ideas*, xxxiii (1972), 365–78.

Burke, Peter, *Popular Culture in Early Modern Europe* (London: Temple Smith, 1978).

Burke, Peter, *A Social History of Knowledge: From Gutenberg to Diderot* (Oxford: Polity, 2000).

Cameron, Euan (ed.), *Early Modern Europe* (Oxford: Oxford University Press, 2001).

Camporesi, Piero (transl. Allan Cameron), *The Anatomy of the Senses: Natural Symbols in Medieval and Early Modern Italy* (Cambridge: Polity Press, 1994).

Carlino, Andrea, *Books of the Body: Anatomical Ritual and Renaissance Learning* (Chicago: University of Chicago Press, 1999).

Céard, Jean, *La Nature et les Prodiges* (Geneva: Droz, 1977).

Cipolla, Carlo M., *Before the Industrial Revolution: European Society and Economy 1000–1700* (London: Routledge, 1993).

Collmann, Herbert L. (ed.), *Ballads & Broadsides Chiefly of the Elizabethan Period and Printed in Black-Letter Most of Which Were Formerly in the Heber Collection and are Now in the Library at Britwell Court Buckinghamshire* (Oxford: Oxford University Press, 1912).

Cook, Harold J., 'Time's Bodies: Crafting the Preparation and Preservation of Marginalia', in Paula Findlen and Pamela Smith (eds), *Merchants and Marvels* (London: Routledge, 2001), 223–47.

Coury, Charles, 'The Teaching of Medicine in France from the Beginning of the Seventeenth Century', in C.D. O'Malley (ed.), *The History of Medical Education* (Berkeley: University of California Press, 1970), 121–72.

Cressy, David, *Travesties and Transgressions in Tudor and Stuart England: Tales of Discord and Dissension* (Oxford: Oxford University Press, 2000).

Crombie, A.C., *Augustine to Galileo* (London: Heinemann Educational, 1979).

Cutter, I.S., and H.R. Viets, *A Short History of Midwifery* (Philadelphia: W.B. Saunders, 1964).

Daston, Lorraine, 'The Nature of Nature in Early Modern Europe', *Configurations*, vi (1998), 149–72.

Daston, Lorraine, 'Marvelous Facts and Miraculous Evidence in Early Modern Europe', in Peter G. Platt (ed.), *Wonders, Marvels, and Monsters in Early Modern Culture* (Newark: University of Delaware Press, 1999), 76–104.

Daston, Lorraine, and Katherine Park, *Wonders and the Order of Nature, 1150–1750* (New York: Zone Books, 1998).

Davies, Jason P., *The Articulation of Roman Religion in the Latin Historians Livy, Tacitus and Ammianus Marcellinus* (PhD, University College London, 1999).

Davies, Jason P., *Rome's Religious History: Livy, Tacitus and Ammianus on their Gods* (Cambridge: Cambridge University Press, 2005).

De Vries, Ad, *Dictionary of Symbols and Imagery* (Amsterdam: North-Holland Publishing Company, 1984).

Dickens, A.G., *Reformation and Society in Sixteenth-Century Europe* (London: Thames and Hudson, 1966).

Douglas, Mary, *Implicit Meanings: Essays in Anthropology* (London: Routledge and Kegan Paul, 1975).

Eisenstein, Elizabeth L., *The Printing Press as an Agent of Change: Communications and Cultural Transformations in Early Modern Europe* (Cambridge: Cambridge University Press, 1979).

Ekong, C.E.U., and B. Rozdilsky, 'Hydranencephaly in Association with Roberts Syndrome', *Canadian Journal of Neurological Science*, v (1978), 253–5.

Evans, E.P., *The Criminal Prosecution and Capital Punishment of Animals* (London: Heinemann, 1906).

Ewinkel, Irene, *De Monstris: Deutung und Funktion von Wundergeburten auf Flugblättern im Deutschland des 16 Jahrhunderts* (Tübingen: Niemeyer, 1995).

Faber, Sjoerd, 'Kindermoord in het Bijzonder in de Achttiende eeuw te Amsterdam', *Bijdragen en Mededelingen Betreffende de Geshciedenis der Nederlanden*, lxxiii (1978), 224–40.

Findlen, Paula, *Possessing Nature: Museums, Collecting, and Scientific Culture in Early Modern Italy* (Berkeley: University of California Press, 1994).

Findlen, Paula, 'Inventing Nature: Commerce, Art and Science in the Early Modern Cabinet of Curiosities', in Paula Findlen and Pamela Smith (eds), *Merchants and Marvels* (London: Routledge, 2001), 297–323.

Fisher, G.J., 'Diploteratology', *Transactions of the Medical Society of the State of New York* (1866), 207–96.

Fishman, R.A. and M. Greer, 'Experimental Obstructive Hydrocephalus', *Archives of Neurology*, viii (1963), 156–61.

Foucault, Michel, *The Order of Things...* (London: Routledge, 1989).

Frazer, James George, *The Golden Bough: A Study in Magic and Religion* (London: Macmillan, 1913).

Freeman, M.V., D.W. Williams, R.N. Schimke, S.A. Temtamy, E. Vachier and J. German, 'The Roberts Syndrome', *Clinical Genetics*, v (1974), 1–16

French, Roger, 'The Anatomical Tradition', in Roy Porter and William F. Bynum (eds), *Companion Encyclopedia of the History of Medicine* (London: Routledge, 1993), 81–101.

French, Roger, *Dissection and Vivisection in the European Renaissance* (Aldershot: Ashgate, 1999).

French, Roger, *Medicine Before Science...* (Cambridge: Cambridge University Press, 2003).

Friedman, John Block, *The Monstrous Races in Medieval Art and Thought* (Cambridge: Harvard University Press, 1981).

Fudge, Erica, 'Monstrous Acts: Bestiality in Early Modern England', *History Today*, l (2000), 20–5.

Gélis, Jacques, *History of Childbirth: Fertility, Pregnancy and Birth in Early Modern Europe* (Oxford: Polity Press, 1991).

Geoffroy Saint-Hilaire, Isidore, *Histoire Générale et Particulière des Anomalies de l'Organisation chez l'Homme et les Animaux...* (Paris: J.B. Baillière, 1832–7).

Gilbert-Barness, E., *Potter's Pathology of the Fetus and Infant* (St Louis: Mosby, 1997).

Gould, George M., and Walter L. Pyle, *Anomalies and Curiosities of Medicine* (New York: Sydenham, 1937).

Gowing, Laura, 'Secret Births and Infanticide in Seventeenth-Century England', *Past & Present*, clvi (1997), 87–115.

Grundfest, T.H., and S. Weisenfeld, 'A Case of Cephalothoracopagus', *New York State Medical Journal*, l (1950), 576–9.

Grundy, H.O., J. Burlbaw, S. Walton and C. Dannar, 'Roberts Syndrome: Antenatal Ultrasound – A Case Report', *Journal of Perinatal Medicine*, xvi (1988), 71–5.

Gupta, R.C., V.K. Gupta and S. Gupta, 'Human Cyclopia with Associated Microstoma and Anencephaly (A Case Report)', *Indian Journal of Ophthalmology*, xxix (1981), 121–3.

Hagelin, Ove, *The Byrth of Mankynde Otherwyse Named The Womans Booke: Embryology Obstetrics Gynaecology Through Four centuries; An Illustrated and Annotated Catalogue of Rare Books in the Swedish Society of Medicine* (Stockholm: Svenska Läkaresällskapet, 1990).

Hall, A. Rupert, 'Medicine in the Early Royal Society', in Allen G. Debus (ed.), *Medicine in Seventeenth Century England* (Berkeley: University of California Press, 1974), 421–52.

Hanafi, Zakiya, *The Monster in the Machine: Magic, Medicine and the Marvelous in the Time of the Scientific Revolution* (Durham: Duke University Press, 2000).

Haneveld, G.T., 'Een Nederlands Schilderij van een Samengegroeide Tweeling (Thoracopagus) uit de 17e Eeuw', *Nederlands Tijdschrift voor Geneeskunde*, cxviii (1974), 801–5.

Harley, David, 'Historians as Demonologists: The Myth of the Midwife-Witch', *Social History of Medicine*, iii (1990), 1–26.

Harper, R.G., K. Kenigsberg, C.G. Sia, D. Horn, D. Stern and V. Bongiovi, 'Xiphopagus Conjoined Twins: A 300-Year Review of the Obstetric, Morphopathologic, Neonatal, and Surgical Parameters', *American Journal of Obstetrics and Gynecology*, cxxxvii (1980), 617–29.

Harrison, Peter, 'Curiosity, Forbidden Knowledge, and the Reformation of Natural Philosophy in Early Modern England', *Isis*, xcii (2001), 265–90.

Hartley, Harold (ed.), *The Royal Society, Its Origins and Founders* (London: The Royal Society, 1960).

Heaton, J.D., 'United Twins', *British Medical Journal*, i (1869), 363.

Hiratsuka, H., H. Tabata, S. Tsuruoka , M. Aoyagi, K. Okada and Y. Inaba, 'Evaluation of Periventricular Hypodensity in Experimental Hydrocephalus by Metrizamide CT Ventriculography', *Journal of Neurosurgury*, lvi (1982), 235–40.

Hoffer, Peter C., and N.E.H. Hull, *Murdering Mothers: Infanticide in England and New England 1558–1803* (New York: New York University Press, 1981).

Hole, Robert, 'Incest, Consanguinity and a Monstrous Birth in Rural England, January 1600', *Social History*, xxv (2000), 183–99.

Holländer, E., *Wunder Wundergeburt und Wundergestalt in Einblattdrucken des Fünfzenhnten bis Achtzehnten Jahrhunderts: Kulturhistorische Studie* (Stuttgart: Ferdinand Enke, 1921).

Houssay, François, *De la Nature, des Causes, des Différences de Monstres d'Après Fortunio Liceti* (Paris: Collection Hippocrate, 1937).

Huizinga, J. (transl. F. Hopman), *The Waning of the Middle Ages: A Study of the Forms of Life, Thought and Art in France and the Netherlands in the Fourteenth and Fifteenth Centuries* (London: Folio Society, 1998).

Jackson, L., A.D. Kline, M.A. Barr and S. Koch, 'De Lange Syndrome: A Clinical Review of 310 Individuals', *American Journal of Medical Genetics*, xlvii (1993), 940–6.

Jarcho, Saul, 'Problems of the Autopsy in 1670 A.D.', *Bulletin of the New York Academy of Medicine*, xlvii (1971), 792–6.

Jimenez, Fidelio A., 'The First Autopsy in the New World', *Bulletin of the New York Academy of Medicine*, liv (1978), 618–19.

Jones, Kenneth Lyons (ed.), *Smith's Recognizable Patterns of Human Malformation* (Philadelphia: W.B. Saunders, 1997).

Kidd, M., and I.M. Modlin, 'Frederik Ruysch: Master Anatomist and Depictor of the Surreality of Death', *Journal of Medical Biography*, vii (1999), 69–77.

Klossowski de Rola, Stanislas, *The Golden Game: Alchemical Engravings of the Seventeenth Century* (London: Thames and Hudson, 1988).

Krietsch, P., 'Zur Geschichte des Pathologischen Museums der Charite Berlin, 2, Mitteilung: Die Sammlung von Missbildungspraparaten ("Monstra")', *Zentralblatt fur Allgemeine Pathologie und Pathologische Anatomie*, cxxxii (1986), 335–47.

Kronick, David A., *A History of Scientific and Technical Periodicals: The Origins and Development of the Scientific and Technological Press 1665–1790* (New York: The Scarecrow Press, Inc., 1962).

Lascault, Gilbert, *Le Monstre dans l'Art Occidental, un Problème Esthétique* (Paris: Klincksieck, 1973).

Lawrence, Christopher, 'The Healing Serpent – The Snake in Medical Iconography', *Ulster Medical Journal*, xlvii (1978), 134–40.

Levitas, A.S., and C.S. Reid, 'An Angel with Down Syndrome in a Sixteenth-Century Flemish Nativity Painting', *American Journal of Medical Genetics*, cxvi A (2003), 399–405.

Livingston, C.R., 'The Provenance of Three Early Broadsheets', *The Library*, series 6, ii (1980), 53–60.

Livingston, C.R., *British Broadside Ballads of the Sixteenth Century: A Catalogue of the Extant Sheets and an Essay* (New York: Garland Publishing, 1991).

Long, Kathleen Perry, 'Sexual Dissonance: Early Modern Scientific Accounts of Hermaphrodites', in Peter G. Platt (ed.), *Wonders, Marvels, and Monsters in Early Modern Culture* (Newark: University of Delaware Press, 1999), 145–63.

Lovejoy, Arthur O., *The Great Chain of Being: A Study in the History of an Idea* (Cambridge: Harvard University Press, 1936).

Luxon, Thomas H., '"Not I, But Christ": Allegory and the Puritan Self', *English Literary History*, lx (1993), 899–937.

MacBain, B., *Prodigy and Expiation: A Study in Religion and Politics in Republican Rome* (Brussels: Collection Latomus, 1982).

Malefijt, Annemarie de Waal, 'Homo Monstrosus', *Scientific American*, ccxix (1968), 112–18.

Malgaigne, J.F. (ed. and transl. W.B. Hamby), *Surgery and Ambroise Paré* (Norman: University of Oklahoma Press, 1965).

Manning, John, *The Emblem* (London: Reaktion Books, 2002).

Martinez-Frias, M.-L., 'Another Way to Interpret the Description of the Monster of Ravenna of the Sixteenth Century', *American Journal of Medical Genetics*, il (1994), 362.

McClellan, James Edward, III, *The International Organization of Science and Learned Societies in the Eighteenth Century* (PhD, Princeton University, 1975).

McClellan, James Edward, III, *Science Reorganized: Scientific Societies in the Eighteenth Century* (New York: Columbia University Press, 1985).

McKeown, Simon, *Monstrous Births: An Illustrative Introduction to Teratology in Early Modern England* (London: Indelible, 1991).

McKie, Douglas, 'The Arrest and Imprisonment of Henry Oldenburg', *Notes and Records*, vi (1948), 28–47.

McKusick, V.A., *Mendelian Inheritance in Man: Catalogs of Human Genes and Genetic Disorders* (Baltimore: Johns Hopkins University Press, 1998).

Moerman, P., E. Verbeken, J.P. Fryns, P. Goddeeris and J.M. Lauweryns, 'The Meckel Syndrome: Pathological and Cytogenetic Observations in Eight Cases', *Human Genetics*, lxii (1982), 240–5.

Morgan, Betty Trebell, *Histoire du Journal des Scavants Depuis 1665 Jusqu'en 1701* (Paris: Presses Universitaires, 1929).

Morley, Henry, *Memoirs of Bartholomew Fair* (Glasgow: G. Routledge and Sons, 1892).

Moscoso, Javier, 'Monsters as Evidence: The Uses of the Abnormal Body During the Early Eighteenth Century', *Journal of the History of Biology*, xxxi (1998), 355–82.

Müller, Uwe, 'Die Leopoldina unter den Präsidenten Bausch, Fehr und Volckamer (1652–1693)', in Benno Parthier and Dietrich von Engelhardt (eds), *350 Jahre Leopoldina – Anspruch und Wirklichkeit: Festschrift der Deutschen Akademie der Naturforscher Leopoldina, 1652–2002* (Halle: Deutsche Akademie der Naturforscher Leopoldina, 2002), 45–93.

Muller-Dietz, H.E., 'Anatomische Praparate in der Petersburg "Kunstkammer"', *Zentralblatt fur Allgemeine Pathologie und Pathologische Anatomie*, cxxxv (1989), 757–67.

Murray, J.T., *English Dramatic Companies, 1558–1642* (New York: Russell and Russell, 1963).

Needham, Joseph, *A History of Embryology* (Cambridge: Cambridge University Press, 1959).

Neverov, Oleg, '"His Majesty's Cabinet" and Peter I's *Kunstkammer*', in Oliver Impey and Arthur Macgregor (eds), *The Origins of Museums: The Cabinet of Curiosities in Sixteenth- and Seventeenth-Century Europe* (Oxford: Clarendon Press, 1985), 54–61.

Newman, H.H., *Twins and Super-Twins: A Study of Twins, Triplets, Quadruplets and Quintuplets* (London: Hutchinson, 1942).

Niccoli, Ottavia, '"Menstruum Quasi Monstruum": Monstrous Births and Menstrual Taboo in the Sixteenth Century', in Edward Muir and Guido Ruggiero (eds), *Sex and Gender in Historical Perspective* (Baltimore: Johns Hopkins University Press, 1990), 1–25.

Niccoli, Ottavia (transl. Lydia G. Cochrane), *Prophecy and People in Renaissance Italy* (Princeton: Princeton University Press, 1990).

Norman, A.V.B., *Wallace Collection Catalogue of Ceramics 1: Pottery, Maiolica, Faience, Stoneware* (London: Trustees of the Wallace Collection, 1976).

Nutton, Vivian, 'The Anatomy of the Soul in Early Renaissance Medicine', in G.R. Dunstan (ed.), *The Human Embryo: Aristotle and the Arabic and European Traditions* (Exeter: University of Exeter Press, 1990), 136–57.

Oaks, Robert F., 'Things Fearful to Name: Sodomy and Buggery in Seventeenth-Century New England', *Journal of Social History*, xii (1978), 268–81.

Olmi, Giuseppe, 'Science-Honour-Metaphor: Italian Cabinets of the Sixteenth and Seventeenth Centuries', in Oliver Impey and Arthur Macgregor (eds), *The Origins of Museums: The Cabinet of Curiosities in Sixteenth- and Seventeenth-Century Europe* (Oxford: Clarendon Press, 1985), 5–16.

Olsen, K.E., and L.A.J.R. Houwen (eds), *Monsters and the Monstrous in Medieval Northwest Europe* (Leuven: Peeters, 2001).

O'Neill, Ynez Violé, 'Michele Savonarola and the *Fera* or Blighted Twin Phenomenon', *Medical History*, xviii (1974), 222–39.

Oostra, R.J., B. Baljet, P.F. Dijkstra and C.M. Hennekam, 'Congenital Anomalies in the Teratological Collection of Museum Vrolik in Amsterdam, The Netherlands, I: Syndromes with Multiple Congenital Abnormalities', *American Journal of Medical Genetics*, lxxvii (1998), 100–15.

Oostra, R.J., B. Baljet, P.F. Dijkstra and R.C. Hennekam, 'Congenital Anomalies in the Teratological Collection of Museum Vrolik in Amsterdam, The Netherlands, II: Skeletal Dysplasias', *American Journal of Medical Genetics*, lxxvii (1998), 116–34.

Oostra, R.J., B. Baljet, B.W. Verbeeten and R.C. Hennekam, 'Congenital Anomalies in the Teratological Collection of Museum Vrolik in Amsterdam, The Netherlands, III: Primary Field Defects, Sequences, and Other Complex Anomalies', *American Journal of Medical Genetics*, lxxx (1998), 46–59.

Oostra, R.J., B. Baljet and R.C. Hennekam, 'Congenital Anomalies in the Teratological Collection of Museum Vrolik in Amsterdam, The Netherlands, IV: Closure Defects of the Neural Tube', *American Journal of Medical Genetics*, lxxx (1998), 60–73.

Oostra, R.J., B. Baljet, B.W. Verbeeten and R.C. Hennekam, 'Congenital Anomalies in the Teratological Collection of Museum Vrolik in Amsterdam, The Netherlands, V: Conjoined and Acardiac Twins', *American Journal of Medical Genetics*, lxxx (1998), 74–89.

Ornstein, Martha, *The Role of Scientific Societies in the Seventeenth Century* (Chicago: University of Chicago Press, 1938).

Pachter, Henry M., *Paracelsus: Magic into Science, Being the True History of the Troubled Life, Adventures, Doctrines, Miraculous Cures, and Prophecies of the Most Renowned, Widely Traveled, Very Learned and Pious Gentleman, Scholar, and Most Highly Experienced and Illustrious Physicus, the Honorable Philippus Theophrastus Aureolus Bombastus ab Hohenheim, Eremita, called Paracelsus...* (New York: Schuman, 1951).

Pagel, Walter, 'The Reaction to Aristotle in Seventeenth-Century Biological Thought: Campanella, van Helmont, Glanvill, Charleton, Harvey, Glisson, Descartes', in E. Ashworth Underwood (ed.), *Science, Medicine and History: Essays on the Evolution of Scientific Thought and Medical Practice Written in Honour of Charles Singer* (London: Oxford University Press, 1953), I, 489–509.

Paget, James, 'Some Rare and New Diseases', *Lancet*, ii (1882), 1017–21.

Park, Katherine, 'The Criminal and the Saintly Body: Autopsy and Dissection in Renaissance Italy', *Renaissance Quarterly*, xlvii (1994), 1–33.

Park, Katherine, and Lorraine J. Daston, 'Unnatural Conceptions: The Study of Monsters in Sixteenth and Seventeenth-Century England and France', *Past & Present*, xcii (1981), 20–54.

Parker, Patricia, *Shakespeare from the Margins: Language, Culture, Context* (Chicago: University of Chicago Press, 1996).

Peignot, Gabriel, *Manuel du Bibliophile* (Dijon: V. Lagier, 1823).

Peña Chavarría, A., and P.G. Shipley, 'The Siamese Twins of Española (The First Known Post-Mortem Examination in the New World)', *Annals of Medical History*, vi (1924), 297–302.

Pfeiffer, R.A., and J. Correll, 'Hemimelia in Brachmann-de Lange Syndrome (BDLS): A Patient with Severe Deficiency of the Upper and Lower Limbs', *American Journal of Medical Genetics*, xlvii (1993), 1014–17.

Pfeiffer, R.A., and H. Zwerner, 'The Roberts Syndrome: Report of a Case Without Anomaly of the Centromeric Region', *Monatsschrift Kinderheilkunde*, cxxx (1982), 296–8.

Platt, Peter G. (ed.), *Wonders, Marvels, and Monsters in Early Modern Culture* (Newark: University of Delaware Press, 1999).

Porter, Roy, 'The Early Royal Society and the Spread of Medical Knowledge', in Roger French and Andrew Wear (eds), *The Medical Revolution of the Seventeenth Century* (Cambridge: Cambridge University Press, 1989), 272–93.

Praz, Mario, *Studies in Seventeenth-Century Imagery* (Rome: Edizione di Storia e Letteratura, 1964).

Purcell, Rosamond Wolff, and Stephen Jay Gould, *Finders, Keepers: Eight Collectors* (London: Pimlico, 1993).

Puschmann, Theodor (ed. and transl. Evan H. Hare), *A History of Medical Education From the Most Remote to the Most Recent Times* (London: H.K. Lewis, 1891).

Razovsky, Helaine, 'Popular Hermeneutics: Monstrous Children in English Renaissance Broadside Ballads', *Early Modern Literary Studies*, 2.3 (1996), 1.1–34, URL: http://purl.oclc.org/emls/02–3/razoball.html, viewed 11 February 2002.

Recklinghausen, F. von, 'Untersuchungen über die Spina Bifida', *Archiv fur Patholigische Anatomie*, cv (1886), 243–330.

Richardson, Ruth, *Death, Dissection and the Destitute* (London: Routledge and Kegan Paul, 1987).

Roberts, J.B., 'A Child with Double Cleft Lip and Palate, Protrusion of the Intermaxillary Portion of the Upper Jaw and Imperfect Development of the Bones of the Four Extremities', *Annals of Surgery*, lxx (1919), 252–3.

Rodriguez, J.I., J. Palacios and S. Razquin, 'Sirenomelia and Anencephaly', *American Journal of Medical Genetics*, xxxix (1991), 25–7.

Rollins, H.E., 'An Analytical Index to the Ballad-Entries (1557–1709) in the Register of the Company of Stationers of London', *Studies in Philology*, xxi (1924), 1–324.

Röpke, W., 'Die Veroffentlichungen der K. Leopoldinische Deutsche Akademie der Naturforscher', *Leopoldina*, i (1926), 151.

Ruggieri, M., and A Polizzi, 'From Aldrovandi's "*Homuncio*" (1592) to Buffon's Girl (1749) and the "Wart Man" of Tilesius (1793): Antique Illustrations of Mosaicism in Neurofibromatosis?', *Journal of Medical Genetetics*, xl (2003), 227–32.

Russell, Daniel, *Emblematic Studies in Renaissance French Culture* (Toronto: Toronto University Press, 1995).

Salgues, J.B., *Des Erreurs et des Préjugés Répandus dans la Société* (Paris: F. Buisson, 1810–13).

Salisbury, Joyce E., *The Beast Within: Animals in the Middle Ages* (New York: Routledge, 1994).

Sanders, Julie, 'Midwifery and the New Science in the Seventeenth Century: Language, Print and Theatre', in Erica Fudge, Ruth Gilbert and Susan Wiseman (eds), *At the Borders of the Human: Beasts, Bodies and Natural Philosophy in the Early Modern Period* (Basingstoke: Macmillan Press, 1999).

Sato, T., K. Kaneko, S. Konuma, I. Sati and T. Tamada, 'Acardiac Anomalies: Review of 88 Cases in Japan', *Asia-Oceana Journal of Obstetrics and Gynaecology*, x (1984), 45–52.

Schama, Simon, *The Embarrassment of Riches: An Interpretation of Dutch Culture in the Golden Age* (Bath: Fontana Press, 1987).

Schenda, Rudolf, 'Das Monstrum von Ravenna: Eine Studie zur Prodigiensliteratur', *Zeitschrift für Volkskunde*, lxvi (1960), 209–15.

Scheurleer, Th. H. Lunsingh, 'Early Dutch Cabinets of Curiosities', in Oliver Impey and Arthur Macgregor (eds), *The Origins of Museums: The Cabinet of Curiosities in Sixteenth- and Seventeenth-Century Europe* (Oxford: Clarendon Press, 1985), 115–20.

Schierhorn, H., 'Die Terata auf der Weltkarte des Richard de Haldingham (um 1280): Versuch einer Deutung', *Gegenbaurs Morphologisches Jahrbuch*, cxxviii (1982), 137–67.

Schutte, Anne Jacobson, '"Such Monstrous Births": A Neglected Aspect of the Antinomian Controversy', *Renaissance Quarterly*, xxxviii (1985), 85–106.

Semonin, Paul, 'Monsters in the Marketplace: The Exhibition of Human Oddities in Early Modern England', in Rosemarie Garland Thomson (ed.), *Freakery: Cultural Spectacles of the Extraordinary Body* (New York: New York University Press, 1996), 69–81.

Shapin, Steven, *A Social History of Truth...* (Chicago: University of Chicago Press, 1994).

Shapiro, Barbara J., *Probability and Certainty in Seventeenth-century England: A Study of the Relationships Between Natural Science, Religion, History, Law, and Literature* (Princeton: Princeton University Press, 1983).

Simonds, J.P., and G.A. Gowen, 'Fetus Amorphus (Report of a Case)', *Surgery Gynecology Obstetrics*, xli (1925), 171–9.

Sinclair, H.M., and A.H.T. Robb-Smith, *A Short History of Anatomical Teaching in Oxford* (Oxford: Oxford University Press, 1950).

Spencer, Rowena, 'Rachipagus Conjoined Twins: They Really do Occur!', *Teratology*, lii (1995), 346–56.

Spencer, Rowena, 'Theoretical and Analytical Embryology of Conjoined Twins, Part I: Embryogenesis', *Clinical Anatomy*, xiii (2000), 36–53.

Spencer, Rowena, 'Theoretical and Analytical Embryology of Conjoined Twins, Part II: Adjustments to Union', *Clinical Anatomy*, xiii (2000), 97–120.

Spencer, Rowena, 'Parasitic Conjoined Twins: External, Internal (Fetuses in Fetu and Teratomas), and Detached (Acardiacs)', *Clinical Anatomy*, xiv (2001), 428–44.

Spiro, Robert K., 'A Backward Glance at the Study of Postmortem Anatomy', *International Surgery*, lvi (1971), 27–40.

Summers, Montague, *The History of Witchcraft and Demonology* (London: Routledge and Kegan Paul, 1926).

Summers, Montague, *The Geography of Witchcraft* (London: Routledge and Kegan Paul, 1927).

Symonds, Deborah A., *Weep Not for Me: Women, Ballads, and Infanticide in Early Modern Scotland* (Pennsylvania: Pennsylvania State University Press, 1997).

Teelucksingh, Jerome, 'The Two-Headed Boy, and Other Medical Marvels' (book review), *Social History of Medicine*, xv (2002), 166–7.

Thijssen, J.M., 'Twins as Monsters: Albertus Magnus's Theory of the Generation of Twins and its Philosophical Context', *Bulletin of the History of Medicine*, lxi (1987), 237–46.

Thomas, Keith, *Religion and the Decline of Magic: Studies in Popular Beliefs in Sixteenth and Seventeenth-Century England* (London: Weidenfeld and Nicolson, 1971).

Thomas, Keith, *Man and the Natural World* (New York: Pantheon, 1983).

Thompson, C.J.S., *The Mystery and Lore of Monsters* (London: Williams and Norgate, 1930).

Thomson, Rosemarie Garland (ed.), *Freakery: Cultural Spectacles of the Extraordinary Body* (New York: New York University Press, 1996).

Thorndike, Lynn, *A History of Magic and Experimental Science* (New York: Columbia University Press, 1941).

Toellner, Richard, 'Im Hain des Akademos auf die Natur Wißbegierig Sein: Vier Ärzte der Freien Reichsstadt Schweinfurt Gründen die *Academia Naturae Curiosorum*', in Benno Parthier and Dietrich von Engelhardt (eds), *350 Jahre Leopoldina – Anspruch und Wirklichkeit: Festschrift der Deutschen Akademie der Naturforscher Leopoldina, 1652–2002* (Halle: Deutsche Akademie der Naturforscher Leopoldina, 2002), 15–43.

Towler, Jean, and Joan Bramall, *Midwives in History and Society* (London: Croom Helm, 1986).

Trolle, Dyre, *The History of Caesarean Section* (Copenhagen: C.A. Reitzel, 1982).

Turnpenny, Peter D., and Robert Hole, 'The First Description of Lethal Pterygium Syndrome with Facial Clefting (Bartsocas-Papas Syndrome) in 1600', *Journal of Medical Genetics*, xxxvii (2000), 314–15.

Urban, M., P. Rogalla, S. Tinschert, P. Krietsch, 'Tetraphocomelia and Bilateral Cleft Lip in a Historical Case of Roberts Syndrome [Virchow, 1898]', *American Journal of Medical Genetics*, lxxii (1997), 307–14.

Van Den Berg, D.J., and U. Francke, 'Roberts Syndrome: A Review of 100 Cases and a New Rating System for Severity', *American Journal of Medical Genetics*, xlvii (1993), 1104–23.

Walsham, Alexandra, 'Sermons in the Sky (Celestial Visions Reported Across Early Modern Europe)', *History Today*, li (2001), 56–63.

Walton, Michael T., R.M. Fineman and P.J.Walton, 'Of Monsters and Prodigies: the Interpretation of Birth Defects in the Sixteenth Century', *American Journal of Medical Genetics*, xlvii (1993), 7–13.

Warnicke, Retha M., *The Rise and Fall of Ann Boleyn…* (Cambridge: Cambridge University Press, 1989).

Watt, Tessa, *Cheap Print and Popular Piety 1550–1640* (Cambridge: Cambridge University Press, 1991).

Webster, Charles, *The Great Instauration: Science, Medicine, and Reform, 1626–1660* (London: Duckworth, 1975).

Whitley, Charles, 'Chroniclers and Antiquaries', in A.W. Ward and A.R. Waller (eds), *The Cambridge History of English and American Literature* (New York: G.P. Putnam, 1907–21).

Wigglesworth, J.S., and D.B. Singer (eds), *Textbook of Fetal and Perinatal Pathology* (Massachusetts: Blackwell Science, 1998).

Williams, A.N., 'Cerebrovascular Disease in Dumas' *The Count of Monte Cristo*', *Journal of the Royal Society of Medicine*, xcvi (2003), 412–14.

Williams, David, *Deformed Discourse: The Function of the Monster in Mediaeval Thought and Literature* (Exeter: University of Exeter Press, 1996).

Willis, Roy Geoffrey, *Man and Beast* (St Albans: Paladin, 1975).

Wilson, Adrian, 'The Ceremony of Childbirth and its Interpretation', in Valerie Fildes (ed.), *Women as Mothers in Pre-Industrial England: Essays in Memory of Dorothy McLaren* (London: Routledge, 1990), 68–107.

Wilson, Adrian, *The Making of Man-Midwifery: Childbirth in England 1660–1770* (London: UCL Press, 1995).

Wilson, Dudley, *Signs and Portents: Monstrous Births from the Middle Ages to the Enlightenment* (London: Routledge, 1993).

Wilson, Philip Kevin, *Surgeon 'Turned' Physician: the Career and Writings of Daniel Turner (1667–1741)* (PhD, University College London, 1992).

Winston, Ken R., 'Craniopagi: Anatomical Characteristics and Classification', *Neurosurgery*, xxi (1987), 769–81.

Woodward, D., 'Some Difficult Confinements in Seventeenth-Century Yorkshire', *Medical History*, xviii (1974), 349–59.

Yates, Frances, *The Rosicrucian Enlightenment* (London: Routledge and Kegan Paul, 1972).

Zanca, A., 'Iconografia Dermatological del XVI Secolo: Un Caso di Neurofibromatosi Multipla Illustrato da Ulisse Aldrovandi', *Archivo Italiano Dermatologia, Venereologia, e Sessuologia*, xl (1975), 119–23.

Zergollern, L., and V. Hitrec, 'Three Siblings with Robert's Syndrome', *Clinical Genetics*, ix (1976), 433–6.

Index

Printed in the United States
By Bookmasters